DATE DUE

APR 1 4 1994	
MAY 2 1994	
SEP 2 8 1994	
MAR - 9 1995	
MAR - 4 1997	
FEB 2 3 1999	
JUL 1 1 2002	

BRODART   Cat. No. 23-221

Alcoholism in North America,
Europe, and Asia

Alcoholism in North America, Europe, and Asia

Edited by

JOHN E. HELZER, M.D.
Department of Psychiatry
The University of Vermont

GLORISA J. CANINO, Ph.D.
School of Medicine
University of Puerto Rico

New York   Oxford
OXFORD UNIVERSITY PRESS
1992

Oxford University Press

Oxford   New York   Toronto
Delhi   Bombay   Calcutta   Madras   Karachi
Kuala Lumpur   Singapore   Hong Kong   Tokyo
Nairobi   Dar es Salaam   Cape Town
Melbourne   Auckland

and associated companies in
Berlin   Ibadan

Library of Congress Cataloging-in-Publication Data
Alcoholism in North America, Europe, and Asia / edited by John E.
Helzer, Glorisa J. Canino.
p.   cm.   ISBN 0-19-505090-8
1. Alcoholism—North America—Epidemiology.
2. Alcoholism—Europe—Epidemiology.
3. Alcoholism—Asia—Epidemiology.
I. Helzer, John E.   II. Canino, Glorisa J.
[DNLM: 1. Alcoholism—epidemiology—Asia.
2. Alcoholism—epidemiology—Europe.
3. Alcoholism—epidemiology—North America.
4. Cross-Cultural Comparison. WM 271 A35714]
RC565.A44638   1991
362.29'22—dc20
DNLM/DLC   for Library of Congress   90-14343

9 8 7 6 5 4 3 2 1

Printed in the United States of America
on acid-free paper

This Book is Dedicated to
John Josiah Helzer
March 23, 1917–March 10, 1991

Steadfast and supportive
throughout his life

Foreword

This volume, edited by Helzer and Canino, is a remarkable accomplishment and should stand as a landmark in the epidemiology of alcoholism and its relationship to culture and psychiatric disorders. The breadth of the initiative is illustrated by the ten different cultural regions, which include a sample standardized to be representative of the U.S. population, along with American Indian and Puerto Rican populations; French and English speaking Canadian groups; German and French groups in Europe; a New Zealand population in the Pacific; and three Asian populations in Taiwan, Korea, and Shanghai, China. If the scope of this study were limited only to each chapter's introductory, historical description of alcohol use and abuse patterns in each culture, it would be a welcome contribution to the alcoholism literature. However, the combination of this material with outstanding quantitative epidemiological data is unprecedented.

The depth of the information contained is demonstrated by the fact that each site uses a common set of diagnostic criteria from the third edition of the American Psychiatric Association, Diagnostic and Statistical Manual (DSM-III), and a common diagnostic assessment instrument—the NIMH Diagnostic Interview Schedule (DIS). Appropriately translated and adapted for use in each culture, this common assessment procedure was used with the more than 48,000 respondents covered in these multiple studies. The unique history of alcohol use in each culture is provided as a context from which correlates are drawn for comparing alcohol use, abuse, and dependence both within and across cultural domains. Although one might be concerned that such an enormous quantitative data base and cultural diversity might result in losing the forest for the trees or in disconnected idiosyncratic analyses, the parallel focus enforced by the editors has precluded this monumental effort from spinning out of control. Instead, the reader is treated to a rich multidisciplinary approach to the study of the complex phenomena of alcoholism in culture. Both anthropological and sociological approaches are reviewed along with the more medically oriented diagnostic specific epidemiological approaches. The full range of psychiatric, psychological, sociological, statistical, interviewing and analytic skills of the investigator are amply reflected in the production of the volume. The language barriers which limit such joint undertakings are noticeably absent. One can only attribute the readability of the product to the remarkable coordinating and editorial skills of Helzer and Canino, who have produced a carefully integrated, multi-authored volume.

Although the reader will readily appreciate the scholarship and readability of the volume, it is helpful to place it in a somewhat broader context to emphasize the value of this work as a historical document. In the mid and late 1970s, there was a comprehensive review of the state of U.S. mental health research, services, and training under the President's Commission on Mental Health, chaired by Mrs. Rosalyn Carter. As part of that review, the status of epidemiological research data for describing the prevalence of alcohol, drug, and mental disorders, as well as the services provided for individuals with these disorders, came under particular scrutiny. The deficiencies in that knowledge base, as well as the promise of new, scientifically credible, diagnostic criteria and measurement instruments, provided support for the initiation, by the National Institute of Mental Health (NIMH), of a new era in psychiatric epidemiological research with the Epidemiologic Catchment Area (ECA) program. The NIMH initiated the development of the Diagnostic Interview Schedule in 1978 to serve as a case identification instrument for broad-scale epidemiological surveys that would use the emerging DSM-III criteria—subsequently published in 1980. I was privileged to coordinate a review of available psychiatric assessment instruments that could be used for diagnosis of mental disorders in community populations. Although none of the instruments met all of the necessary criteria for such a study, the Renard Diagnostic Interview of Helzer and Robins appeared to provide the best conceptual base. Hence in 1978, Lee Robins of Washington University was awarded a NIMH contract to work jointly with Robert Spitzer and Janet Williams, who led the DSM-III development, to produce the NIMH Diagnostic Interview Schedule. This interview became the diagnostic or "case identification" assessment instrument for the ECA.

The success of the ECA collaborative research model may be measured not only by the almost 200 publications that have emerged thus far, but also by the extent to which the methods have been used worldwide. The latter accomplishment is a credit to Lee Robins and John Helzer, who established a training center for the DIS that enabled investigators from many countries to learn how the instrument works and how it could be reliably administered in their own cultures. A model for translating the instrument into other languages was also provided by Marvin Karno and his associates at UCLA in the first translation of the instrument into Spanish for the UCLA Hispanic ECA sample. Several of the authors of this volume came to St. Louis for training in the DIS, and the successful adaptations to other cultures are exemplified in the findings produced for this volume—the first of its kind to pull together data from such a wide range of studies in one comprehensive work. The research and this book itself are excellent examples of how a timely scientific innovation such as the NIMH-DIS can have a ripple effect throughout the entire world.

This study serves as an example of a prototypical cross-cultural epidemiological approach which was built on the research shoulders of pioneers in the field such as Alexander Leighton and Jane Murphy with their more anthropologically based cross-cultural studies. Other previous cross-cultural efforts are represented by the US/UK study and International Pilot Study of Schizophrenia sponsored by the World Health Organization. However, the sheer scope and number of individuals covered in this volume points to a future that could well revolutionize psychiatric epidemiology and its relationship to clinical practice and research throughout the world.

In 1978, at about the same time as we at NIMH were initiating the ECA, the parent Alcohol, Drug Abuse, Mental Health Association (ADAMHA) administrator Dr. Gerald Klerman, initiated a cooperative agreement on diagnosis and classification with the World Health Organization, Division of Mental Health, directed by Dr. Norman Sartorius. By means of numerous small and several large conferences or workshops in the late 1970s and early 1980s, WHO obtained a consensus that the DSM-III model of using explicit diagnostic criteria was a scientifically valid and useful innovation that should be adopted worldwide. Although the existing criteria for diagnostic categories were presumed to vary across the many nations who used ICD-9 and are signatories to the WHO treaty, the consensus process was set in motion for arriving at a new set of common criteria for the ICD-10, which would be a part of the official nomenclature within each of the member countries.

Following the example of the ECA, the ADAMHA and WHO collaborators in the WHO/ADAMHA Cooperative Agreement began simultaneous development and testing of three diagnostic assessment instruments that would incorporate the ICD-10 diagnostic criteria for research when they are officially released in the next few years. The assessment instruments will include the Composite International Diagnostic Interview (CIDI), which uses as its core and format the NIMH Diagnostic Interview Schedule that has been so successfully used in studies described here. In addition the Schedules for Clinical Assessment in Neuropsychiatry (SCAN), based on the Present State Examination (PSE), will be released. Early versions of this more clinical technique have been used in many research studies around the world, including the International Pilot Study for Schizophrenia and the US/UK study. Finally, the International Personality Disorders Examination (IPDE), which was based on the Personality Disorders Examination (PDE) of Loranger in the United States, has now been studied in multiple countries to assess this difficult area of psychiatric morbidity.

With the emergence of the ICD-10 and multiple psychiatric assessment tools for epidemiological and clinical research, volumes such as the one we have here may become more commonplace in the future. In future cross-cultural studies, it may also be possible to test etiological hypotheses on the relative contributions of environment, genetics, and other biological factors to the occurrence of alcoholism, drug abuse, and mental disorders around the world. Hence, the current volume should be seen not only as a landmark accomplishment, but as a harbinger of a new generation of cross-cultural studies which will follow in the next decade. This is a most valuable stepping-off point, which I commend to scientists, clinicians, and lay readers alike in their efforts to understand one of the most prevalent and socially disruptive of the mental and behavioral disorders.

Rockville, Maryland   Darrel A. Regier, M.D., M.P.H.
November, 1991

Preface

It is rare for authors to have an opportunity as unique as the one described in this book. This study is based on a set of fortuitous circumstances that grew out of the Epidemiologic Catchment Area (ECA) survey, itself a fortuitous occurrence.

For decades a large general population survey of carefully defined psychiatric disorders had been contemplated at the National Institutes of Mental Health, but for a variety of reasons had not become a reality. The recommendations of President Carter's Commission on Mental Health, chaired by Rosalyn Carter, enabled Darrel Reigier and others at NIMH to amass the funding and commitment necessary for a major population survey. They began by commissioning the development of the Diagnostic Interview Schedule (DIS) as the instrument for the primary clinical data collection. The DIS was to be based on DSM-III, and its development occurred just as DSM-III was being completed.

When DSM-III was published in 1980, it gained almost instant popularity throughout the world. As the wide use of the Feighner criteria and the Research Diagnostic Criteria (RDC) had already demonstrated, the development of a highly specific set of diagnostic definitions for the major mental illnesses was clearly an idea whose time had come.

Interviewing for the ECA also began in 1980, and a number of factors ensured that it too would gain worldwide attention. First, it was the largest general population survey of mental illness ever done. Second, its aim was to measure population rates of psychiatric illnesses in the United States as defined in clinical settings. This differed from many previous surveys that generated rates of "impairment," but not of specific disorders as a clinician would recognize them. Third, the ECA captured attention because of its use of the Diagnostic Interview Schedule. In addition to being based on DSM-III, the DIS was designed so that it could be administered by non-clinicians, thus making it cost-effective for large-scale epidemiologic work.

This broad visibility helped to refocus attention on psychiatric epidemiology as a necessary discipline for determining the prevalence and distribution of mental illness, assessing the adequacy of psychiatric services, and studying the etiology of illness. One consequence was that several other countries became interested in gathering epidemiologic data for their own needs. Since the ECA had been a major stimulus for these projects, it naturally became the model that these "spinoff" surveys would be patterned after. Thus, in the 1980s a number of population surveys in various parts of the world were started, utilizing the DSM-III criteria as the basis for the diagnostic assessment, the DIS interview to gather the clinical data, and population sampling methods similar to those used in the ECA.

However, there was another similarity between these efforts and the ECA that was especially important in our later ability to make valid cross-national comparisons. Since the DIS was developed largely in St. Louis, one of the ECA sites, it naturally fell to the St. Louis group to provide interview training to the other ECA participants. We established a training program that, because of the continued interest in the interview, has continued to the present day. When investigators in other countries became interested in replicating the ECA, they typically came to St. Louis to obtain training in the administration of the DIS. At that time they had an opportunity to become better acquainted with the DSM-III terms and constructs that were the basis of the interview, and to learn how these were expressed in specific DIS questions. This enabled them to be faithful to those same constructs when they made translations of the interview for use in their own countries. As we discuss in Chapter 2, there are many features of the DIS that facilitate its translation, but this unique situation of uniform training by the original developers of the interview helped to preserve its consistent use not only in the ECA survey itself, but in the subsequent efforts in other countries as well.

The opportunity to develop this book stemmed from this fortuitous set of circumstances. The editors approached all the investigators they were aware of who had used the DIS in large population surveys in the early to mid-1980s to propose a cross-national comparison. The relevant surveys were broadly geographically distributed so that we were able to include widely separated areas of the world. The participating sites fell conveniently into three geographic regions: North America, Europe, and Asia and the Pacific. We pilot-tested a variety of comparison methods in a series of symposia, involving many of the authors in this book, presented over a three-year period at annual meetings of the American Psychiatric Association. In order to take advantage of the similarity of the data sets, the comparison method we evolved was to initiate a set of analyses using the ECA data. This set of analyses, including the computer programs and output and the resulting data tables, was sent to all the other sites. Each site replicated the analysis using their own data and developing their own data tables in the same or similar format. Each site was free to do additional analyses on its own as well. This process is described in Chapter 5.

We begin the introductory section of the book with a general discussion of cross-national comparisons in psychiatry and the constraints that have made such efforts difficult. Chapter 2 discusses the development of the DIS and its adaptation for other cultures in more detail, including translation issues. In Chapter 3, Jane Murphy discusses anthropological and sociological approaches to cross-national comparison as a context for the more clinical approach utilized here. In Chapter 4, Tom Babor reviews the considerable previous cross-national work on alcoholism. This chapter helps to highlight the particular importance of the highly coordinated effort in the present volume. In Chapter 5, Leaf and his coauthors review methodological issues in psychiatric epidemiology and summarize the methods used in the various surveys presented here.

Chapters 6 through 15 are reports from each of the ten countries or cultural regions that participated in this effort. Each set of authors was asked to begin with a discussion of the history of alcohol use in their culture and a review of contemporary mores regarding alcohol. Next they present results from their own epidemiologic survey. In order to ensure some degree of uniformity in the latter, each group was asked to replicate a basic set of analyses that were initiated with the ECA data and distributed to the other participants. Not all were able to accomplish all of these analyses, and some went beyond the basic set to examine other issues as well, but by and large this basic outline has been followed and is directly comparable across chapters.

In Chapter 16, we discuss the very important question of the appropriateness of applying a set of diagnostic criteria (the DSM-III) developed in the United States to a wide variety of cultural contexts, particularly for the study of alcoholism, an illness that is likely to be strongly influenced by cultural context. We follow this discussion with an attempt to summarize the results from the surveys reported in Chapters 6 through 15 to see what this effort teaches us about biological, social, and cultural influences in alcoholism and about future prospects in the field of cross-cultural psychiatric epidemiology.

Burlington, Vermont   J. E. H.
November, 1991   G. J. C.

Contents

III   Europe

IV   Asia and the Pacific

V   Conclusions

Contributors

Lynn Ackerson, M.S.
Department of Psychiatry
University of Colorado Health
  Sciences Center
4200 East Ninth Street
Denver, Colorado 80262

Thomas F. Babor, Ph.D.
Department of Psychiatry
University of Connecticut Health
  Center
Farmington, Connecticut 06032

Anna E. Baron, Ph.D.
Department of Psychiatry
University of Colorado Health
  Sciences Center
4200 East Ninth Street
Denver, Colorado 80262

Roger C. Bland, M.D.
Chairman, Department of Psychiatry
University of Alberta
Faculty of Medicine
1E 1.01 Mackenzie Centre
8440 - 112th Street
Edmonton, Alberta T6G 2B7,
  Canada

Denyse Boivin
Hospital St. Francois D'Assise
10 Rue de L'espinay
Quebec G1L 3L5, Canada

Thomas Bronisch, M.D.
Max-Planck-Institut for Psychiatrie
Kraepelinstrasse 10
8000 Munchen 40
West Germany

Kathleen Bucholz, Ph.D.
Department of Psychiatry
Washington University Medical
  Center
216 South Kingshighway Boulevard
P.O. Box 14109
St. Louis, Missouri 63178

Audrey Burnam, Ph.D.
The Rand Corporation
1700 Main Street
Santa Monica, California 90401

John A. Bushnell, Ph.D.
Department of Community Health
Christchurch School of Medicine
University of Otago
P.O. Box 4345
Christchurch, New Zealand

Raul Caetano, M.D., Ph.D.
Alcohol Research Group
1816 Scenic Avenue
Berkeley, California 94709

Glorisa J. Canino, Ph.D.
Director, Behavioral Sciences
*   Research Institute*
University of Puerto Rico
Medical Sciences Campus
G.P.O. Box 365067
San Juan, Puerto Rico 00936-5067

William Clark, M.D.
R.R.1, Box 482
Woolwich, Maine 04579

Marilyn Fernandez, Ph.D.
Pacific/Asian American Mental
*   Health Research Center*
University of Illinois
Chicago, Illinois 60607

John E. Helzer, M.D.
Chairman, Department of Psychiatry
University of Vermont College of
*   Medicine*
Burlington, Vermont 05405

Andrew R. Hornblow, Ph.D.
Professor of Community Health
Christchurch School of Medicine
P.O. Box 4345
Christchurch, New Zealand

Hai-Gwo Hwu, M.D.
Department of Psychiatry
National Taiwan University Hospital
#1 Chang-Te Street
Taipei, Taiwan, China

Peter R. Joyce, M.B., Ch.B.,
*   **Ph.D.**
Professor of Psychological Medicine
Christchurch School of Medicine
P.O. Box 4345
Christchurch, New Zealand

Philip J. Leaf, Ph.D.
Department of Mental Hygiene
Johns Hopkins University
624 North Broadway
Baltimore, Maryland 21205

Chung Kyoon Lee, M.D.
Professor and Chairman
Department of Neuropsychiatry
Seoul National University Hospital
#18 Yeongun-Dong, Chrongro-Gu
Seoul 110, Korea

William T. Liu, Ph.D.
Pacific/Asian American Mental
*   Health Research Center*
University of Illinois
Chicago, Illinois 60607

Ching-Tung Lung, Ph.D.
Pacific/Asian American Mental
*   Health Research Center*
University of Illinois
Chicago, Illinois 60607

Spero M. Manson, Ph.D.
National Center for American Indian
*   & Alaska Native Mental Health*
*   Research*
Department of Psychiatry
University of Colorado Health
*   Sciences Center*
4200 East Ninth Avenue
Denver, Colorado 80262

Jane M. Murphy, Ph.D.
Massachusetts General Hospital
703 Warren Building
Boston, Massachusetts 02114

Gordon Neligh, M.D.
Department of Psychiatry
University of Colorado Health
*   Sciences Center*
4200 East Ninth Street
Denver, Colorado 80262

Stephen C. Newman, M.D.
Mental Health Services
Alberta Social Services and
*   Community Health*
4th Floor, South Tower
Seventh Street Plaza
10030 107th Street
Edmonton, Alberta T5J 3E4,
*   Canada*

Mark A. Oakley-Browne, M.B., Ch.B.
Department of Psychological Medicine
Christchurch School of Medicine
P.O. Box 4345
Christchurch, New Zealand

Helene Orn, B.Ed.
Mental Health Division
Alberta Social Services and
  Community Health
4th Floor, South Tower
10030 107th Street
Edmonton, Alberta T5J 3E4,
  Canada

Guang-Ya Qu, M.D.
Shanghai Institute of Mental Health
  and Shanghai Hospital
600 Wan Pin Nan Lu
Shanghai, China

Simone Radouco-Thomas, Ph.D.
Hospital St. Francois D'Assise
10 Rue de L'espinay
Quebec G1L 3L5, Canada

Lee N. Robins, Ph.D.
Department of Psychiatry
Washington University School of
  Medicine
4940 Audubon Avenue
St. Louis, Missouri 63110

James H. Shore, M.D.
Chairman, Department of Psychiatry
University of Colorado Health
  Sciences Center
4200 East Ninth Street
Denver, Colorado 80262

Chang-Hua Wang, M.D.
Shanghai Institute of Mental Health
  and Shanghai Hospital
Shanghai, China

J. Elisabeth Wells
Department of Community Health
Christchurch School of Medicine
P.O. Box 4345
Christchurch, New Zealand

Hans-Ulrich Wittchen, Ph.D.
Max-Planck-Institut for Psychiatrie
Kraepelinstrasse 10
8000 Munchen 40
West Germany

Amy Wolfson
Department of Psychology
Washington University
St. Louis, Missouri 63110

Zheng-Yi Xia, M.D.
Shanghai Institute of Mental Health
  and Shanghai Hospital
600 Wan Pin Nan Lu
Shanghai, China

Chang-Lin Xu, M.D.
Shanghai Institute of Mental Health
  and Shanghai Hospital
600 Wan Pin Nan Lu
Shanghai, China

Eng-Kung Yeh, M.D.
c/o C.P. Yeh
3918 Amy Avenue
Garland, Texas 75043

Elena S.H. Yu, Ph.D.
Graduate School of Public Health
San Diego University
San Diego, California 92182

Ming-Yuan Zhang, M.D.
Shanghai Institute of Mental Health
  and Shanghai Hospital
Shanghai, China

[I] Introduction

[1] Epidemiology and Cross-National Comparisons

JOHN E. HELZER AND GLORISA J. CANINO

Comparison of illness rates across national boundaries or cultural groups can lead to a better understanding of risk, protective, and etiological factors involved in specific mental disorders. Conceptually this is relatively straightforward: Prevalence or incidence rates of a particular disorder are compared across groups to look for similarities and differences. Similarities suggest that cultural differences between the groups may have little impact on the occurrence of the illness. Conversely, when cross-cultural differences in illness rates are found, additional differences in social or cultural variables are sought to see if they correlate with the rate differences. Such correlates provide clues for further etiological investigation.

As straightforward as this may sound in theory, many practical problems arise in the execution of cross-national comparisons, especially in the area of mental disorders. First, nationwide estimates for specific psychiatric disorders are available in only a few countries, are typically based only on cases coming to medical attention, and may be difficult for investigators to gain access to. As a substitute, the epidemiologist will often seek national or regional data on "secondary indicators," variables that are available for the total population and that might be used as substitute indicators of illness rates. A brief review of a secondary indicator for alcoholism illustrates the problems in this strategy.

Per capita alcohol consumption, the total amount of alcoholic beverages consumed by a population in a year, is hypothesized by Ledermann (1956) to be an indicator of the number of alcoholics in that population. An estimate of per capita consumption is generally readily available, since the governmental unit that taxes the production or sale of alcohol has a financial incentive to maintain statistics on the volume of all legally produced alcoholic beverages. However, there are two problems with this indicator. First, not everyone agrees that Ledermann's hypothesis that the consumption of alcohol by the total population is an index of the number of alcoholics. Second, there may be inaccuracies in the per capita consumption data and the degree and type of inaccuracy are likely to vary from one country to the next. For example, in Korea (Chapter 14), considerable unregistered (and untaxed) alcohol production takes place in private homes for personal consumption. Thus, the use of official per capita consumption as a cross-national secondary indicator is reduced (Kreitman, 1977).

But there is an even more serious problem. Even if we were able to accurately measure and compare per capita consumption, and we could be certain this secondary indicator was in fact an accurate gauge of the prevalence of alcoholism, these data have another drawback in that they cannot be correlated with characteristics of specific individuals within the population. They can be used to generate hypotheses about associations between overall consumption (or illness prevalence) and other known characteristics of the country or region, such as the degree of religiosity or national drinking customs. But we cannot be certain that variables appearing to be associated at the population level are in fact associated at the individual level. For this, personal information on specific individuals is needed.

There have been many attempts to make cross-national illness comparisons using personal interview data, but here there are problems also, mainly in the way illnesses are defined and ill persons are identified. It is clear that even large cross-national differences in estimated illness rates can arise from relatively minor differences in illness definition or study methodology (Cooper et al., 1972). If cases are defined differently from one culture to the next, or if ascertainment or method of examination differ, cross-cultural comparisons are frustrated.

Definitional consistency has not always been important in psychiatry. For example, in the United States, from the time of Kraepelinian emphasis on diagnostic classification at the turn of this century, psychiatry evolved toward a deemphasis of diagnosis. By the middle of the century, psychopathology was widely conceptualized as a continuum from wellness, through mild illness, to frank psychosis. Describing American psychiatry, Lorr (1966) said that "formal diagnosis is actually ignored as relatively unimportant and outmoded, or disparaged as nondynamic and useless." In this atmosphere, consistency in the identification of specific disorders was not a major concern.

However, the past two decades have seen a dramatic revival of Kraepelinian ideas with renewed interest in the reliable identification of discrete diagnostic categories. The recognition of the importance of definitional consistency, which is now almost worldwide, has led to the widespread adoption of highly specific definitions, such as those of DSM-III (APA, 1980), DSM-IIIR (APA, 1987), and the ICD-10 (World Health Organization, 1987). Well-defined criteria of this sort, which emphasize observable behavior and its quantification rather than unconscious processes or interpretations of behavior, improve the consistency of diagnosis between cases and diagnostic agreement between clinicians (Helzer et al., 1977; Spitzer, 1983; Grove et al., 1981; Helzer, 1983).

Recent Advances in Assessment

This renewed emphasis on discrete diagnoses has influenced epidemiologic studies, largely through the development of structured interview instruments based on highly detailed, "operational," diagnostic criteria. Structured interviews promote the application of specified criteria to epidemiologic work in two ways. First, they help ensure the consistent use of criteria across the entire research population. Contemporary diagnostic criteria, like those contained in the DSM-III, are so detailed that they virtually require an interview guide in order to be certain that questions about all the symptoms have been asked and have been taken into account in arriving at a diagnosis. Furthermore, even well-defined diagnostic systems may still leave room for a considerable degree of variability in symptom definition or ascertainment (Helzer & Coryell, 1983). An interview that specifies symptom questions for the individual criteria items helps reduce this variability.

The other way in which highly structured interviews advance psychiatric epidemiology is through a vehicle for applying uniform diagnostic criteria to large populations. Since we lack laboratory tests, the best method we have for making a diagnosis in psychiatry is a careful examination by a trained psychiatric clinician. But it is generally impractical to apply such effort-intensive methods to the hundreds or thousands of individuals who might be examined in an epidemiologic study. Therefore, it has been difficult to gather detailed clinical information on such large numbers of subjects. The method pioneered by the studies presented in this volume, and discussed in detail in the following chapter, relies on a highly structured interview that enables lay or nonclinician examiners to gather the data that clinicians use in making psychiatric diagnoses.

This trend toward more precise diagnostic methods, which has had such a strong impact on general psychiatric epidemiology, also has important implications for cross-cultural epidemiology. Partly because of the difficulty in interpreting differences in illness rates when illness definitions are so variable or indistinct, cross-cultural comparisons of population samples have been relatively infrequent (see Chapter 4) and often difficult to interpret. Comparisons have more typically been undertaken at an individual, or ethnographic, level as discussed in Chapter 3.

To the degree that definitional consistency transcends national borders, cross-national comparison of illness rates becomes more feasible, since variations in rates attributable to differences in illness definition are reduced. For example, the current American Diagnostic and Statistical Manual (DSM-III) is known and used virtually worldwide, and in many countries has become the de facto national diagnostic system (Mezzich, 1985). A major reason for the international success of DSM-III lies in the objectivity of its illness definitions. Since it is an "operational" diagnostic system, DSM-III is easier to apply consistently than the more descriptive criteria of DSM-II or the current International Classification of Disease (ICD-9). Both the widespread adoption of DSM-III and its objectivity facilitate the evolution of cross-cultural psychiatric epidemiology from the ethnographic to the population level.

In this volume, we have drawn together from various parts of the world investigators applying this relatively precise set of diagnostic criteria and a highly structured interview based on DSM-III, the Diagnostic Interview Schedule (DIS), to the study of alcohol abuse and dependence, largely in general population samples. The studies presented here are all based on personal interview data, and for several of the studies, the numbers of persons interviewed are in the thousands.

Remaining Methodological Constraints

Large population surveys using personal interviews based on objective diagnostic criteria rectify many of the past difficulties in making cross-national comparisons. But such an approach does not eliminate all of the problems in cross-cultural epidemiology. First, although it is clear that structured interviews and objective criteria enhance diagnostic reliability, by no means do they make clinical diagnosis in psychiatry a perfectly reliable process (Helzer et al., 1977). Second, while previous research has shown that diagnoses based on clinical data gathered by lay examiners are similar to those clinicians make in the same subjects (Helzer et al., 1981), these similarities are greater in identified patients than they are in respondents drawn from the general population (Anthony et al., 1985; Helzer et al., 1985).

It is also important to recognize that some diagnostic categories are more "specifiable" than others. Mood states such as depression and dysthymia, for example, are highly personal experiences, even within the same culture. Although there may be a typical constellation of symptoms that constitutes the syndrome of affective illness, the depressive mood state itself may not necessarily be manifested consistently from one person to the next, or indeed in any readily observable way. Possibly because of this, interrater agreement on the various types of depressive illnesses has been difficult to achieve, even when the variation in the clinical information obtained is minimized by using highly specific definitions and structured interviews.

Conversely, other diagnostic categories, such as the substance use disorders, are easier to agree on because virtually all of the manifestations are readily externally observable. Most studies of interrater reliability of psychiatric diagnosis have demonstrated that the levels of agreement for the substance use disorders are generally quite high (Robins, 1981).

Constraints in Cross-Cultural Research

In a cross-cultural context we face the additional problem of whether psychopathological constructs developed and validated in one culture are applicable and valid in others. Additionally, even though underlying psychopathology may be similar cross-culturally, the expression of specific symptoms may vary (Murphy, 1976). This may be even more true of alcohol abuse and dependence, as defined in DSM-III, since much of the definition is based on societal response to the individual. Ironically, the characteristics that improve the reliability of this definition within a single culture may reduce its cross-cultural consistency.

Since it is largely a physiological event, the manifestations of drunkenness are presumably much the same from one culture to the next. However, the social and legal problems that befall the alcohol abuser depend greatly on social context. A few examples can be drawn from symptoms used in the alcoholism section of the DIS interview. Alcohol-related traffic accidents and arrests for driving while intoxicated are not likely to be an important social manifestation of alcoholism in societies where the vast majority of drinkers do not own cars. In societies that are strongly patriarchal, the family may not be as likely to complain about the father's excessive drinking as they are in societies where family structure is more egalitarian. Physician warnings about excessive drinking are less likely to be given in societies where visits to physicians are a rare event. Alarcón (1983) questions the cross-cultural applicability of some of the DSM-III diagnostic categories, especially to third world countries, and suggests an additional "psychocultural" axis for DSM-III containing criteria to aid in the description of symptom clusters across cultures.

There may also be important aspects of the clinical expression of alcoholism in some cultures that the DIS does not ascertain, and the expression of the disorder may appear to be more similar than it really is. It is therefore important that the judgments about what constitutes a psychiatric disorder and presumed symptoms be derived in part from the experience and perceptions of the subject population (Manson, Shore, Bloom, 1985). This process of adaptation of the taxonomy of DSM-III to another culture (the Hopi Indians of the United States) has been described by Manson et al. (Chapter 8), who used a combination of ethnographic and empirical methods.

Some of the other investigators contributing chapters to this book have not addressed directly the applicability of DSM-III criteria of alcoholism to their particular culture. However, all of them have elected to use the DIS because they felt DSM-III was applicable. Furthermore, as discussed in individual chapters, most of the study sites represented here have not only translated, but have validated or adapted the DIS for use in their specific culture. Lastly, a recently published survey of twenty-four countries, discussed in Chapter 16, attests to the widespread cross-national acceptance and perceived appropriateness of the DSM-III illness definitions.

Interview Translation

Language shapes the world we experience and interacts with culture. Translating a psychiatric interview from one language to another is, therefore, a complex task. To a degree, it involves translating one culture's view of the world to another. But the translation process can also help identify the cultural inequivalencies discussed above.

Good translation requires an attempt at both semantic and cultural equivalence. Various translation methods can be used, but the salient steps, followed by many of the studies included here, have been summarized by Brislin (1970):

1. An initial translation is "back translated" by a second bilingual who has no knowledge of the original interview. The latter is then compared with the back translation to see if the original intent of the question items has been retained.
2. Bilingual subjects are used as respondents, answering first in one of the languages and then in the other so that responses to the "same" questions can be compared.
3. A bilingual committee compares the translated instrument to the original.
4. The translation is pretested to examine its overall intelligibility and revised as necessary.

Even this elaborate strategy has limitations. Its success will depend greatly on the efficacy of the bilingual committee. For example, questions that seem to backtranslate perfectly may lose some of their original intent in translation. Yu et al. (1984) reported difficulties in the use of backtranslation in translating the DIS to Chinese. These related to the lack of comparability in verb tenses, divergence between spoken and written forms in the Chinese language, and difficulties with the back-translation of some of the idiomatic expressions in the DIS. But difficulties of this kind can usually be corrected by bilingual experts (Bravo et al., 1987).

Linguistic complexities in the original instrument can also produce translation difficulties. Brislin (1970) has suggested guidelines for wording of the original questions to facilitate subsequent translations. Some of these guidelines are the use of short, simple sentences of less than sixteen words, employment of the active rather than passive voice, avoidance of colloquialisms, avoidance of subjunctives, and the use of specific rather than general terms.

However, as with many instruments, the DIS was not originally developed with translation in mind, and as a result these features are often lacking (Karno et al., 1983; Yu et al., 1984). Furthermore, observing such guidelines can actually be a drawback for the original instrument. For example, colloquialisms sometimes convey meaning more effectively than more formal wording does. Bilingual committees can often resolve these problems. Such a group in the Puerto Rico survey (Chapter 9) reduced the complexity and length of many of the original DIS questions simply by subdividing them into shorter questions in the translation. This was done without changing the content or intention of the items so that comparability between the translation and the original DIS was preserved. Field trials of this translation helped to identify other questions that were too lengthy or cognitively complex for many Puerto Rican respondents with low educational achievement.

Translation also helps to identify items that lack relevance in the new culture, a problem highlighted by Gaviria (1985). For example, questions in the DIS alcohol section ask about alcohol-related traffic offenses and job loss due to alcohol. In cultures where automobiles are rare and jobs are often given by the State for life, these items will not be relevant for most respondents. Their likelihood of meeting a diagnostic threshold could be reduced because there are fewer criterion items for which they are at risk. However, where many more items are included in the criteria than are necessary for diagnosis, as is the case with the DSM-III, this is less of a difficulty. If necessary, items that are more culturally relevant can be added to the instrument, so as to make the odds of reaching the diagnostic threshold more even across cultures while at the same time improving the applicability of the instrument to the new culture.

Continuous variables can also be affected by cultural differences. Again, Yu et al. (1984) report differences in quantification equivalencies and types of liquor mentioned in the DIS (a fifth of liquor, a six pack of beer, and 7 or more glasses of wine) compared to China. A literal translation of the instrument in this case would not suffice. An adaptation of the items by knowledgeable bilinguals is necessary in order to maintain the original intent.

Even when the best translation or adaptation methods are used, the clinical constructs on which the instrument is based must be applicable to the new culture. Otherwise, the meaning ascribed to symptom items by respondents may systematically vary cross-nationally. The more different the cultures being compared, the more likely such variation becomes. The widespread adoption of DSM-III in various countries around the world is testament to its robustness in this regard.

Compromise and Solution

At present there is no perfect method for comparing rates of psychiatric disorder across widely diverse cultures. As we have just seen, there are many practical difficulties in attempting to apply the same set of illness definitions across all cultures. On the other hand, if the concepts and definitions of illness are unique to each culture, there is no basis for comparison at all, since differences may simply be ones of definition. If the etiology and pathophysiology of psychiatric illnesses were known, the task would be much more straightforward. Clinical definitions in each culture could be constructed in such a way that the same etiological spectrum was identified. But, of course, a major reason for cross-national comparisons is to search for etiological clues, and the whole enterprise would become unnecessary if etiology were already known. The compromise employed by the investigators here is to use the illness concepts and definitions embodied in a single set of diagnostic criteria (DSM-III), but to adapt a structured interview based on those criteria (the DIS) to their own cultural setting and language.

There are many practical advantages to this method. As detailed in subsequent chapters, the same coding structure and computer diagnostic programs are used in each study, thus making it easy to communicate with one another about the illness variables and to maintain uniformity in the data analysis. In fact, in the studies presented here, there is considerably more similarity in the clinical variables than in many of the social ones. Some of the latter variables, such as marital status, are included in the DIS also. But many key social variables, such as socioeconomic status, are not, and finding consistent definitions of these constructs that can be applied to each of the data sets is more difficult.

We feel there are many conceptual advantages to the epidemiologic methods used here in that they offer a balance between similarity and flexibility in the diagnostic assignment of cases. The DSM-III definitions provide a fairly definitive framework for the illness constructs, and the DIS provides a means of applying those constructs in a general population setting. The translation process permits adapting the original application to other cultural contexts. In a review of psychiatric epidemiology, Shapiro and Stromgren (1979) discuss the need for greater standardization of diagnostic methods. They point out that the cumulative impact of research done throughout the world is "considerably reduced by the fact that results of the various studies are not comparable because of differences in diagnosis and assessment methods . . ."

Because of these noncomparabilities, prior attempts at cross-cultural comparisons in psychiatry have often and rightly been viewed with skepticism. The methods we have used in order to achieve greater consistency are by no means a panacea, and as the prior discussion makes clear, there are still many pitfalls in the fascinating but complex area of cross-cultural research. Research in any field is an evolutionary process, and we feel the efforts taken here are a step in an appropriate direction.

References

Alarcón, R. D. (1983). A Latin-America perspective on DSM-III. *Am. J. Psychiatry* 140:102–5.

American Psychiatric Association, Committee on Nomenclature and Statistics (1980). *Diagnostic and Statistical Manual of Mental Disorders—Edition 3 (DSM-III)*. Washington, D.C.: American Psychiatric Association.

American Psychiatric Association, Committee on Nomenclature and Statistics (1987). *Diagnostic and Statistical Manual of Mental Disorders Revised Edition (DSM-III-R)*. Washington, D.C.: American Psychiatric Association.

Anthony, J. C.; Folstein, M.; Romanski, A. J.; VonKorff, M. R.; Nestadt, G. N.; Chahal, R.; Merchant, A.; Brown, C. H.; Shapiro, S.; Kramer, M.; and Gruenberg, E. M. (1985). Comparison of lay Diagnostic Interview Schedule and a standardized psychiatric diagnosis: Experience in eastern Baltimore. *Arch. Gen. Psychiatry* 42.667–75.

Bravo, M.; Canino, G.; and Bird, H. (1987). El DIS en español: Su tradiccion y adaptacion en Puerto Rico. *Acta Psiquiatr. Psicol. Am. Lat.* 33:27–42.

Brislin, R. W. (1970). Back translation for cross-cultural research. *J. Cross-Cultural Psychol.* 3:185–216.

Cooper, J. E.; Kendall, R. E.; Gurland, B. J.; Sharpe, L.; Copeland, J. R. M.; and Simon, R. (1972). *Psychiatric Diagnosis in New York and London*. New York: Oxford University Press.

Gaviria, F. M.; Pathak, D. S.; Flaherty, J. A.; Winthrop, R. M.; Martinez, H.; Garcia-Pacheco, C.; Richman, J.; and Birz, S. (1985). Developing instruments for cross-cultural research. Presented at the American Psychiatric Convention, Dallas, Texas, May.

Grove, W. M.; Andreasen, N. C.; McDonald, P.; Keller, M. B.; and Shapiro, R. W. (1981). Reliability studies of psychiatric diagnosis: Theory and practice. *Arch. Gen. Psychiatry* 38:408–13.

Helzer, J. E. (1983). Standardized interviews in psychiatry. *Psychiatric Developments* 2:161–78.

Helzer, J. E.; Clayton, P. J.; Pambakian, R.; Reich, T.; Woodruff, R. A., Jr.; and Reveley, M. A. (1977). Reliability of psychiatric diagnosis. II. The test–retest reliability of diagnostic classification. *Arch. Gen. Psychiatry* 34:145–49.

Helzer, J. E.; and Coryell, W. (1983) More on DSM-III: How consistent are precise criteria? Editorial, *Biol. Psychiatry* 18;1201–3.

Helzer, J. E.; Robins, L. N.; Croughan, J. L.; and Welner, A. (1981). Renard Diagnostic Interview: Its reliability and procedural validity with physicians and lay interviewers. *Arch. Gen. Psychiatry* 38:381–89.

Helzer, J. E.; Robins, L. N.; McEvoy, L. T.; Spitznagel, E. L.; Stoltzman, R. K.; Farmer, A.; and Brockington, I. F. (1985). Results of the St. Louis ECA physician reexamination: A study of the Diagnostic Interview Schedule. *Arch. Gen. Psychiatry* 42:657–66.

Karno, M.; Burnam, A.; Escobar, J. I.; Hough, R.; and Eaton, W. W. (1983). Development of the Spanish Language Version of the National Institute of Mental Health Diagnostic Interview Schedule. *Arch. Gen. Psychiatry* 40:1183–88.

Kreitman, N. (1977). Three themes in the epidemiology of alcoholism. In G. Edwards and M. Grant (eds.), *Alcoholism: New Knowledge and New Responses.* London: Croom Helm, pp. 48-59.

Ledermann, S. (1956). Alcool, alcoolisme, alcoolisation: Donnees Scientifiques de Caractere Physiologique Economique et Social [Alcohol, alcoholism, alcoholization: Scientific data of economic and social psychological character]. (Institut National d'Etudes Demographiques, Travaux et Documents; Cahier No. 29). Paris: Presses Universitaires de France.

Lorr, M. (ed.) (1966). *Explorations in Typing Psychotics.* New York: Pergamon.

Manson, S. M.; Shore, J. H.; and Bloom, J. D. (1985). The depressive experience in American Indian communities: A challenge for psychiatric theory and diagnosis. In A. Kleinman and B. Good (eds.), *Culture and Depression.* Berkeley, California: University of California Press.

Mezzich, J. E.; Fabrega, H.; Mezzich, A. C.; and Coffman, G. A. (1985). International experience with DSM-III. *J. Nerv. Ment. Dis.* 173:738–41.

Murphy, J. M. (1976). Psychiatric labeling in cross-cultural perspective. *Science* 191:1019–21.

Robins, L. N. (1981). The diagnosis of alcoholism after DSM-III. In R. E. Meyer; B. C. Glueck; J. E. O'Brien; T. F. Babor; J. H. Jaffe; and J. R. Stabenau (eds.), *Evaluation of the Alcoholic: Implications of Research, Theory and Treatment,* NIAA Research Monograph 5, DHHS Pub. No. (ADM) 81–1033, pp. 85–102.

Shapiro, R. W., and Stromgren, E. (1979). The relevance of epidemiological methods, techniques, and findings for biological psychiatry. In H. M. vanPraag (ed.), *Handbook for Biological Psychiatry, Part I.* New York: Marcel Dekker, Inc.

Spitzer, R. L. (1983). Psychiatry diagnosis: Are clinicians still necessary? *Compr. Psychiatry* 24:399–411.

World Health Organization (1987) *Tenth Revision of the International Classification of Diseases (ICD-10).* Geneva: World Health Organization.

Yu, E.; Zhang, M.; Xia, Z.; and Liu, W. T. (1984). Instrument translation in cross-cultural research: Issues and dilemmas. Paper presented at the First Symposium on Cross-Cultural Psychiatric Epidemiology, Chinese University of Hong Kong, Shatin, Hong Kong, May 10–12.

[2] Development of the Diagnostic Interview Schedule

JOHN E. HELZER

The ECA Survey

In the late 1970s, Darrel Regier and his colleagues at the National Institute of Mental Health (NIMH) started a multicenter psychiatric epidemiologic study in the United States, the Epidemiologic Catchment Area (ECA) Survey (Regier et al., 1984). The scope of this effort was huge. Plans called for several thousand face-to-face interviews to be conducted in five sites across the United States. Respondents were to be interviewed regarding their lifetime and recent history of psychiatric symptoms, utilization of health care services, perceived barriers to care, use of psychotropic medication, and recent untoward life events. There was also to be a follow-up interview 1 year after the index examination in order to estimate incidence of psychiatric disorder. It was apparent that it would be financially impractical to use psychiatrists as interviewers for an effort of this magnitude, and that it was therefore necessary to develop an interview instrument that would enable nonclinician (lay) interviewers to gather the clinical and other data needed to make psychiatric diagnoses.

This was a new approach to psychiatric epidemiology. The collection of epidemiologic data to assess psychiatric morbidity in individuals has taken many forms, including mailed questionnaires, interviewer-administered scales that are not diagnostically based, unstructured or semistructured "clinical" examinations by a psychiatrist, structured interviews utilizing screening questions for each diagnosis with a full examination only for those who pass through the screening "cut-off", and two-stage surveys in which only a portion of the sample is given a full examination.

The idea behind the ECA was to conduct a large-scale epidemiologic survey, using an instrument that could be administered by nonclinicians and that would generate specific psychiatric diagnoses according to well-defined criteria derived from clinical settings. This would maximize concordance with prior clinical knowledge and make the epidemiologic findings more clinically germane.

There was also a desire to minimize the use of previously popular screening questions and ask all symptom questions of every respondent. This would mean a longer interview but it would offer significant advantages, such as the opportunity to estimate prevalence of specific symptoms or symptom clusters, to attempt to relate these to the personal characteristics of individual respondents, to assess the distribution of the severity of individual disorders based on the number of positive symptoms, and to vary diagnostic thresholds.

In order to meet these goals, Regier and his colleagues contracted for a new epidemiologic interview to be developed for this project. The resulting instrument was the Diagnostic Interview Schedule or DIS (Robins et al., 1981a,b).

The Evolution of the DIS

The immediate predecessor of the DIS was the Renard Diagnostic Interview (RDI) (Helzer et al., 1981), a fully structured instrument for lay or clinician interviewers designed around the "Feighner" diagnostic criteria (Feighner et al., 1972), the most widely used psychiatric taxonomy at the time. After reviewing a variety of existing instruments, NIMH asked the authors of the RDI to develop a new interview that would preserve the specific questions and probes of the RDI and its completeness of coverage and coding, but one that would add a distinction between current and past diagnoses. New questions were to be added for the as yet unpublished DSM-III (APA, 1980) as well as for the Research Diagnostic Criteria (RDC) (Spitzer et al. 1975), since several previous studies had used the latter and it would be advantageous to be able to compare their prevalence rates with rates from the general population.

To create the new interview, the authors and a group of consultants reviewed the draft of the DSM-III to decide which of its diagnoses to include in the DIS. The diagnoses selected were those likely to be of greatest public health relevance and those for which criteria appeared to be sufficiently specific (see Chapter 5). Two diagnoses, generalized anxiety and post-traumatic stress disorder, were added after the ECA was already underway and thus were not included in most of the surveys in this volume. The Folstein-McHugh Mini-Mental State Examination (1975) was incorporated to provide a cross-sectional assessment of cognitive function.

A major challenge in the development of the DIS was to decide how the presence of psychiatric symptoms could be assessed by a lay (not clinically trained) interviewer. The design we used was as follows. First, a standard question is asked, for example: "Have you ever been bothered

by dizziness?" If the respondent answers positively, the clinical significance of the symptom is assessed by a standard set of probes, asking: 1) if
the symptom was reported to a physician or other health professional,
2) if the respondent has taken medication for the symptom more than
once, or 3) if the symptom has caused considerable interference with the
respondent's life and functioning. If none of these has occurred, the
symptom is considered not clinically significant, is given a unique code,
and pursued no further. Obviously, some symptoms, for example, suicide attempts, are considered intrinsically significant.

The next step is to learn whether there was always a physical explanation for the symptom. Two kinds of physical explanations are considered: 1) side effects of alcohol, medication, or illicit drugs, or 2) a physical illness or condition. If one or both of these physical explanations
always accounted for the symptom, it is not considered a possible manifestation of (a nonsubstance related) psychiatric disorder. A complex set
of probes is used to make this assessment, and only symptoms that had
no known physical cause are counted as possible psychiatric symptoms.

Through the probe structure, the DIS overcomes one of the chief
limitations of earlier lay interviewer surveys—their failure to distinguish
possible psychiatric symptoms from the ordinary discomforts of everyday life and from signs of physical illness. A typical example of the effect
of pruning initial positive responses is dizziness. In the St. Louis ECA
survey, dizziness was reported as having occurred at some time by
24 percent of the population, but after using the probes to rule out
occurrences that were not clinically significant and those explained by
nonpsychiatric causes, there were only 4 percent in whom it constituted
a possible psychiatric symptom.

Use of the DIS in Cross-National Research

The principles observed in developing the DIS for the ECA survey
enhance its utility for cross-national surveys as well. For example, since it
can be used by lay interviewers, financial constraints on the ascertainment of epidemiologic samples are reduced. The wide symptom coverage and the fact that all symptoms are asked of every respondent make it
possible to compare the symptomatic expression of disorders, not just
their rate of occurrence, and where diagnostic prevalences do vary, to
evaluate component differences. This also permits an examination of
risk factors at the symptom or subsyndromal level, rather than only at
the diagnostic level. The investigator can also experiment with different
diagnostic thresholds.

The interview also offers the opportunity of examining diagnoses
dimensionally or categorically rather than only the latter. This is particularly important in psychiatry, in which there are seldom biological mark-

ers against which to validate categories. It could be even more important in cross-national research, since meaningful categorical thresholds may vary considerably from one culture to the next, even if the underlying dimensions appear to be conceptually similar.

Because the interview is so highly structured, translation is facilitated. Translators are dealing with specific terms and phrases rather than more open-ended clinical concepts or judgments that leave greater latitude for translation. Furthermore, translations of the interview are diagnostically scored using the algorithms originally developed for the DIS. This ensures diagnostic consistency once the primary data have been collected. The computer diagnostic scoring program includes a series of thirty-five test cases, so that its comparability on local computer hardware can·be demonstrated before it is used to score collected data.

The DIS Alcohol Section

As with other interview segments, the alcohol section in the DIS focuses primarily, but not exclusively, on those symptom items specified in the DSM-III criteria. The section opens with a question about whether the respondent has ever been intoxicated and the age at which this first occurred. Lifelong abstainers are skipped out of the section. There are a few questions about quantity and frequency of alcohol use followed by a series of items about alcohol related social, medical, and legal problems that might have occurred at any time in the subject's life. Respondents who deny all such problems and do not have a history of heavy drinking are not asked the few remaining more serious alcohol-related complications such as withdrawal symptoms and medical complications. In all there are about thirty symptom questions in the alcohol section of the DIS.

As in other diagnostic sections, those who acknowledge alcohol symptoms are asked the ages of first and most recent occurrence of symptoms. For those who meet diagnostic criteria, these two ages are defined as the onset and recency of the disorder, respectively. Alcoholism is also one of the few sections of the interview where no probe questions are asked. The symptoms are all serious enough that they can be considered clinically significant, and they are phrased in relation to alcohol use so that probes regarding causation are unnecessary. Copies of the alcohol section Version III of the DIS and of the SAS (SAS Institute, 1982) computer program statements used to score it for DSM-III alcohol abuse and dependence appear in Appendices I and II. (Version III was the edition of the DIS used for the ECA survey. The most recent edition is Version IIIR, which incorporates the more recently published DSM-IIIR diagnostic criteria.)

Before its use in the ECA survey, the DIS was tested in a mostly clinical population so as to examine its utility as a diagnostic instrument. The primary intent was to see whether it was feasible to use nonclinician examiners to gather clinical data sufficient to make psychiatric diagnoses. Two hundred and sixteen inpatients, outpatients, and nonpatients were each examined twice, once by a lay interviewer using the DIS and once by a psychiatrist. The latter began with the DIS, but then was allowed to pursue any diagnostic uncertainties with additional clinical questions in a free-form manner (Robins et al., 1981a; Robins et al., 1982). The results were encouraging and indicated that lay/physician diagnostic agreement using this instrument was comparable to agreement between psychiatrists in a previous study of an interview designed exclusively for clinicians (Helzer et al., 1977). Results for alcohol diagnoses were especially good, and the kappa statistic (a measure that corrects for chance agreement) was 86 for DSM-III defined alcohol abuse and dependence. In only 3 percent of the cases were the psychiatrists in doubt about the diagnosis of alcoholism after completing the DIS. Agreement remained high regardless of the age, sex, or patient status of the respondent; there was also good agreement with diagnoses appearing in the patient's medical charts.

For practical reasons, this initial study of the DIS had to be completed mostly on identified patients. In order to test the DIS in the general population, a physician comparison study was done as part of the ECA project itself. This was accomplished by having psychiatrists reexamine approximately 400 of the lay-interviewed population respondents. The physicians readministered the DIS and also conducted a separate clinical examination using a diagnostic checklist based on DSM-III (Helzer et al., 1985).

Results showed lower agreement rates than in the previous clinical study, an expected result since psychiatric cases in the general population can be expected to be milder and more difficult to agree on. For most diagnoses, though, results were still quite acceptable. Alcohol abuse and dependence showed the best agreements of all those tested; the kappa was .63 and the y statistic was .73. (The latter statistic controls both for chance agreement and for the low diagnostic base rates expected in a general population survey.) Furthermore, there was no evidence of any bias in the alcoholism prevalence estimate.

Recently, we have examined the predictive validity of the lay and physician examinations using information collected at the ECA 1-year follow-up examination. We tested lay interviewer DIS diagnoses and physician DSM-III Checklist diagnoses anterospectively to see which better predicted outcomes at 1 year. Results varied by diagnosis, but overall we found that the lay and physician diagnoses predicted follow-up status approximately equally (Helzer et al., 1987).

Methodological Limitations

Taken together, these studies suggest that it is feasible to use nonclinician examiners to gather the clinical data necessary to make specific psychiatric diagnoses in general population surveys, and that the diagnosis of alcoholism is one of the most reliable of all. However, in evaluating results presented in this volume, the reader must keep in mind certain limitations in the data. First, findings are based on personal interview only; the respondent serves as the sole informant regarding his own past history of psychiatric symptoms. Thus, the data depends on the individual's willingness to report prior symptoms and behaviors candidly, and on his ability to recall past events accurately. This differs from some previous epidemiologic efforts in psychiatry in which, in addition to self report data, investigators also had access to informants who knew the subject well, records or reports from caregivers, and/or various public records such as those pertaining to health service utilization. For the most part, the sample sizes in the studies reported here make such additional information infeasible to obtain, particularly since few in the general population will have any record of treatment for emotional disorders.

Another limitation is the fact that the surveys contained here are all reporting prevalence of disorder rather than incidence. Prevalence is based on the count of all persons who are or have been ill during a specified time period. In contrast, incidence counts only those who have developed a new illness during the specified period. In epidemiologic research, the investigator searches for etiological clues by looking for social or personal factors that correlate with rates of illness, that is, illness risk factors. In this volume we will be comparing risk factors between various cultural and ethnic groups. However, the search for etiological risk factors is more appropriately done using incidence rather than prevalence rates, since prevalence correlates may be more strongly associated with the duration of illness than its cause.

One advantage of the present data in regard to the incidence versus prevalence issue is that the DIS focuses primarily on what is called "lifetime prevalence"; respondents are asked to report for each symptom if it has ever occurred in their lifetime. A lifetime diagnosis provides a history of psychiatric disorder over the individual's entire life span. Thus, the confounding of the occurrence of illness and its duration mentioned in the previous paragraph is less of a problem. But one unresolved question regarding lifetime prevalence is whether an individual is able to accurately recall symptoms that occurred only many years ago.

Lastly, we may question whether population respondents are likely to be candid when asked to report on personal behaviors of a sensitive nature, such as alcohol-related social or legal problems. A recent review of the literature concluded that self-reports of alcohol use and symptoms are generally valid (Midanik, 1982). For example, collateral reports were not found to provide better consumption information. This replicated earlier work by Guze et al. (1963) who found that discrepancies between alcoholics and their relatives were almost always a positive report of drinking by the former and a negative report by the latter. A recent study used several strategies to estimate reliability and validity of alcohol consumption reported in a household survey, and found both to be high (Williams, Aitken, and Malin, 1985). It has also been suggested that the perceived lack of candor in self reports of drinking by alcoholics may be due to situational demand characteristics (Hesselbrock et al., 1983) that would not apply in the relatively anonymous context of epidemiologic surveys. In general, estimates of reliability and validity of alcoholics' self reports have been good and suggest that such data can generally be used with confidence.

References

American Psychiatric Association, Committee on Nomenclature and Statistics (1980). *Diagnostic and Statistical Manual of Mental Disorder—Edition 3 (DSM-III)*. Washington, D.C.

Feighner, J. P.; Robins, E.; Guze, S. B.; Woodruff, R. A.; Winokur, G.; and Munoz, R. (1972). Diagnostic criteria for use in psychiatric research. *Arch. Gen. Psychiatry* 26, 57–63.

Folstein, M. F.; Folstein, S. E.; and McHugh, P. R. (1975). "Mini-Mental State": A practical method for grading cognitive state of patients for the clinician. *J. Psychiatr. Res.* 12:189–98.

Guze, S. B.; Tuason, V. B.; Steward, M. A.; and Picken, B. (1963). The drinking history: A comparison of reports by subjects and their relatives. *Q. J. Stud. Alcohol* 24:249–60.

Helzer, J. E.; Clayton, P. J.; Pambakian, R.; Reich, T.; Woodruff, R. A. Jr.; and Reveley, M. A. (1977). Reliability of psychiatric diagnosis. II. The test/retest reliability of diagnostic classification. *Arch. Gen. Psychiatry* 34:129–33.

Helzer, J. E.; Robins, L. N.; McEvoy, L. T.; Spitznagel, E. L.; Stoltzman, R. K.; Farmer, A.; and Brockington, I. F. (1985). A comparison of clinical and DIS diagnoses: Physician reexamination of lay interviewed cases in the general population. *Arch. Gen. Psychiatry* 42:657–66.

Helzer, J. E.; Robins, L. N.; Croughan, J. L.; and Welner, A. (1981). Renard Diagnostic Interview: Its reliability and procedural validity with physicians and lay interviewers. *Arch. Gen. Psychiatry* 38:393–98.

Helzer, J. E.; Spitznagel, E. L.; and McEvoy, L. (1987). The predictive validity of lay DIS diagnoses in the general population: A comparison with physician examiners. *Arch. Gen. Psychiatry* 44:1069–77.

Hesselbrock, M.; Babor, T. F.; Hesselbrock, V.; Meyer, R. E.; and Workman, K. (1983). "Never believe an alcoholic"? On the validity of self-report measures of alcohol dependence and related constructs. *Int. J. Addict.* 18:593–609.

Midanik, L. I. (1982). Over-reports of recent alcohol consumption in a clinical population: A validity study. *Drug and Alcohol Dependence* 9:101–10.

Regier, D. A.; Meyers, J. K.; Kramer, M.; Robins, L. N.; Blazer, D. G.; Hough, R. L.; Eaton, W. W.; and Locke, B. Z. (1984). The NIMH Epidemiologic Catchment Area program: Historical context, major objectives, and study population characteristics. *Arch. Gen. Psychiatry* 41:934–41.

Robins, L. N.; Helzer, J. E.; Croughan, J. L.; Williams, J. B. W.; and Spitzer, R. L. (1981a). NIMH Diagnostic Interview Schedule, Version III. Rockville, Md.: NIMH, Public Health Service (HHS), Publication ADM-T-42-3 (5-81, 8-81).

Robins, L. N.; Helzer, J. E.; Croughan, J. L.; and Ratcliff, K. S. (1981b). The NIMH Diagnostic Interview Schedule: Its history, characteristics, and validity. *Arch. Gen. Psychiatry* 38:381–89.

Robins, L. N.; Helzer, J. E.; Ratcliff, K. S.; and Seyfried, W. (1982). Validity of the Diagnostic Interview Schedule, Version II:DSM-III diagnoses. *Psychol. Med.* 12:855–70.

SAS Institute (1982). *Statistical Analysis System (SAS) User's Guide: 1982 Edition.* Cary, North Carolina: SAS Institute, Inc.

Spitzer, R. L.; Endicott, J.; and Robins, E. (1975). *Research Diagnostic Criteria (Instrument No. 58).* New York: Biometrics Research Division, New York State Psychiatric Institute.

Williams, G. D.; Aitken, S. S.; and Malin, H. (1985). Reliability of self-reported alcohol consumption in a general population survey. *J. Stud. Alcohol* 46:223–27.

[3] Contributions of Anthropology and Sociology to Alcohol Epidemiology

JANE M. MURPHY

Culturally speaking, alcohol is not a neutral topic. As far as is known, all contemporary societies have knowledge of alcohol, either through their own fermentation and distilling techniques, or through contact with areas where alcoholic beverages are produced. Yet groups of people bound together by a shared belief system and a common cultural heritage often hold distinctive views about drinking (Marshall, 1979; Heath, 1986a, 1986b). Among some groups, the use of alcohol is highly valued for the ideologic and integrative role it plays in religious ceremonies and social festivals. Among others, its use is severely proscribed and sometimes legally prohibited.

Also, considerable evidence has been accumulated indicating that rates of alcohol abuse may vary across different cultural groups (Lex, 1985). While it has frequently been observed that men are at greater risk than women, early attention to the influence of sociocultural factors was drawn by information about high rates of alcohol abuse among Irish Catholic men and low rates among Jewish men (Bales, 1946; Snyder, 1958). The cultural pluralism of a nation like the United States has given rise to studies that indicate marked differences in behaviors that may have influence on rates of abuse. The dominant pattern among some fundamentalist religious enclaves is total abstinence. On the other hand, while some Native American Indian groups also practice abstinence, others are known for very high rates of public drunkenness and a wide variety of alcohol-related problems.

A number of hypotheses about the way in which sociocultural factors might contribute to such differences have been put forward (Pittman &

Funds for the preparation of the paper were derived from NIMH Grant MH39576. Grateful appreciation is also expressed to Dr. Barbara Lex for guidance to the recent literature.

Snyder, 1962; Bennett & Ames, 1985; Babor, 1986). Some of these focus on the relationships between different cultural groups, usually in terms of the disadvantages and stresses of minority status. These deal with issues about cultural change and modernization, about conflict and confusion in cultural values, and about modes of adaptation to marginality, such as social cohesion versus social fractionation in the face of persecution.

Other hypotheses focus on factors within a culture. These concern questions about the influence of different types and degrees of social organization; about cultural values regarding altered states of consciousness, especially as they may play a role in rites of passage and other ceremonial rituals; about cultural patterns for alleviating anxiety; about levels of religious orthodoxy; about variations in socioeconomic security; and about a wide range of cultural practices concerning what, when, where, and with whom people drink.

It seems probable that, at the present time, awareness is nearly universal that abuse of alcohol has damaging consequences and that it takes a heavy toll regarding both the quality and length of life. Even where cultural beliefs and practices seem to protect some individuals from excessive drinking the recognition of potential ill-effects contributes to the view that alcoholism is now a health concern in many societies.

At the same time, the etiologies of alcohol disorders remain largely unknown, as do the means of preventing and controlling them. It is highly likely that alcoholism is a complex disorder with many factors contributing to its origins, course, and outcome. Sound research is thus needed along a broad front that includes investigation of genetic, biochemical, and psychological factors, as well as the social and cultural factors that may have an effect upon the epidemiology of alcohol disorders. Nevertheless, existing findings about the wide variation in patterns of consumption in different social groups as well as differences in rates of abuse suggest that alcohol epidemiology may be one of the most promising and fruitful areas for cross-cultural research.

World Ethnography

Cross-cultural research is customarily recognized as having been developed within the discipline of anthropology. Based on materials from ethnographic field studies, an extensive library of descriptive information known as the Human Relations Area File (HRAF) has been built up for use in comparative investigations (Murdock, 1967). Ethnographic studies—as the name indicates—are concerned with constructing a picture of an ethnic group by describing the beliefs and practices that make up its pattern of life and that distinguish it from other groups.

Typically an ethnography is a report prepared by an anthropologist who has lived for a period of time with a given cultural group, and who, using the techniques of participant-observation and key-informant interviewing, describes the group's pattern of subsistence, religious orientation, ceremonials, art, technology, habitat, everyday activities, and the basic assumptions that constitute the group's philosophical ethos. The goal of ethnography is to give an unbiased account of the values and lifestyle of a group as they are perceived and experienced within the group, in contrast to being filtered through what may be the prejudices of an outsider.

At the present time, the HRAF contains ethnographic data about several hundreds of cultural groups, mainly groups who are nonliterate and who are non-Western in philosophical orientation. Until recently it was rare for anthropologists to undertake ethnographic studies that were specifically and exclusively concerned with the cultural use of alcohol in such societies (Heath, 1975 and 1987). Nevertheless, the library contains a large amount of incidental information concerning values and attitudes about alcohol as well as patterns of its use. Access to this information is made possible through the cataloguing used in maintaining the HRAF.

Consistent with the fact that a topic like alcohol use and abuse invites interdisciplinary research, one of the earliest cross-cultural studies to make use of this anthropology-based library was carried out by a sociologist and centered on alcohol. Based on fifty-six societies about which information was considered to be adequate, this comparative study suggested that "the primary function of alcoholic beverages in all societies is the reduction of anxiety" (Horton, 1943, p. 223). Other studies of this type followed in which alcohol was perceived as serving still other functions, such as conviviality, and in which drunkenness was related to various types of cultural contexts.

Ethnography and Epidemiology

This type of cross-cultural research did not in and of itself lay the foundation for comparative investigation of the epidemiology of alcohol abuse. Epidemiologic studies require counting instances of something for a numerator and counting members of a population for a denominator. The instances that make up the numerator are usually those pathological behaviors and processes that separate the few from the many. Ethnography, on the other hand, is mainly concerned with identifying uniformities in cultural values and practices. The emphasis is on "the many" and not "the few," and on "use" rather than "abuse."

A lively interdisciplinary controversy has recently taken place about "problem deflation" and "problem amplification" as they relate to differences between ethnography and epidemiology in alcohol research (Room, 1984; Heath, 1987). It has been suggested that ethnographic studies tend to minimize the "problem" aspects of alcohol use in non-Western areas. On the other hand, planners and policymakers who are concerned with national development in these same areas and who have been influenced by epidemiologic evidence tend to emphasize what they perceive to be a growing number of "problems" related to alcohol abuse.

The minimization of problem drinking by anthropologists can be seen to flow from various methodologic and theoretical orientations. In keeping with the fact that ethnography focuses on the dominant patterns of cultural behavior, anthropologists "generally focus on the majority, who drink moderately or with impunity" and deal with alcohol "as it is used in the normal course of workaday affairs in integral communities" (Heath, 1987, p. 105). Ethnographic evidence has also been influenced by the functionalist school of thought, which tends to concentrate on the features of a sociocultural group that display stability and equilibrium. Everything that exists is seen as having a function, and an often-cited function of drinking is "the maintenance of social cohesion" (Room, 1984, p. 171).

In addition, "problem deflation" probably reflects the "principle of cultural relativity," which has been a fundamental premise in much of the anthropologic work in this area (Waddell, 1981). While excessive use of alcohol may lead to social, legal, and medical problems in industrialized societies, it can be argued that these are not necessarily the consequences of it in a non-Western area. An example of the relativist point of view is provided by Heath (1986a, p. 16) who, in generalizing about nonliterate societies, has said that "few have anything that might be called 'alcoholism' or even frequent 'drinking problems,' even when drinking and drunkenness are common." His ethnographic work with the Camba of eastern Bolivia (Heath, 1958) indicated that "virtually all the Camba drink to the point of passing out, at least twice a month" (Heath, 1975, p. 14). Using a 178-proof drink that is stronger in alcoholic concentration than most of the types of beverages used in other populations, Camba men drink in a ritualistic manner at social ceremonies, often continuing to drink for a day or more (Heath, 1971). Yet ethnographic observations of this group led to the conclusion that "there is no one among them who suffers any economic, social, or psychological problems in relation to alcohol, nor are there fights, insults, or other aggressive acts in connection with drinking" (Heath, 1975, p. 14).

Looking back on the history of ethnography, it seems as though there would have been value if more effort had been directed toward determining whether the groups studied had a concept of alcohol abuse, and especially whether there was a culturally standardized definition of abuse. Anthropological work of this latter type as it applies to the concept of insanity seems to have provided useful background information for cross-cultural studies of schizophrenia (Edgerton, 1966; Murphy, 1976). In one of the few studies of this type pertaining to alcohol, Kaplan and Johnson (1964) point out that the concept of "crazy drunkenness" is used by some Navajos to identify what they perceive to be a psychopathologic syndrome.

My own early effort to find out if an Eskimo group in the Bering Sea area had concepts of abnormal behavior that approximated psychiatric illness pointed to a clear-cut idea that alcohol could be abused and that adverse consequences might be involved (Murphy, 1972). Work with this group of Eskimos, who reside on St. Lawrence Island, also emphasized the importance of historical circumstances that may contribute to variations in attitudes and behaviors about alcohol use that need to be given attention when considering broad generalizations about cultural patterns.

The U.S. Indian Health Service (1977, p. 1) "considers that alcoholism is one of the most significant and urgent health problems facing the Indian and Alaskan Native people today." While there is considerable variation, several indicators of alcohol-related problems among these groups "reveal rates of alcohol abuse and alcoholism that are several times greater than those for the general population" (Lex, 1985, p. 152). In the mid-1950s when I worked in Alaska, such problems were already common. The St. Lawrence Eskimos, however, were distinctive in that they had been able in recent years to avoid the kinds of problems seen among other native groups in Alaska.

In the latter part of the eighteenth century, it had been customary for whaling ships to stop at St. Lawrence Island and to provide Eskimos with alcoholic beverages in trade, or to some extent, in payment for help in whaling (Hughes, 1960). In 1878, these Eskimos experienced a "Great Starvation" during which the population was decimated. It is probable that this event had multiple causes. In the eyes of many Eskimos who later reconstructed its history, one cause was seen to be the failure of the group to lay in an adequate supply of walrus meat, due to the fact that many of the hunters had been in a prolonged alcoholic debauch. For at least 40 years leading up to the time of my work there, the St. Lawrence Eskimos had lived under a strict and self-imposed prohibition against the use of alcohol. Most of the younger Eskimos of my acquaintance had no experience with alcohol, but the concepts of inebriation and abuse were part of the cognitive orientation that both explained and maintained prohibition (Murphy & Leighton, 1965).

It seems fair to say that ethnographic estimates of epidemiologic rates are subject to many sources of inaccuracy, not the least of which is the fact that they tend to be derived from the observations of a single person often with relatively little attention to problems of sampling. Being based on the interpretations of one individual, ethnographic generalizations tend also to reflect that person's orientation, or changes in orientation, despite the overall intent of presenting an unbiased and nonprejudicial picture of a cultural group. Honigmann (1980), for example, describes the differences in his presentation of drinking patterns in three Alaskan communities and relates them partly to his own attitudinal changes across an early, middle, and last study.

These comments about ethnography as a poor source for epidemiologic rates do not mean that studies of this kind cannot make a contribution to cross-cultural alcohol epidemiology. Ethnography remains a uniquely valuable approach for gathering data about cultural definitions of normal and abnormal behavior. If a cultural group is found to have a concept of alcohol abuse such as is conveyed in the idea of "crazy drunkenness" or in the behavior of instituting prohibition to guard against economic reverses, ethnographic studies can also lead to information about the indicators people in a given culture use to identify hazardous attributes of drinking, as well as giving data about ways to inquire about alcohol abuse so as to make such inquiry culturally appropriate and meaningful.

Ethnohistory is becoming more central among the methods of anthropology, and its application in alcohol studies will augment cross-sectional investigations by disclosing the circumstances under which attitudes and behaviors change over time. Insofar as epidemiologic studies of pathological behaviors can be enhanced by parallel investigations of the drinking patterns of those who do not become abusers, ethnographic studies that focus on the many who use alcohol without injury will continue to be needed. Lastly, ethnographic studies can provide an important qualitative base for interpreting epidemiologic findings and for generating culturally-sensible hypotheses.

Contributions to Survey Technology

It was also largely in the hands of sociologists that some of the more directly pertinent methods for epidemiologic research were developed (Merton & Lazarsfeld, 1950). From sociology came techniques for population sampling, thus addressing the denominator problem, and techniques for constructing questionnaires and carrying out systematic personal interviews about variations in behavior, thus addressing some aspects of the numerator problem.

Surveys involving structured interviews with subjects selected as probability samples of populations are now a well-known means of gathering information on a wide variety of human topics. The topics range from demographic issues, such as those that make up a census enumeration, to political issues that are involved in public opinion polling. Such surveys are predicated on the view that there are numerous features of human behavior and attitudes that can only be known by asking people questions and recording responses. Furthermore, if comparisons are to be drawn, people need to be asked the same questions, and be asked to respond by means of categories that are also the same for each person. The technology for constructing such systematic interviews is well developed, and there are established canons about the formulation of unambiguous questions, about probing routines, and about the training of lay interviewers.

Survey methods of this type have been used in a large number of investigations that concern health and illness, including studies of the epidemiology of psychiatric disorders (Srole et al., 1962; Berkman & Breslow, 1983). When structured interviews administered by persons not trained in clinical psychiatry were first used, the results were viewed with suspicion. In part this seems to have stemmed from the fact that psychoanalytic psychiatry suggested that most people were unaware of the crucial features of their own psychopathology. Since the most important aspects of intrapsychic dynamics were thought to be unconscious, many clinical psychiatrists believed that responses to simple, direct questions about psychiatric symptoms were uninformative. While suspicion about the meaning of answers to such questions has not completely abated, it has diminished. Although psychiatric syndromes are not necessarily equal in being accessible to questioning, it is now widely accepted that if it is desirable to know whether a person is depressed or not, for example, it is useful to ask questions about lowered mood, poor spirits, sleep disturbance, appetite loss, and so on.

Where alcohol studies are concerned, skepticism has taken a somewhat different turn. It has been thought that people selected as sample members would not report faithfully about alcohol use and abuse, not because they were unconscious of their own behavior, but because they would not want to admit it to an interviewer who happened to knock on their door. Resistance to giving accurate information about drinking was thought to be the stance many sample members would take—especially those with drinking problems—due to the social censure that surrounds alcoholism.

The survey method has, however, been used in a number of population studies of alcohol abuse. The results are unequivocal on one point. It is that variation has always been found in the responses people give to questions about the frequency and quantity of their drinking. Thus it is clear that denial is not universal. Furthermore, as such survey information has increased, the variations in such self-report data about drinking seem to make sense in that they correlate reasonably well with other types of evidence about rates of alcohol abuse in different segments of the population and in different regions of the country. While more work is needed, the available indicators of the reliability and validity of responses given in systematic surveys encourage the view that the personal interview can be an important tool for advancing cross-cultural studies of alcohol abuse.

Several sociological surveys of alcohol use have now been carried out in various states and among national samples of the U.S. (Mulford, 1968; Cahalan, 1970; Clark & Midanik, 1982). They offer consistent evidence that men are at higher risk than women. Variations in terms of residence in different regions of the country, socioeconomic status, and ethnic background have also been reported. The possibly protective influence of being a fairly orthodox Jew has stood up in this survey work, and, increasingly, similar influence is seen to stem from being a practicing Methodist or Baptist.

Recent Advances and Current Issues

Over the last 20 years, a major characteristic of alcohol studies is the degree to which they have become interdisciplinary. If not actually the product of joint effort on the part of researchers from different disciplines, many recent studies at least use interdisciplinary methods. While psychiatrists may have been slow to engage in epidemiologic studies of alcoholism and alcohol abuse (Kreitman, 1984), the collaboration of anthropologists, sociologists, and psychologists has been fundamental to a number of research endeavors (Jessor et al., 1968; Levy & Kunitz, 1974; Klausner & Foulks, 1982; Bennett & Ames, 1985). A feature of these collaborative studies is the sharing and cross-fertilization of ethnographic and survey methods. The researchers engaged in recent studies have also become much more knowledgeable about the alcohol field as a whole, especially the genetic and biological aspects of alcoholism, than was true of the earlier generations of ethnographers and survey analysts.

At the same time, innovative methods for gathering and checking information about alcohol use have been developed. For example, an investigation of religion and ethnicity that confirmed survey findings about Jewish and Irish contrasts was carried out in an emergency room using breathalyzer tests (Wechsler et al., 1970 and 1972). It has been suggested that the use of a hand-held battery-operated breath monitor might also prove to be an effective addition to ethnographic studies as would also improved techniques for determining the alcohol content of indigenous beverages (Lex, 1986). Other methods that are beginning to take their place in alcohol research are drinking diaries and increased use of consumption indicators, such as bar bills and inventory records.

Not only are new methods being used but also new interests are being expressed. Among these is concern to improve understanding about the functioning of self-help groups such as Alcoholics Anonymous (Madsen, 1974). Another is to clarify which types of treatment may be especially appropriate for certain cultural groups (Jilek-Aall, 1974).

The expansion of anthropological and sociological research on alcohol has been encouraged by the establishment in 1970 of the National

Institute on Alcohol Abuse and Alcoholism (NIAAA) and its program of postdoctoral programs for these disciplines (Heath, 1987). Similar encouragement has come from such "invisible colleges" as that which emanates from the Rutgers Center of Alcohol Studies and the Alcohol and Drug Study Group. Several encyclopedic reviews of anthropological studies of alcohol constitute an on-going archive of the field (Heath, 1975, 1986a, 1986b, 1987).

Despite these advances, a persistent issue is the difficulty in establishing an adequate definition of alcohol abuse for comparative studies. While it appears that persons can and will report drinking practices and problems, important questions have been raised about how to analyze information on differing quantities and frequencies of drinking so as to identify alcohol abuse in a consistent way that is meaningful in both clinical and cultural terms.

Comparability regarding the definition of disorder is not a unique problem to alcohol studies. It has pervaded the field of cross-cultural psychiatry generally. Where schizophrenia is concerned, however, significant progress has been made through the use of standardized personal interviews and the application of specified criteria for defining the disorder. The International Pilot Study of Schizophrenia has shown, for example, that patients diagnosed as schizophrenic tend to give interview material that displays similar symptomatic manifestations in widely scattered cultural areas around the world and that a standard definition of schizophrenia employed for research purposes in this study is surprisingly comparable to the diagnostic criteria customarily employed by psychiatrists in these different areas (World Health Organization, 1973).

Similarly, prospects for a thrust forward regarding cross-cultural alcohol studies relates to the considerable consensus about definitions that has been achieved for the presentation of alcohol disorders in the World Health Organization's *International Classification of Disorders* (ICD-9) (World Health Organization, 1977), and the American Psychiatric Association's *Diagnostic and Statistical Manual of Mental Disorders* (DSM-III) (American Psychiatric Association, 1980).

Addressing the need for improved definitions, WHO established a committee of experts to prepare a glossary for the mental disorder section of ICD that gives fuller diagnostic descriptions than heretofore, thus paving the way for more reliable assessments (World Health Organization, 1978). The architects of DSM-III went even further in that the diagnostic categories are defined by operational criteria. Where DSM-I, for example, defined alcoholism solely as a "well established addiction to alcohol" (American Psychiatric Association, 1952), DSM-III gives multiple indicators of abuse, specifies durational criteria for abusive consumption, and requires that impairment in social or occupational functioning be in evidence and that the disturbance has been present for at least a month.

By virtue of having available specified criteria reflecting the consensus of a large psychiatric community, it has been possible to design a schedule for a personal interview through which information relevant to the operational definitions of disorders can be collected. The NIMH Diagnostic Interview Schedule (DIS) was developed for a large multi-site study in the United States known as the Epidemiologic Catchment Area (ECA) program (Robins et al., 1981; Regier et al., 1984). Through the DIS, as explained by Helzer in Chapter 2, a foundation is being laid for a new type of large-scale multinational research that may give crucial information about alcohol abuse. There remain, however, questions about the appropriateness of DSM-III alcohol abuse criteria for investigations in other cultures. Although these definitional criteria have been accepted for a nation of great cultural diversity, it would be a mistake to assume that the criteria are universally applicable. Furthermore the DIS was originally prepared in English and has needed to be translated into other languages not only for use among non-English speakers in the U.S. but also for use in other countries.

While tests of the cultural relevance of the alcohol section of the DIS will undoubtedly increase in number, it is of interest that in a U.S. study of monolingual and bilingual Spanish-speaking patients, among whom a Spanish translation of the DIS was assessed, the agreement between the DIS and clinical diagnoses was higher for alcohol abuse than that for any other diagnosis (Karno et al., 1983). Such information suggests that methods are now available for productive international research on the psychosocial and cultural correlates of alcohol disorders.

References

American Psychiatric Association (1952). *Diagnostic and Statistical Manual: Mental Disorders* (First Edition). Washington, D.C.: American Psychiatric Association.

American Psychiatric Association (1980). *Diagnostic and Statistical Manual: Mental Disorders* (Third Edition). Washington, D.C.: American Psychiatric Association.

Babor, T. F. (ed.) (1986). *Alcohol and Culture: Comparative Perspectives from Europe and America.* The New York Academy of Sciences, New York.

Bales, R. F. (1946). *Quart. J. Stud. Alcohol* 6:480.

Bennett, L. A., and Ames, G. M. (eds.) (1985). *The American Experience with Alcohol: Contrasting Cultural Perspectives.* New York: Plenum Press.

Berkman, L. F., and Breslow, L. (1983). *Health and Ways of Living: The Alameda County Study.* New York: Oxford University Press.

Cahalan, D. (1970). *Problem Drinkers.* San Francisco: Jossey-Bass, Inc.

Clark, W., and Midanik, L. (1982). *Alcohol Consumption and Related Problems,* Alcohol and Health Monograph No. 1. Rockville, Md.: National Institute of Alcohol Abuse and Alcoholism, 3.

Edgerton, R. B. (1966). *Am. Anthropology* 68:408.

Heath, D. B. (1958). *Quart. J. Stud. Alcohol* 79:491.

Heath, D. B. (1971). *Hum. Organization* 30:179.

Heath, D. B. (1975). In R. Gibbins, Y. Israel, H. Kalant, R. Popham, W. Schmidt, and R.

Smart (eds.), *Research Advances in Alcohol and Drug Problems*. New York: John Wiley & Sons, 2:1.

Heath, D. B. (1986a). *Transcult. Psychiatr. Res. Rev.* 23:1, 7.

Heath, D. B. (1986b). *Transcult. Psychiatr. Res. Rev.* 23:2, 103.

Heath, D. B. (1987). *Ann. Rev. Anthropol.* 16:99.

Honigmann, J. J. (1980). In J. Hamer and J. Steinbring (eds)., *Alcohol and Native Peoples of the North*. Washington, D.C.: University Press of America.

Horton, D. J. (1943). *Quart. J. Stud. Alcohol* 4:199.

Hughes, C. C. (Murphy, J. M., collaborator) (1960). *An Eskimo Village in the Modern World*. Ithaca: Cornell University Press.

Jessor, R.; Graves, T. D.; Hanson, R. C.; and Jessor, S. L. (1968). *Society, Personality, and Deviant Behavior: A Study of a Tri-Ethnic Community*. New York: Holt, Rinehart and Winston.

Jilek-Aall, L. (1974). *Canadian Psychiatric Assoc. J.* 19:357.

Kaplan, B., and Johnson, D. (1964). In Kiev, A. (ed). *Magic, Faith and Healing*. New York: The Free Press of Glencoe.

Karno, M.; Burnam, M. A.; Escogar, J. I.; Hough, R. L.; and Eaton, W. W. (1983). *Arch. Gen. Psychiatry* 40:1183.

Klausner, S. Z., and Foulks, E. F. (1982). *Eskimo Capitalists: Oil, Politics, and Alcohol*. Allanheld, N.J.: Osman Publishers.

Kreitman, N. (1984). *Soc. Psychiatry* 19:153.

Levy, J. E., and Kunitz, S. J. (1974). *Indian Drinking: Navajo Practices and Anglo-American Theories*. New York: John Wiley & Sons, Inc.

Lex, B. W. (1985). In J. Mendelson and N. Mello (eds)., *The Diagnosis and Treatment of Alcoholism*. New York: McGraw-Hill, 89.

Lex, B. W. (1986). *Med. Anthropol.* 17:95.

Madsen, W. (1974). *The American Alcoholic: The Nature-Nurture Controversy in Alcoholic Research and Therapy*. Springfield, Ill.. Charles C. Thomas.

Marshall, M. (ed.) (1979). *Beliefs, Behaviors, and Alcoholic Beverages: A Cross-Cultural Survey*. Ann Arbor: University of Michigan Press.

Merton, R. K., and Lazarsfeld, P. F. (eds.) (1950). *Continuities in Social Research*. New York: Free Press.

Mulford, H. A. (1968). In Spitzer, S. P., and Denzin, N. K. (eds.), *The Mental Patient: Studies in the Sociology of Deviance*. New York: McGraw-Hill.

Murdock, G. P. (1967). *Ethnographic Atlas*. Pittsburgh: University of Pittsburgh Press.

Murphy, J. M. (1972). In Lebra, W. P. (ed.), *Transcultural Research in Mental Health*. Honolulu: University of Hawaii Press, 213.

Murphy, J. M. (1976). *Science* 191:1019.

Murphy, J. M., and Leighton, A. H. (1965). In Murphy, J. M., and Leighton, A. H. (eds). *Approaches to Cross-Cultural Psychiatry*. Ithaca: Cornell University Press, 64.

Pittman, D. J., and Snyder, C. R. (eds.) (1962). *Society, Culture, and Drinking Patterns*. New York: John Wiley & Sons, Inc.

Regier, D. A.; Myers, J. K.; Kramer, M.; Robins, L. N.; Blazer, D. G.; Hough, R. L.; Eaton, W. W.; and Locke, B. Z. (1984). *Arch. Gen. Psychiatry* 41:934.

Robins, L. N.; Helzer, J. E.; Croughan, J.; and Ratcliff, K. S. (1981). *Arch. Gen. Psychiatry* 38:381.

Room, R. (1984). *Current Anthropology* 25:169.

Snyder, C. R. (1958). *Alcohol and the Jews: A Cultural Study of Drinking and Sobriety*. New Brunswick, N.J.: Publications Division, Rugters Center for Alcohol Studies.

Srole, L.; Langner, T. S.; Michael, S. T.; Opler, M. K.; and Rennie, T. A. C. (1962). *Mental Health in the Metropolis: The Midtown Manhattan Study*. New York: McGraw-Hill.

United States Indian Health Service, Task Force on Alcoholism (1977). *Alcoholism: A High Priority Health Problem*. Washington, D.C.: Indian Health Service.

Waddell, J. O. (1981). In D. B. Heath, J. O. Waddell, and M. D. Topper (eds.), *Cultural*

Factors in Alcohol Research and Treatment of Drinking Problems. Journal of Studies on Alcohol suppl. 9:18.

Wechsler, H.; Demone, H. W., Jr.; Thum, D.; and Kasey, E. H. (1970). *J. Health Hum. Behav.* 11:21.

Wechsler, H.; Thum, D.; Demone, H. W., Jr.; and Dwinnell, J. (1972). *Quart. J. Stud. Alcohol* 33:132.

World Health Organization (1973). *Report of the International Pilot Study of Schizophrenia.* Geneva: World Health Organization.

World Health Organization (1977). *Manual of the International Statistical Classification of Diseases, Injuries, and Causes of Death* (Ninth Revision). Geneva; World Health Organization.

World Health Organization (1978). *Mental Disorders: Glossary and Guide to Their Classification in Accordance with the Ninth Revision of the International Classification of Diseases.* Geneva: World Health Organization.

[4] Cross-Cultural Research on Alcohol: A Quoi Bon?

Thomas F. Babor

One of the most important developments in alcohol studies in recent years is the realization that this relatively young and disparate field is outgrowing the watertight compartments in which its youth was spent. As the fund of knowledge grows and improvements are made in methods of inquiry, it has become increasingly evident that there are a multitude of questions that cannot be answered within the self-imposed limits of single disciplines.

The social and natural sciences are both crucial to an understanding of drinking behavior. Natural scientists tend to be reductionist, assuming that complex phenomena can be broken down into simpler components and that one must begin by studying these basic units. Social scientists eschew reductionism, arguing that the whole is often greater than the sum of its parts. Despite the lack of mature theoretical systems, social scientists have focused on multivariate descriptions of alcohol-related phenomena, tending to reject the emphasis of the natural sciences on rudiments.

Except in the most reductionistic and superficial terms, the drinking behavior of individuals cannot be understood without constant reference to the cultural and social environments in which they have developed and within which they have to live. This means that while genetics, biology, chemistry, and pharmacology all have their place in the field of alcohol studies, the social and behavioral sciences have an equally important role to play, especially with respect to integrating and applying the findings of the various scientific disciplines.

With this general assumption in mind, the present chapter will survey what is perhaps the most difficult, ambitious, and hazardous type of alcohol research; cross-cultural comparisons of drinking behavior. The purpose of this review is to show how this area of social research has evolved over the years, what findings have emerged, how their findings have contributed to the development of theory, and how these theories have resulted in some practical applications to the prevention and treatment of alcohol-related problems.

33

Before examining the contributions of cross-cultural research to alcohol studies, it is important to clarify the meaning of some important terms. Leighton and Murphy (1965) have defined culture as an abstraction that refers to the pattern of life exhibited by a social group. This "way of life" is sufficiently cohesive to constitute the basis for a society. Another common definition of culture is the learned beliefs and behaviors shared by a group of individuals over time. Culture has meaning only in relation to human groups. These social units have been variously defined by age, sex, socioeconomic status, ethnicity, race, religion, and national identity, as well as by combinations of these overlapping social categories. Once these units have been specified, cross-cultural comparative research has typically compared cultural groups in terms of drinking behavior, to identify differences that might be explained by cultural variables or to identify commonalities that might suggest universal aspects of drinking (Babor, 1986).

Despite the intuitive logic of cross-cultural comparisons of drinking behavior, the term *culture* has been rarely defined or made explicit in such research. Heath (1987), remarking on the use of the word at a recent conference on cultural studies of drinking, concluded that at least four different definitions of culture were employed by the group of social scientists convened to discuss their research. Some spoke of culture in a historical sense, giving emphasis to social heritage or tradition. Others used the word culture in a descriptive sense, emphasizing enumeration of cultural content. A third meaning referred to normative rules or ways of living, while a final sense was in terms of normative rules or values plus behavior. While lack of a common definition of culture has not dissuaded social researchers from cross-cultural comparisons of drinking, alcohol researchers' relative lack of interest in the content and process of culture has probably impeded the development of integrated theory and social explanations of drinking problems.

To understand what contributions emerge when social scientists from many different countries study large numbers of variables in many different cultures, it is crucial to examine the broad territory of cross-cultural analysis as it has been applied to alcohol research. Room (1988) has attempted to map the territory of cross-cultural analysis by examining the different traditions of data collection that have developed in the past 3 decades. These include general theoretical analyses of alcohol and culture (e.g., MacAndrew and Edgerton's (1969) book *Drunken Comportment*); holocultural studies, such as Horton's (1943) analysis of anxiety and drunkenness in fifty-six tribal societies; cross-cultural diagnostic studies, which have typically focused on either culture-bound symptomatological differences or common syndromes within different clinical samples (Westermeyer, 1974); within-country ethnic comparisons (see Lex, 1987); cross-national surveys of drinking practices, attitudes, or problem indicators (e.g., Ritson, 1985; Makela, 1986); and comparisons of cross-national trends in drinking problems and alcohol control policies (Makela et al., 1981). Because this literature has been reviewed elsewhere (Heath, 1987; Room, 1988), including several of the introductory chapters to this volume, the present chapter will limit itself to the more practical task of illustrating how sociocultural research has contributed to an understanding of drinking behavior and its consequences.

These contributions can be characterized in terms of four broad topics: 1) understanding of macro-level variables affecting longitudinal trends in incidence and prevalence; 2) elucidation of basic mechanisms in human drinking behavior; 3) testing the generalizability of otherwise culture-bound theories; and 4) stimulating action-oriented research in the service of public health. While this categorization is by no means complete, it should provide a representative survey of the applications of sociocultural analysis to the field of alcohol studies.

Macrolevel Variables

When rates of cirrhosis mortality, alcoholism, heavy drinking, per capita consumption, and alcohol-related problems are compared cross-nationally and over historical periods, a number of insights can be obtained into the macrolevel variables that affect long-term trends in the evolution of drinking patterns and problems. Thus, one contribution cross-cultural, and more specifically, cross-national comparisons have made to the understanding of drinking behavior is to provide a view of the "big picture." In this case, the big picture is the panoramic view of how social, historic, and economic factors affect societal drinking patterns, as well as the incidence and prevalence of alcohol-related problems.

Per Capita Consumption and Alcohol-Related Problems

Cross-national differences in cirrhosis mortality have been linked to per capita consumption in different countries. Skog (1985), for example, has used cross-national consumption estimates to identify the "wetness" of drinking cultures as a key variable in the epidemiology of liver cirrhosis. Before him, Ledermann (1964) used cross-national comparisons of longitudinal trends in drinking to identify demographic and economic determinants of drinking problems. These associations are subject to a variety of interpretations; they have increased our awareness of the possible economic, political, demographic, historical, and sociocultural forces that influence consumption levels and the manifestation of alcohol-related problems.

Many of the longitudinal techniques perfected in earlier national studies of alcohol consumption were brought together in the International Study of Alcohol Control Experiences (ISACE). The goal of

ISACE was to study the social history of postwar alcohol control policy in seven societies: California, Finland, Ireland, the Netherlands, Ontario, Poland, and Switzerland (Makela et al., 1981; Osterberg, 1986), and to assess the influence of alcohol control policy on alcohol consumption and its consequences. Changes in alcohol-related problems were studied not only in relation to alcohol consumption, but also in relation to societal perception of social problems and the influence these perceptions have on alcohol problem statistics. Although ISACE found evidence of a general correlation between average per capita consumption and liver cirrhosis, the association was by no means consistent with respect to other types of problems. According to Osterberg, analysis of the alcohol problems statistics indicated that:

> Each society has certain specific social circumstances and drinking habits, and the mixture of alcohol-related problems thus varies accordingly. . . . Even in a given cultural setting, however, the relationship between consumption level and problems is by no means a simple one. First of all, the cultural patterns of drinking and drunken behavior do change. Second, many other factors besides actual drinking behavior determine the rate and seriousness of alcohol problems. Urban ecology influences the probability that public drunkenness will result in social conflicts; medical technology has an impact on the incidence of fatal delirium, and so on.
>
> (Osterberg, 1986, pp. 17–18).

Another important finding of the ISACE study was that during the postwar period, cultural perceptions of alcohol problems changed radically in every society studied. "Alcohol problems tended to be redefined as medical problems. Behavior that had earlier been looked upon as reprehensible conduct and dealt with by social and legal authorities was redefined as a symptom of an underlying disease which had to be treated" (Osterberg, 1986, p. 18). What these findings indicate is that the "alcoholism movement" in the United States may have been less responsible for the "medicalization" of alcohol-related problems than the broader social and economic changes that were typical of all industrialized societies during this period.

The ISACE study is unique in the annals of cross-cultural research on alcohol in its emphasis on both the process and the quantitative aspects of the relationship between alcohol and culture. In addition to providing a view of the "big picture," it also gave evidence of how pieces of the alcohol puzzle fit together to form a dynamic, ever-changing whole whose boundaries are constantly being defined by an interplay between external and internal forces.

Patterns of Drinking and Types of Alcohol Problems

Another contribution of cross-cultural research has been to increase understanding of international variations in drinking patterns and beverage preferences. Historical and epidemiological evidence has been marshalled to explain the development of different patterns of drinking that appear to be linked to types of alcoholism. Historical analysis, ethnographic research, and epidemiological surveys provide some support for the notion that patterns of drinking differ markedly between the wine-producing countries, typified by France, and those industrialized countries, such as the United States, where beer and distilled liquors are the preferred beverages (Sulkunen, 1976).

In the wine-producing Mediterranean countries of Spain, Portugal, Italy, France, and Greece, the pattern of drinking and the type of alcoholism has historically been associated with the use of wine as a dietary supplement, as well as a social lubricant, medicine, and stimulant for manual workers. Drunkenness is considered uncommon in relation to the high level of daily consumption. Drinking tends to be integrated into daily activities and rituals. Wine is typically consumed in moderation by a large segment of the population, and it is used more for its social and presumed nutritional value than for its psychological effects. Children are introduced to alcohol gradually and naturally. There are few legal restrictions on the availability of alcoholic beverages. Because alcohol has been closely connected with the economic and cultural development of these countries since ancient times, it is not surprising that their drinking customs are both numerous and complex.

How did the southern European nations come to develop a set of drinking customs and a pattern of alcoholism that differ in major respects from those of other countries? To understand the development of national drinking cultures, it is necessary to know something about the social, economic, and geographic forces that determine the history of drinking in a particular society. Cultural geography, for example, has shown that wine production is strongly affected by soil conditions and climate (Wagner, 1974). Historically, people drink what is produced locally. This may explain why there is so much diversity in the drinking customs and problems of the different European countries, despite their common cultural and economic heritage. Traditionally, the European nations, which consume approximately half the world's alcohol, have specialized in the production of wine, beer, or spirits. Because of its moderate climate and abundance of sunny days, southern Europe excels in wine production. Not surprisingly, Portugal, Spain, France, and Italy are among the world's leaders in wine consumption. Similarly, central European countries like Germany, Austria, and the United Kingdom, where conditions favor the production of barley and hops, have developed a preference for beer as their national alcoholic beverage. Finally, the northern countries, where only grains and fruits are economical to grow, are partial to the use of distilled spirits.

While geographic differences are not the sole explanation for the emergence of wine-drinking, beer-drinking, and spirits-drinking cultures, statistical comparisons of national beverage preferences have been useful, identifying factors that influence aggregate alcohol consumption as well as the social problems associated with different culturally-patterned drinking practices (Makela, 1978; Sulkunen, 1976). When other variables, such as economic fluctuations, technological development, political forces, and demographic trends are studied in relation to the historical variations in alcohol-related indicators, major contributions have been made to our understanding of the factors that control the societal or aggregate level of alcohol use.

Geography and climate are enabling conditions that interact with social and economic factors over the course of history. In ancient Rome, alcoholic beverages were, for the most part, produced locally using rudimentary procedures suited to the agricultural products of a particular region. With the collapse of the Roman Empire, Catholic religious institutions, particularly the monasteries, became the repositories of the brewing and wine-making techniques developed in the ancient world (Seward, 1982). In addition to the need for wine to celebrate Mass, medieval monks produced and sold large quantities of wine to support the monastic movement that flowered in the twelfth century. The abbeys of Austria, Italy, Spain, Switzerland, Portugal, and Hungary all cultivated the grape. In France, the monks developed the burgundies, bordeaux, and champagnes that graced the finest tables of medieval Europe. French monks perfected the art of sparkling champagne, were probably the first to fortify sherry, and brought distillation into widespread use on the European continent (Dion, 1977; Seward, 1982).

The beginning of western European drinking customs emerged out of the Dark Ages with the tremendous changes in agriculture, trade, and population that took place during the twelfth and thirteenth centuries. Distillation was introduced to Europe around 1250. From the beginning, spirits drinking became associated with a number of religious rituals and medical customs. By the sixteenth century, flavored liqueurs became popular among the aristocracy as an after dinner drink. By the beginning of the seventeenth century, the drinking habits of the different European countries were defined by customs and rituals that would be familiar to the contemporary observer.

Since the late nineteenth century, France and the wine-producing countries have consistently led the world in per capita alcohol consumption. One national survey conducted in 1974 (Armyr et al., 1982) estimated that 43 percent of the adult population of France drinks wine daily, or almost daily. In addition to wine, the French, Swiss, and Italians also consume significant amounts of distilled alcohol.

Given the pervasive use of alcoholic beverages in the wine-producing countries, it is not surprising that they lead the world in many indicators alcohol-related health problems. Although international statistics must be interpreted cautiously, there is some agreement that the French, for example, rank among the highest in alcohol-related liver cirrhosis, cancer, and traffic accidents. The rate of alcohol dependence is also assumed to be extremely high (Armyr et al., 1982).

In contrast to the wine-drinking countries of the Mediterranean and other temperate climates, the use of distilled spirits tends to be concentrated in the northern periphery of Europe. What distinguishes the drinking patterns of countries such as Norway, Sweden, Finland, and Poland is the separation of drinking from dietary functions, the deliberate use of alcohol to produce intoxication, and the concentration of heavy drinking in a relatively small portion of the male population. In a comparative study of attitudes toward drinking and drunkenness in four Scandinavian countries, Makela (1986) found that situational norms are similar among these countries. This study revealed three characteristic features of the traditional Nordic drinking culture: 1) drinking and work are kept strictly separate; 2) drinking is still not integrated with daily meals, as in the Mediterranean countries; and 3) there is a clear demarcation between nondrinking situations and situations where drinking to intoxication is culturally accepted. The traditional uses of alcohol in spirits-drinking countries have contributed to a pattern of drinking problems characterized by alcohol-related accidents, social disruption, and public intoxication.

The predominantly beer-drinking countries of Germany, Austria, Belgium, the United States, and the United Kingdom are less amenable to classification because per capita consumption tends to be intermediate between the wine-drinking and spirits-drinking countries. These countries tend to have more diversified drinking customs, and have been increasing their per capita consumption by adding drinking customs and beverage types from other countries.

According to Makela (1986), the historically dominant functions of alcohol present in each society play an important role in the drinking patterns and alcohol-related problems that are manifested in that society. By suggesting what these dominant functions are, and how they evolve over time, cross-cultural analysis has made important contributions, not only to our understanding of the distribution and determinants of alcohol problems at the societal level, but also to the explanation of why problem drinkers differ among themselves.

Basic Mechanisms in Human Drinking Behavior

Another contribution cross-cultural research has made to alcohol studies has been to broaden our understanding of the basic biological, psychological and social mechanisms that control human drinking behavior. Among the many factors social researchers have studied using cross-cultural analysis are biological vulnerability to alcohol, personality predispositions, and the role of social learning processes, such as socialization and acculturation, in the development of drinking practices.

Biological Vulnerability

Drinking patterns are perpetuated by tradition and cultural practice, yet are not merely cultural inventions. To the extent that some complex social behaviors, such as incest taboos, may be under a degree of genetic control, certain drinking behaviors and dependence symptoms may be shaped by a special kind of evolution in which genes and culture work together.

If alcoholism were predominantly under genetic control, those predisposed to it would be capable of learning only one set of drinking behaviors and the basic structure of drinking patterns would be similar. Not even the most ardent genetic theorists suggest that alcoholics are genetic automatons, although early in this century biologists espoused a form of genetic determinism that argued that genes governed not only anatomy but also drinking behavior.

One line of cross-cultural research that has broadened our understanding of biological and genetic mechanisms is the study of the so-called "flushing response" to alcohol. In an influential study, Wolff (1972) investigated objective correlates of face flushing and alcohol use in several ethnic groups. Orientals (Japanese, Taiwanese, and Koreans) showed a higher incidence of face flushing, greater changes in optical density, greater increases in blood pressure, and a greater variety of intoxication symptoms. Other researchers have confirmed that Asians are more likely to flush after consuming alcohol (Park et al., 1984; Ewing et al., 1974), supporting the hypothesis that Asians may metabolize alcohol more rapidly than Caucasians. This produces an accumulation of acetaldehyde, which in turn could result in dysphoria, increased heart rate, and other symptoms observed in Oriental drinkers. For example, Park et al. (1984) found that there were more fast flushers (flush after one or fewer drinks) among Chinese in Taiwan than among Koreans, a factor that could account for the lower alcohol consumption by Chinese. Researchers engaged in this line of cross-cultural investigation have attempted to explain the apparent relation between alcohol reactivity and rates of alcohol consumption by means of a possible interaction between physiological variables and cultural orientation (Sue & Nakamura, 1984).

The mechanisms of the genetic component in alcoholism have not been developed into a systematic theory, perhaps because of the reluctance of natural scientists to venture into explanations of complex behavior, or perhaps because the biological data are inadequate to the task. Genetically determined influences that are triggered under certain cultural conditions and physiologically based acquired needs (e.g., dependence) are two of the biologically based constructs that must be integrated with the sociocultural data before a comprehensive biopsychosocial theory of alcoholism can be advanced. It has become a truism that genetically determined behaviors need not be universally displayed. But the research suggests that genes may bias the choice an individual makes, rendering it more likely that one behavior will be favored over an alternative.

Personality, Psychopathology, and Patterns of Alcoholism

The interaction between sociocultural and personality factors in the development of alcoholism has been discussed extensively by E. M. Jellinek (1960). He argued that culture influences the manifestation of alcohol problems by creating a set of enabling conditions for those with predisposing personality traits. Jellinek (1962) suggested that the concept of alcoholism has different meanings throughout the world as a consequence of cultural differences in the way alcoholics drink, the symptoms they develop, the consequences they experience, and the various etiologies of their disorder. In England, Scandinavia, and North America, the terms alcoholic and alcoholism tend to be associated with the "steady symptomatic excessive drinker," that is, a drinker whose impaired control over drinking is a consequence of an underlying psychological problem. This view of alcoholism may not be universal, however, as suggested by public attitudes and medical concepts in the predominantly wine-drinking nations of southern Europe and South America. The French conception of alcoholism is considered to be typical of this alternative conception. According to Jellinek (1962, p. 384): "There is in the French literature on alcoholism frequent mention of *l'alcoolisme sans ivresse* (alcoholism without drunkenness); that is, it is asserted that a drinker can become alcoholic without ever showing signs of intoxication."

The absence of intoxication is not the only characteristic distinguishing this "inveterate" drinker. Whereas psychological problems and personality disturbance are presumed to underlie symptomatic drinking in the "Anglo-Saxon" countries, social customs and economic incentives are seen as the major influences in French alcoholism. Termed "gamma" and "delta" alcoholics, respectively, these varieties of alcoholism can be found in every nation of drinkers. But because one variety or the other tends to predominate, the alcoholism label brings with it a set of meanings consistent with the prevailing cultural view.

Despite widespread acceptance of the gamma-delta distinction in the international classification of alcoholics, this typological theory has inspired little cross-cultural research (Babor & Dolinsky, 1988). A comparative study of French-speaking and English-speaking Canadian alcoholics conducted by Negrete (1973) showed that Anglo-Protestants differed from French Catholics on indicators of poor social functioning, such as unemployment, marital adjustment, and legal problems. In addition to having poorer social performance, personality disorder seemed to be more prevalent among the Anglo Protestants. These findings were interpreted as evidence in favor of the gamma-delta distinction. In another study supporting the gamma-delta classification, Babor et al. (1974) compared French and American alcoholics on self-report measures of drinking patterns and alcohol-related problems. Although both groups reported consuming approximately the same average amounts of alcohol, the Americans drank in a more periodic fashion, reported more frequent intoxication, and experienced more legal and familial complications.

In a sequel to this study, reported in this volume and elsewhere (Babor et al., 1987; Hesselbrock et al., 1984), Babor and colleagues compared samples of French, French-Canadian, and American alcoholics in terms of the prevalence of psychiatric disorder and its contribution to the severity and patterning of alcoholism. The data showed that antecedent psychopathology, particularly antisocial personality (ASP) characteristics, are associated with a pattern of male alcoholism characterized by early onset, more rapid course, and more serious alcohol-related symptomatology. This relationship was consistent across samples of American, French, and French-Canadian alcoholics. The fact that the Americans reported a higher prevalence of ASP may account for the general impression that American alcoholics epitomize the gamma pattern of alcoholism.

In a related comparative study of French, French-Canadian, and American alcoholics, Babor et al. (1986) found consistent cross-national differences in the way alcoholics conceptualize the term "alcoholism," and how they perceive its generalized victim, the alcoholic. In contrast to French alcoholics, Americans characterized alcoholism more as a disease, with emotional difficulties playing a prominent role in its etiology. The Americans also characterized alcoholics more as periodic drinkers who have impaired control over their drinking. French-Canadian alcoholics scored in the intermediate range between the French and Americans, except in their ratings of emotional difficulties (where they scored closer to the Americans) and willpower (where they scored closer to the French). Interestingly, analysis of selected correlates of the French and American attitude ratings indicated that endorsement of these concepts was not related to the amounts of previous treatment received by these patients. There was evidence among male alcoholics, however, that degree of alcohol dependence correlated positively with attitudes about impaired control and emotional difficulties. These findings suggest that concepts of alcoholism, at least among alcoholics, are related more to their actual symptomatology than to exposure to treatment ideology, which tends to be strongly imbued with the disease concept of alcoholism.

Socialization

The process by which societal members inculcate society's culture in others is referred to as "socialization." While much socialization takes place during childhood, alcohol researchers have focused on adolescence as a crucial period for the learning of drinking behavior. One line of socialization research employing cross-cultural comparative methods was undertaken to study the generality of developmental stages in the initiation of alcohol and drug use. Choosing societies that differ widely in the prevalence of alcohol-related problems and drinking patterns (France, Israel, and the United States), Adler and Kandel (1981) found similar initiation sequences in all three countries. The use of legal drugs was found to be closely related to the use of illegal drugs. Involvement in illicit drugs was preceded by the use of legal drugs, with alcohol playing a crucial role in the developmental sequence. Beer and wine were found to be entry drugs into substance use, followed by cigarettes, hard liquor, marihuana and then other illicit drugs.

In a related study based on household surveys of urban youths in France, Israel, and the United States, Adler and Kandel (1982) found that in all three countries, interpersonal influences were more powerful predictors of adolescent alcohol use than demographic characteristics, attitudes, or academic behavior. However, cross-cultural differences appeared in the relative importance of parental modeling versus peer influences. Parents were more important role models in Israel than in the other two countries, while peers were more important in the United States. In Israel, parents not only have a direct influence on their children by acting as role models; they also have an indirect influence through the kinds of adolescents their children select as friends. One of the most striking findings of the study was the strength of peer effects in the United States compared to the other two countries.

These findings are consistent with earlier, less systematic comparative studies of Jewish drinking conducted by Bales (1946) and Snyder (1978). The moderation that has been found to characterize alcohol use among Jews is assumed to result from the socialization of drinking in family situations where it is imbued with religious connotations. Here alcohol use is governed by prescribed rituals that do not permit drinking to intoxication. In contrast, the use of alcohol in countries like Ireland and the United States has been characterized by a cultural emphasis on escapism, hedonism, and pleasure seeking, all utilitarian functions according to Bales (1946).

Acculturation

Acculturation refers to the way that indigenous drinking patterns change when an individual or group moves from one cultural setting to another. Acculturation has been studied in terms of intergenerational differences within immigrant ethnic groups that have different degrees of exposure to a dominant cultural group, and by comparing persons of similar age who have adopted differentially to their new environment as a function of different ethnic identities. Lolli et al. (1958) found that Italian-Americans added new drinking practices to the traditional European dietary uses of wine. In a similar study of three generations of Italian Americans, Blane (1977) found that there were decreases in the frequency of drinking by men across generations, but increases in the amounts consumed per occasion. The results indicated that by the third generation Italian-American drinking had become a distinct pattern, combining elements of Italian and American drinking.

Gordon (1978) found that recent immigrants to the United States from the Dominican Republic developed strong norms of moderation in association with aspirations for economic improvement. Caetano and Medina Mora (1988) compared drinking patterns and alcohol problems in persons of Mexican descent. One group was composed of Mexicans who recently migrated to the United States, the other of Mexican-Americans, and a third of persons living in Mexico. The study was designed to evaluate the impact of American culture on the drinking patterns of Mexican immigrants. Acculturation was associated with a decrease in the rate of abstention among women, and with an increase in the frequency of drinking by men. Interestingly, acculturation was associated with a decrease in the prevalence of alcohol problems among men, and with an increase in problems among women.

In what is perhaps one of the most creative studies of acculturation, Greeley et al. (1980) studied differences among four American ethnic groups in order to trace the persistence of problem drinking across generations. Interviews were conducted with random samples of urban Americans of Italian, Jewish, Irish, and Swedish descent. One parent and one adolescent were interviewed within each family, and retrospective information was also obtained about grandparents' drinking habits. Consistent with other studies, Greeley et al. found that there were sharply differentiated drinking subcultures, particularly in the grandparental generation. The Irish were found to be heavy drinkers with the most drinking problems, while the Italians tended to be heavy drinkers with minimal problems. The Swedes, despite their high abstinence rate, were more likely to have problems when they drink, and the Jews least likely to have problems. While the same patterns were observed in the parental generation, among adolescents there were fewer differences in quantity and frequency of drinking, but similar ethnic variations with respect to drinking problems.

These results are consistent with other acculturation studies and suggest that there are problem drinking subcultures that differ among various ethnic groups. Subcultural differences tend to persist across generational lines, in spite of a general trend toward the assimilation of ethnic subcultures into the mainstream of American society. This apparent resistance to assimilation of drinking customs is explained by the influence of socialization, which includes modeling of parental drinking behavior, the quality of the parent-child relationship, power and support within the family, and the teaching of ethnic drinking customs. When drinking patterns do change, it is difficult to predict whether they will become more or less problematic in terms of the physical, social, and psychological consequences related to drinking in a given society.

Testing the Generalizability of Otherwise Culture-Bound Theories

One important aim of alcohol research is to formulate and test theories that explain the nature and consequences of drinking. Investigations based on single samples, especially national or subcultural samples whose representativeness is unknown, are a poor basis for scientific inference. Replication using multiple samples recruited from different cultural settings increases the credibility of generalizations to the extent that hypothesized relationships can be demonstrated consistently. In the past, cross-cultural research using clinical as well as general population samples has been lacking in theory-based hypotheses, conceptual sophistication, and suitable research instruments (Westermeyer, 1974; Babor, 1986). In the last decade, there have been significant advances in all of these areas, thereby permitting better research using cross-national data sets. In particular, the development of structured interviews and standardized questionnaires provides a means of measuring common concepts of psychopathology and drinking across cultural and national boundaries.

Traditionally, social researchers have pursued this goal by using the comparative method to identify differences in drinking behavior and symptom patterns that can be attributed to cultural factors, as well as common features of alcohol use that transcend cultural boundaries and thereby imply universal aspects of man's relation to alcohol (Babor, 1986). Two contributions cross-cultural research has made to the identification of pancultural universals are in the areas of development stages of drinking problems and the characteristics of the alcohol dependence syndrome.

Developmental Stages of Drinking Problems

It has long been assumed that alcoholics pass through a prescribed and predictable sequence of developmental stages during the natural course of chronic alcoholism. One of the most influential stage theories of alcoholism was proposed by Jellinek (1962), who divided the course of alcoholism into prodromal, crucial, and chronic phases. Because Jellinek's stage theory was based primarily on his analysis of American alcoholics affiliated with Alcoholics Anonymous, several researchers have attempted to replicate his findings in alcoholic samples from other drinking cultures. Park (1962) compared the drinking histories of 806 Finnish alcoholics with those reported by 192 English alcoholics. Similarities were found between the two groups in the age sequence in which alcoholism symptoms were manifested and in the frequency with which they occurred. Nevertheless, differences were observed in the greater rapidity of progression by the Finnish alcoholics, and the greater heterogeneity of symptomatology among the English alcoholics. In a similar study of symptom progression in French alcoholics, Babor et al. (1972) found some support for the Jellinek stages, but great variability in the prevalence of symptoms. Because of limitations in methodology and sampling procedures, these studies provide little more than suggestive evidence for the generalizability of Jellinek's stage theory to other cultures. To evaluate these hypotheses properly, prospective studies would be required with comparable data collected in several different cultural settings.

An example of this approach to testing the generalizability of developmental theory is the Collaborative Alcohol-Related Longitudinal Project (Fillmore et al., 1988). In this project, data sets from more than thirty longitudinal studies are being pooled in order to test the hypothesis that the incidence and chronicity of drinking patterns vary as a function of age and are equivalent across birth cohorts, historical periods, and cultures. Initial results indicate that the incidence of unwanted drinking behaviors declines substantially with age among men, after attaining their highest levels in the period of late adolescence. By comparing data sets obtained from different countries and historical periods, this study may explain how alcohol problems are related to universal aspects of human development, and why drinking problems subside spontaneously in a significant proportion of men and women as they grow older.

The Alcohol Dependence Syndrome

Although the concept of dependence is not new to the international nomenclature of alcohol-related disorders, it has only attracted systematic research attention in the past two decades. To address a perceived need for improved nomenclature and better diagnostic procedures, the World Health Organization convened a group of experts to develop a provisional definition of alcohol dependence for international discussion and investigation. What emerged from the expert committee was a recommendation to conceptualize alcohol dependence as one of a variety of alcohol-related disabilities. As a core syndrome, dependence was characterized in terms of a matrix of cognitive, behavioral, and psychological symptoms that interact reciprocally to perpetuate harmful drinking (Edwards et al., 1976). In addition to the large body of experimental and clinical research this theoretical concept has inspired (Edwards, 1986), the dependence syndrome concept has stimulated social researchers to investigate the cross-cultural generalizability of its provisional elements.

In one of the first studies testing the hypothesis that the syndrome elements are similar across cultural boundaries, Babor et al. (1987) asked recently detoxified alcoholics in France and the United States to rate the frequency of dependence symptoms on a specially designed rating instrument. There was a strong tendency for dependence symptoms to covary, with a high degree of internal consistency in both patient samples. Additional support for the syndrome hypothesis was provided by factor analysis, which indicated that the dependence elements formed a dimension that was independent of alcohol-related problems.

In contrast to the study of dependence symptoms in clinical samples, in which all alcohol-related symptoms would be expected to be highly intercorrelated, Saunders and Aasland (1987) analyzed the internal consistency of thirteen items measuring the frequency of dependence symptoms in a broad range of nonalcoholic drinkers sampled from medical settings in six countries (Bulgaria, Kenya, Mexico, Norway, Australia, and the United States). Item-to-total score correlations were high across all samples, with the overall reliability coefficients of internal consistency (Chronbach's alpha) in the exceptionally high range between .80 (Australia) and .98 (Mexico).

These data are consistent with the hypothesis that dependence symptoms are relatively invariant regardless of cultural influences or exposure to Western notions of a traditional disease concept that is heavily emphasized in American-style treatment settings. The fact that the same dependence items tend to cluster together regardless of exposure to treatment ideology, culturally conditioned drinking patterns, or severity of alcohol-related problems suggests that the alcohol dependence syndrome may be a biobehavioral universal. Cross-national studies of depression and schizophrenia (Jablensky et al., 1981; World Health Organization, 1973) have identified syndromes that are remarkably similar, regardless of cultural differences in the meaning of and societal response to mental disorder. Although the evidence is very preliminary in the case of alcohol dependence, it suggests that there may be a common core syndrome of symptoms and behaviors that could provide a basis for reliable international classification of alcohol use disorders.

Action Research

A relatively new area of cross-cultural research has developed under a mission oriented approach to social science that can be best described as "action research." Formulated within a public health perspective and typically coordinated by an international health agency like the World Health Organization (WHO), action research attempts to apply social science methods to the amelioration or solution of social problems. This type of research is best exemplified by three recent WHO-sponsored collaborative projects.

The first, aptly termed the Community Response to Alcohol-Related Problems Project, was initiated in 1976 in three collaborating centers located in Zambia, Scotland, and Mexico. Its purpose was to develop approaches for coordinated research and action to deal with alcohol-related problems at the community level in different cultural settings (Rootman & Moser, 1984; Ritson, 1985). This was accomplished as much by attending to the process as to the content of cross-national research.

In the first phase of the study, drinking patterns, alcohol-related problems, attitudes toward drinking, and the ways in which the community could respond to problematic drinking were studied by means of general population surveys in different rural and urban communities in each country. In addition, staff and clientele of a wide variety of health and social service agencies were studied. Although cross-cultural comparison was not a major objective of this study, the findings provided valuable insights into the differing societal implications of drinking in developing and developed countries. Even though the abstention rate was significantly higher in Mexico and Zambia, the pattern of heavy drinking in those countries gave rise to a greater number of personal and social problems than in Scotland. The countries also differed in the acceptance of drinking by women and young adults, with Scotland being the most permissive and the developing countries the least permissive. Not only did the study produce guidelines and procedures for planning community response programs, it also generated valuable information about how and where problem drinkers seek help in different cultural settings (Rootman & Moser, 1984). For example, the Scottish public favored professional intervention for alcohol-related problems, but were remarkably reticent about consulting anyone with regard to their problems. In contrast, a much wider range of nonspecialist resources were listed by the Mexicans and Zambians, who were much more likely to seek help from family members.

In part to address the need for a better knowledge base for community responses to alcohol-related problems, WHO initiated a second international collaborative project in 1982 designed to improve the identification and early treatment of drinkers with harmful alcohol consumption (Saunders & Aasland, 1987). Conducted simultaneously in Mexico, Australia, Bulgaria, Kenya, Norway, and the United States, this research led to the development of a simple culture-free screening instrument capable of identifying persons with early alcohol problems and hazardous levels of alcohol consumption. The instrument was developed on the basis of an extensive validation study that evaluated 1,905 patients recruited from various health facilities in the six collaborating centers. The study demonstrated that a common screening instrument could be employed in both developing and developed countries, and that the absolute level of alcohol consumption that presents a significant elevation in the relative risk of alcohol problems (30 grams) is similar regardless of cultural setting.

A third international collaborative project designed primarily for its practical applications is the WHO-ADAMHA Program on the Diagnosis and Classification of Mental Disorders, Alcohol- and Drug-Related Problems (Sartorius, 1985). In addition to the development of new diagnostic criteria for alcohol dependence and abuse, this project is currently testing two new assessment instruments that will be made available to epidemiologists, clinicians, and clinical researchers for various applications. The first instrument, the WHO Composite International Diagnostic Interview (CIDI), is a general purpose, structured diagnostic instrument that has been modeled after the Diagnostic Interview Schedule and the Present State Examination. The second instrument, the Schedules for Clinical Assessment in Neuropsychiatry, is a revised version of the Present State Examination which for the first time contains sections for the diagnosis of alcohol and drug use disorders. Both instruments will provide diagnostic classification according to the latest versions of the International Classification of Diseases (ICD-10) and the revised Diagnostic and Statistical Manual of the American Psychiatric Association (DSM-III-R). While the CIDI is designed primarily for epidemiological studies, the SCAN is an extensive system for gathering clinical data from psychiatric patients. With the introduction of these two diagnostic interviews under the auspices of WHO, it is likely that the next generation of cross-national studies will benefit from the standardization of diagnostic criteria and interview techniques.

Conclusions

As this review indicates, there is an increasing demand for practical and theoretical knowledge about sociocultural aspects of drinking and alcohol problems that has accentuated the need for systematic comparative research. Despite several decades of tangible progress toward this goal, legitimate questions can be raised about whether the social sciences are ready for these tasks. In general, the theoretical underpinnings of even recent efforts of cross-cultural and cross-national comparison are poor and fragmentary. Very little has been done within the various social science disciplines to develop the tools of analysis and assessment procedures required to integrate data at widely different levels of comparability. Finally, only a few scattered beginnings have been made to ensure adequate data bases for systematic comparisons across the societies of the world.

Fortunately, technical developments and other trends may accelerate movement toward better cross-cultural research. First, improvements in statistical models and computer technology will facilitate the collation and processing of population level as well as individual data from different cultures. Second, the trend toward the standardization of sample surveys and interview schedules will provide comparative data even when the original goal of data collection was for purely local description. Third, alcohol studies in many countries have attracted sufficient numbers of social scientists interested in international comparisons to provide for the first time an adequate infrastructure of resources, career professionals and professional organizations.

After more than a century of descriptive comparisons and global generalizations, alcohol researchers are just beginning to recognize the potential applications, as well as the practical limitations, of their trade for theory development and policy planning at both the national and international levels.

References

Adler, I., and Kandel, D. B. (1981). Cross-cultural perspectives on developmental stages in adolescent drug use. *J. Stud. Alcohol* 42:701–15.

Adler, I., and Kandel, D. B. (1982). A cross-cultural comparison of sociopsychological factors in alcohol use among adolescents in Israel, France, and the United States. *J. Youth Adolesc.* 11:89–113.

Armyr, G.; Elmer, A.; and Herz, U. (1982). *Alcohol in the World of the 80s.* Stockholm: Sober Forlags AB.

Babor, T. F. (1986). Taking stock: Method and theory in cross-national research on alcohol. In T. F. Babor (ed.), *Alcohol and Culture: Comparative Perspectives from Europe and America.* Annals of the New York Academy of Sciences 472:1–9.

Babor, T. F., and Dolinsky, Z. S. (1988). Alcoholic typologies: Historical evolution and empirical evaluation of some common classification schemes. In R. M. Rase and J. Barrett (eds.), *Alcoholism: Origins and Outcome.* New York: Raven Press, pp. 245–66.

Babor, T. F.; Hesselbrock, M. H.; Radouco-Thomas, S.; Benard, J. Y.; Ferrant, J. P.; and Choquette, K. (1986). Concepts of alcoholism among American, French and French-Canadian alcoholics. *Ann. N.Y. Acad. Sci.* 472:82–93.

Babor, T. F.; Lauerman, R.; and Cooney, N. (1987). In search of the alcohol dependence syndrome: A cross-national study of its structure and validity. In P. Paakkanen and P. Sulkunen (eds.), *Cultural Studies on Drinking and Drinking Problems, Report on a Conference.* Helsinki: Social Research Institute of Alcohol Studies.

Babor, T. F.; Martinay, C.; Benard, J. Y.; Ferrant, J. P.; and Wolfson, A. (1987). Homme alcoolique, femme alcoolique: Etude comparative sur l'alcoolisme feminin. (Male alcoholic, female alcoholic: A comparative study on female alcoholism.) *Bulletin de la Societe Francaise d'Alcoologie* 9(1):20–30.

Babor, T. F.; McCabe, T. R.; Masanes, P.; and Ferrant, J. P. (1974). Patterns of alcoholism in France and America: A comparative study. In M. E. Chafetz (ed.), *Alcoholism: A Multilevel Problem.* Washington, D.C.: U.S. Government Printing Office.

Babor, T. F.; Masanes, P.; and Ferrant, J. P. (1972). Enquete sur le type, la frequence et l'ordre chronologique d'apparition des symptomes de l'alcoolisme. *La Revue de l'Alcoolisme* 8:23–36.

Bales, R. F. (1946). Cultural differences in rates of alcoholism. *Quarterly Journal of Studies on Alcohol* 4:480–99.

Blane, H. T. (1977). Acculturation and drinking in an Italian American community. *J. Stud. Alcohol* 38:1324–46.

Caetano, R., and Medina Mora, M. E. (1988). Acculturation and drinking among people of Mexican descent in Mexico and the U.S. *Journal of Studies on Alcohol.* 49:5.

Dion, R. (1977). *Histoire de la Vigne et du Vin en France.* France: Flammarion.

Edwards, C.; Gross, M. M.; Keller, M.; and Moser, J. (1976). Alcohol-related problems in the disability perspective. *Jour. Stud. Alcohol* 37;1360–82.

Edwards, G. (1986). the Alcohol Dependence Syndrome: A concept as stimulus to enquiry. *British Journal of Addiction* 81:171–83.

Ewing, J. A.; Rouse, B. A.; and Pellizzari, E. D. (1974). Alcohol sensitivity and ethnic background. *Am. J. Psychiatry* 131(2):206–10.

Fillmore, K. M.; Grant, M.; Hartka, E.; Johnstone, B. M.; Sawyer, S.; Speiglman, R.; and Temple, M. T. (1988). Collaborative longitudinal research on alcohol problems. *Br. J. Addict.* 83:441–44.

Gordon, A. J. (1978). Hispanic drinking after migration: The case of Dominicans. *Med. Anthropol.* 2:61–84.

Greeley, A. M.; McCready, W. C.; and Theisen, G. (1980). *Ethnic Drinking Subcultures.* New York: J. F. Bergin Publishers.

Heath, D. B. (1987). Cultural studies on drinking: Definitional problems. In P. Paakkanen and P. Sulkunen (eds.), *Cultural Studies on Drinking and Drinking Problems, Report on a Conference.* Helsinki: Social Research Institute of Alcohol Studies, 1987.

Hesselbrock, M.; Hesselbrock, V.; Babor, T.; Stabenau, J.; Meyer, R.; and Weidenman, M. (1984). Antisocial behavior, psychopathology, and problem drinking in the natural history of alcoholism. In D. Goodwin, K. Van Dusen, and S. Mednick (eds.), *Longitudinal Studies of Alcoholism.* Nijhoff Publishing Co., pp. 197–14.

Horton, D. (1943). The functions of alcohol in primitive societies: A cross-cultural study. *Q. J. Stud. Alcohol* 4:199–320.

Jablensky, A.; Sartorius, N.; Gulbinat, W.; and Ernberg, C. (1981). Characteristics of depressive patients contacting psychiatric services in four cultures. *Acta Psychiatr. Scand.* 63:367.

Jellinek, E. M. (1962). Cultural differences in the meaning of alcoholism. In D. J. Pittman and C. R. Snyder (eds.), *Society, Culture and Drinking Patterns.* Carbondale, Ill: Southern Illinois University Press.

Jellinek, E. M. (1960). *The Disease Concept of Alcoholism.* New Haven, Conn.: College and University Press.

Ledermann, S. (1964). *Alcool, Alcoolisme, Alcoolisation.* Presses Universitaries de France.

Leighton, A. H., and Murphy, J. M. (1965). Cross-cultural psychiatry. In J. M. Murphy, and A. H. Leighton (eds.), *Approaches to Cross-Cultural Psychiatry.* Ithaca, N.Y.: Cornell University Press.

Lex, B. W. (1987). Review of alcohol problems in ethnic minority groups. *J. Consult. Clin. Psychol.* 55:293–300.

Lolli, G.; Serianni, E.; Golder, G. M.; and Luzzato-Fegis, P. (1958). *Alcohol in Italian Culture.* Glencoe, Ill: Free Press.

MacAndrew, C., and Edgerton, R. B. (1969). *Drunken Comportment: A Social Explanation.* Chicago, Ill: Aldine.

Makela, K. (1986). Attitudes Toward Drinking and Drunkenness in Four Scandinavian Countries. In T. F. Babor (ed.), *Alcohol and Culture: Comparative Perspectives from Europe and America,* vol. 472. New York: New York Academy of Sciences pp. 21–32.

Makela, K. (1978). Level of consumption and social consequences of drinking. In Y. Israel,

F. B. Glaser, H. Kalant, R. E. Popham, W. Schmidt, and R. G. Smart (eds.), *Research Advances in Alcohol and Drug Problems,* vol. 4. New York: Plenum, pp. 303–48.

Makela, K.; Room, R.; Single, E.; Sulkunen, P.; and Walsh, B. (1973). *Alcohol, Society, and the State.* Toronto: Addiction Research Foundation, 1981.

Negrete, J. C. (1973). Cultural influences and social performance of alcoholics. A comparative study. *Q. J. Stud. Alcohol.* 34:905–16.

Osterberg, E. (1986). Alcohol-related problems in cross-national perspective results of the ISACE study. In T. F. Babor (ed.), *Alcohol and Culture: Comparative Perspectives from Europe and America,* vol. 472. New York: New York Academy of Sciences, pp. 10–20.

Park, P. (1962). Drinking experiences of 806 Finnish alcoholics in comparison with similar experiences of 192 English alcoholics. *Acta Psychiatr. Scand.* 38:227–46.

Park, J. Y.; Huang, Y. H.; Nagoshi, C. T.; Yen, S.; Johnson, R.; Ching, C. A.; and Bowman, K. (1984). The flushing response to alcohol use among Koreans and Taiwanese. *J. Stud. Alcohol* 45:481–85.

Ritson, E. B. (1985). *Community Response to Alcohol-Related Problems.* Public Health Papers No. 81. Geneva: World Health Organization.

Room, R. (1988). Cross-cultural research in alcohol studies: Research tradition and analytical issues. In L. Towle and T. Harford, (eds.), *Cultural Influences and Drinking patterns: A Focus on Hispanic and Japanese Populations.* NIAAA Research Monograph No 19, Dept. of Health and Human Services. Washington, D.C.: U.S. Government Printing Office.

Rootman, I., and Moser, J. (1984). *Guidelines for Investigating Alcohol Problems and Developing Appropriate Responses.* WHO Offset Publication No. 81. Geneva: World Health Organization.

Sartorius, N. (1985). *Mental Disorders, Alcohol- and Drug-related Problems—International Perspective on Their Diagnosis and Classification.* Int. Congress Theories #669, Excerpta Medica, Amsterdam, The Netherlands.

Saunders, J. B., and Aasland, O. G. (1987). WHO Collaborative Project on Identification and Treatment of Persons with Harmful Alcohol Consumption. WHO/PMH/DAT/86.3. Geneva: World Health Organization.

Seward, D. (1982). *Les Moines et le Vin.* Paris: Pygmalion/Gerard Watelet.

Skog, O. J. (1985). The collectivity of drinking cultures. A theory of the distribution of alcohol consumption. *Br. J. Addict.* 80:83–99.

Snyder, C. R. (1978). *Alcohol and the Jews.* Carbondale: Southern Illinois University Press.

Stivers, R. (1976). *A Hair of the Dog: Irish Drinking and American Stereotype.* University Park: Pennsylvania State University Press.

Sue, S., and Nakamura, C. Y. (1984). An integrative model of physiological and social/psychological factors in alcohol consumption among Chinese and Japanese Americans. *Journal of Drug Issues* 14:349–64.

Sulkunen, P. (1976). Drinking patterns and the level of alcohol consumption. An international overview. In R. J. Gibbins, et al. (eds.), *Research Advances in Alcohol and Drug Problems,* vol. 3. New York: Wiley.

Wagner, P. (1974). Wines, grape vines and climate. *Sci. Am.* 230:107–15.

Westermeyer, J. (1974). Alcoholism from the cross-cultural perspective: A review and critique of clinical studies. *A. J. Drug Alcohol Abuse* 1:89–105.

Wolff, P. (1972). Ethnic differences in alcohol sensitivity. *Science* 125:449–51.

World Health Organization (1973). Report of the international pilot study of schizophrenia, vol. 1. Geneva: World Health Organization.

[5] Recent Advances in the Investigation of the Epidemiology of Alcohol Abuse and Addiction

PHILIP J. LEAF, HAI-GWO HWU,
AND GLORISA J. CANINO

During the past decade, there has been increased interest in psychiatric nosology and epidemiology, stimulated to a great extent by the revision of the Diagnostic and Statistical Manual of the American Psychiatric Association (APA, 1980; APA, 1987) and by the Epidemiologic Catchment Area (ECA) Project, a five-site epidemiologic study undertaken by the National Institute of Mental Health and five universities (Eaton and Kessler, 1985; Robins et al., 1985; Myers et al., 1984). The diversity of contributions to this volume indicates that interest in the epidemiology of specific psychiatric disorders has not been limited to the United States. The existence of studies utilizing a common research instrument represents an exciting development in psychiatric epidemiology. The contribution that these studies make to our understanding of the etiology and consequences of alcohol-related disorders suggests that there is much to be gained by applying this methodology to other contexts.

By studying the lifetime prevalence and correlates of alcoholism, we obtain a better understanding of the clinical manifestations of this disorder, the extent to which different clinical patterns exist in different communities or among different subpopulations, and the extent to which they have common correlates and consequences in different countries and for individuals with different ethnic or cultural backgrounds. This information can guide both treatment and public health initiatives by providing information concerning chronicity and impaired functioning. In terms of control, the more we understand the differing nature of disorders, the better able we are to identify those individuals at risk.

Methodologic Advances

The studies described in this volume highlight two important advances in our approach to examining and interpreting variations in the rates and correlates of alcoholism and other psychiatric disorders. The first advance is our recognition of the need to examine the prevalence and correlates of the disorder in defined populations. In the past, much of our knowledge concerning alcoholism and other psychiatric disorders has been gained from the examination of individuals seeking or receiving treatment. However, few individuals with alcohol-related disorders are in treatment at any point in time, and it is likely that a substantial proportion of individuals with alcohol-related disorders never receive medical treatment (Leaf & Bruce, 1987). Studies that focus on patients, therefore, provide only limited information concerning the distribution of alcohol-related disorders in the population and data collected only from individuals in treatment are likely to introduce significant bias into our studies (Cohen and Cohen, 1984). Because availability of services effects use, this bias is likely to be particularly troubling when one attempts to compare data collected from individuals living in communities with greatly different health care systems.

The second important advance is the examination of specific diagnostic criteria using the DIS, a structured interview to identify specific diagnostic criteria. In the past, studies of alcoholism in the community have focused primarily on quantity of consumption or counts of symptoms commonly related to alcoholism. Although symptom scales assess many of the symptoms commonly found in individuals with alcohol-related disorders, these scales do not necessarily sample from all symptoms used in establishing the existence of alcohol abuse or dependence. Few large-scale community studies have been conducted of alcohol-related disorders because of the costs involved in having clinicians interviewing large numbers of individuals, most of whom would not meet criteria of any psychiatric disorder. The procedures used in the studies reporting in this volume, however, allow for the interviewing of large numbers of individuals using the same criteria employed by clinicians but using trained lay interviewers rather than clinical interviewers. As a result, studies of psychiatric disorders are now feasible in a community context, both in developed and developing countries.

In this chapter, we review the methodology that forms the basis for the investigations described in detail in this volume. The availability of comparable data from different countries, cultures, and economic systems represents a unique opportunity for the investigation of the prevalence and correlates of alcohol abuse and dependence. However, these developments do not constitute an amulet that guarantees insight regardless of the skill with which they are applied. In interpreting the following research reports, it is important to understand the strengths and the limitations of the research strategy being utilized.

Community-based Studies

Conducting community-based studies of alcoholism or other psychiatric disorders requires interviewing a great many individuals. The major advance of the ECA Projects referred to earlier has been the development of a research instrument and a methodology that allows researchers to investigate the existence of psychiatric disorders in large numbers of individuals at a cost that can be sustained in even many of the less affluent countries of the world.

The goal of epidemiologic research is to develop estimates of the prevalence and the identification of correlates and risk factors of alcoholism. These disorders are relatively uncommon in many countries or subgroups, requiring large samples for the generation of estimates of prevalence and the identification of correlates and risk factors. It is important, therefore, to identify the specific target populations of interest.

Most of the research reported in this volume is interested in rates of disorder for specific countries or political units. The researchers use a variety of procedures in their attempts to obtain random samples of respondents. The ECA projects in the United States provide the most extensive coverage, including individuals living in institutional settings (Leaf et al., 1984). Projects in other countries focus primarily on non-institutionalized individuals, although at least one of these projects is currently in the process of augmenting existing community data with information from institutionalized individuals.

The test of any survey is the extent to which the sampling procedures utilized ensure that all individuals in the universe of interest, in this case a specific geographic area, have some known probability of being selected into the sample. Problems encountered in developing a sampling frame include obtaining a list of potential respondents and ensuring random selection within strata or clusters of sampling units. Two basic procedures are used in the studies discussed. The most common is to first sample geographic areas such as census tracts or communities, then sample smaller geographic units such as blocks, then households, and finally an individual within a household. To the extent that these sampling units are clustered or stratified to reduce costs of the study, statistical analyses of prevalence rates need to take the effects of this clustering into account when calculating the confidence intervals around rates.

A second strategy involves sampling households or even individuals directly from some list. Although this procedure has the advantage of locating households prior to selecting a sample, lists are often inaccurate, because people move and buildings become uninhabitable or turn from residential use to business use. The use of either strategy requires considerable effort to ensure that the survey population closely resembles the desired target population.

Study Designs

The projects described in this volume use a variety of procedures to obtain samples. Several of the studies described in this volume use data from residents of households, psychiatric hospitals, jails, and nursing homes. None use simple random sampling procedures. We now provide a brief overview of the regions studied. The purpose of these descriptions is to provide the reader with sufficient understanding of the procedures used at each site to interpret the analyses described later in this volume. In many cases, detailed discussions of the specific procedures used at each site are available elsewhere, as referenced in the individual chapters. An overview of the general population-based studies described in this volume is presented in Table 5–1. Two of the chapters (8 and 11) are based on special, nongeneral population samples and are thus not included in Table 5-1.

U.S. EPIDEMIOLOGIC CATCHMENT AREA (ECA) PROJECTS.   The initial ECA site, New Haven, was established by researchers at Yale University in 1978, followed by Eastern Baltimore (Johns Hopkins University), St. Louis (Washington University), Piedmont, North Carolina (Duke University), and Los Angeles (UCLA).

The ECA Project consists of surveys in five communities using comparable interview schedules and study designs. However, the communities studied vary considerably in size and population. The only criteria put forth by NIMH in structuring the sampling frame was that the designated study areas had to consist of one or more community mental health center catchment areas. A detailed description of the stratified cluster samples used in this study are presented in Holzer et al. (1985), and the institutional sampling frames are described in Leaf et al. (1985).

The *New Haven ECA* consists of New Haven and the surrounding twelve towns that constitute the catchment area for the Connecticut Mental Health Center. The *Eastern Baltimore ECA* consists of three contiguous mental health center catchment areas within the City of Baltimore. The *St. Louis ECA* consists of three noncontiguous mental health center catchment areas; one in the inner city of St. Louis, one in a suburb adjacent to the city, and the third in a more rural area. The *Piedmont ECA* consists of five counties in North Carolina, four of which are rural. The *Los Angeles ECA* consists of two noncontiguous mental health center

Table 5-1 Description of Study Sites

	U.S. ECA Studies	Canada	Puerto Rico	Korea	Taiwan	New Zealand	Shanghai	West Germany
Date of survey	1980–83	1983–84	1984	1984	1982	1986	1982	1981
Age range studied	18+	18+	17–64	18–65	18+	18–64	18+	24–64
Areas studied	Parts of five cities-multiple rural counties	City	Island	Nation	City	Metropolitan Region	Part of City	Part of City
Completed interviews	3,004–5,034 per site (total = 20,862)	1,200	1,551	5,100	5,005	1,498	3,804	501 or 455
Completion rate	68–79% per site	66–72%	91%	82%	61%	70%	98%	76.3
Oversamples	Age 65+ (some sites) Blacks (St. Louis)	None	None	None (all eligible residents of household interviewed)	None	Women 18–44 years old	None	Probable cases

catchment areas in Los Angeles County, one of which is predominately hispanic.

All of the ECA sites use multistage sampling procedures to identify households in their respective communities and use procedures developed by Kish (1965) to ensure random selection of respondents within households. The Eastern Baltimore ECA included an oversample of elderly by interviewing all individuals ages 65 or older in sampled households. The New Haven and Piedmont ECAs included an oversample of elderly but selected these individuals from additional households. Blacks were oversampled in the St. Louis ECA. At all ECA sites, the respondent cohort was weighted back to the 1980 United States Census.

These ECA sites do not constitute a probability sample of all the communities in the United States. Furthermore, all five are in close proximity to major medical centers. On the other hand, the communities studied differ in terms of geographic location, characteristics of the population, and urbanicity, and represent considerable diversity in factors that might affect the incidence, prevalence, or treatment of psychiatric disorders. Therefore, the ECA Project allows for testing the consistency of rates and risk factors.

EDMONTON, ALBERTA, CANADA.   This project was conducted between October 1982 and May 1986 and used a two-stage design, sampling residences located within the city of Edmonton from a computerized residential listing, and then selecting one respondent per household using the method proposed by Kish (1965). The results were weighted back to data from the 1981 national census.

PUERTO RICO.   This project used a multistage sampling procedure based on the 1980 Census Population and Housing Census of Puerto Rico. Individuals ages 17–64 were selected within households using the Kish procedures. Data was weighted based on the 1980 census.

TAIWAN.   This study uses a multistage stratified cluster sample from types of communities, city, township, and rural. Interviews were conducted in eight administrative districts of Taipei, in two townships (one close to Taipei and one isolated), and in six rural communities. In all three samples, census tracts were randomly selected and then a roster of inhabitants obtained from each District Household Registration Office. Districts in Taipei were stratified into three levels in terms of educational level and economic activities, with additional sampling equivalent down to blocks. Information concerning the name, age, sex, marital status, education, occupation, and address of potential respondents was also recorded. Initial attempts to obtain interviews in Taipei encountered a considerable nonresponse, and sampling was done with replacements. The nonresponse reported in the table is overestimated because it includes nonresponse due to inaccuracies in the registration lists. This is the only study in this volume that used sampling with replacement.

SHANGHAI.   This study was undertaken in 1982 in one of the ten administrative districts of the City of Shanghai. A multistage sample was conducted using lists of households from two of the nine Street Committees in the district, and then selecting an individual ages 18–64 from each samples household. The response rate for this survey was 98 percent, the highest of any of the studies described in this volume.

KOREA.   This study was conducted from January 4, 1984 to February 23, 1984 and involved two multistage probability samples: one for Seoul and one for rural areas. A difference between this study and the others described in this volume is that all residents ages 18–64 were interviewed in households selected for participation.

WEST GERMANY.   Data for this study are from the second wave of interviews, with a sample originally studied in 1974. Respondents were ages 18–55 at the time of the original sample. The original sample was stratified in order to produce an enriched sample of "probable cases" and only individuals ages 24–65 were eligible for the second survey. Responses from this survey were weighted to reflect the demographic distribution for the responses of the original survey.

NEW ZEALAND.   The interviewing for this study was done from April to December 1986. A three-stage sample was drawn of persons 18–64 years old living in the Christchurch metropolitan region, including the central city, suburbs, and the semirural margin of the city. Because of a particular interest in eating disorders and depression, an oversample of young women was done. For two out of three selected dwellings, any occupant age 18–64 was eligible. But for every third dwelling, only women ages 18–44 were eligible. Data were weighted back to the 1986 census for the household sampling frame. No institutional sample was included. Overall completion rate was 70 percent.

Cross-Site Coordination of Analyses

Each of the chapters in this volume attempts to strike a balance between 1) independent exploration and implications of the findings for the particular cultural context, and 2) coordination of analyses with the other sites for the purpose of cross-national comparison. The latter is more difficult to achieve due to difficulties in communication and coordination between investigators scattered around the world. Obviously cross-site coordination was greatly facilitated by use of the same interview instrument (the DIS), the same illness definitions (DSM-III), the same computerized diagnostic and scoring programs, and similar sampling designs. However, the particular analyses that were to be done in common still had to be specified. This was accomplished by originating the analyses in one site (St. Louis) on a single data set (the ECA data) and constructing tables based on these analyses. The analytic programs, raw data, and the constructed tables were then sent to the other sites where the same process was replicated. The generation of the ideas for analysis came largely through meetings of a cross-cultural consortium of the investigators organized by Dr. Helzer at the annual conferences of the American Psychiatric Association.

This process worked well for the illness and demographic variables contained in the DIS. However, some of the social and demographic variables that are worth examining in relation to illness were either not contained in the DIS, or had to be altered to suit local needs. An example of this is occupational status. This is difficult to compare cross-nationally because similar occupations may vary greatly in status, depending on the culture. To solve this problem, the St. Louis group ranked occupations according to their level of prestige in the United States, then trichotomized the prestige scores. Those who were unemployed at the time of interview were assigned the prestige score of their most recent job. Each site did the same for their own cultural context. Thus for most chapters we are able to report associations between alcoholism and a trichotomized occupational status.

Statistical Analyses

None of the studies described in this volume use simple random sampling procedures to identify respondents, so the standard tests of statistical significance reported by some of the students probably are usually nonconservative (Kessler et al., 1984; Leaf et al., 1985). This is because many of the procedures used clustering procedures to decrease the cost of interviewing, and individuals living near each other are often more similar than individuals living at a greater distance.

Almost all surveys involved weighting of data so that the characteristics of the respondents reflected known characteristics of the target population. In most cases, these characteristics were obtained from a government sponsored census. The West German study weighted data back to reflect the characteristics of the original sample. This poststratification procedure represents an attempt to correct for nonresponse. It assumes that nonresponse is not related to the primary variable of interest, alcoholism, and that certain subpopulations are more difficult to interview and are thus underrepresented among those providing data.

Many of the projects described in this volume adjust for deviations from simple random samples introduced by weighting and sampling procedures by using computer programs that estimate the effects of these factors and take these estimates into account when calculating the statistical significance of results. Although the poststratification procedures improve the fit between estimates generated from the samples and the known characteristics of the sampling frames (Holt & Smith, 1979), they also influence the interrelationships observed in the data. Poststratification attempts to take into account nonresponse and inadequacies in the sampling frame but assumes that the data used for standardization accurately represents the true characteristics of the study area. When design-based statistical procedures are not used to assess the statistical significance of relationships, these statistical tests are usually nonconservative.

The Diagnostic Interview Schedule

The ECA Projects in the U.S. demonstrated that large-scale epidemiologic studies of specific psychiatric disorders could be conducted without clinically trained interviewers. The procedures and instrument developed for use in the ECA study allow for the identification of cases in a community context. The fact that these procedures have been used successfully in a diverse set of communities suggests that the DIS and the use of community survey techniques can serve as the foundation for important cross-national comparisons. Because the administration of the DIS does not require clinically trained interviewers, it is possible to conduct studies of alcoholism and other psychiatric disorders without the need for large numbers of highly trained clinical interviews, a luxury that even the most affluent research centers can scarcely afford.

Although survey research techniques have been applied in a wide variety of settings including epidemiologic studies (Weissman et al., 1986), the research possibilities opened by the development of the DIS cannot be underestimated. Developed to examine diagnostic criteria established by the American Psychiatric Associations Diagnostic and Statistical Manual, Third Edition (DSM-III), the DIS allows for the assessment of a number of psychiatric disorders in large surveys using a single diagnostic interview. The DIS represents an important advance in psychiatric epidemiology because it represents the first time a structured interview schedule had been developed for administration by nonclinicians that employed the same diagnostic criteria and algorithms as those used by clinicians.

A detailed discussion of the development and reliability of this instrument is beyond the scope of this chapter, although the DIS has been the subject of extensive scrutiny (Anthony et al., 1985, Helzer et al., 1985; Robins et al., 1981, Robins et al., 1985). Instead, we will present a general overview of the instrument, referring the reader to other sources where appropriate.

In developing the DIS, two goals had to be met. First, an instrument was required that utilized the same diagnostic criteria as clinicians, DSM-III. Second, the instrument had to be administrable in a large epidemiologic survey. Since a survey of sufficient size to produce stable estimates of the prevalence of psychiatric disorders would require 3,000 or more interviews, it was clear that this type of project would require lay interviewers rather than trained clinicians.

As noted in Chapter 2, the DIS is based on the Renard Diagnostic Interview (RDI) (Helzer et al., 1981), a structured instrument developed at Washington University to make diagnoses on the basis of the Feighner (1972) criteria. The authors of this instrument were contracted by NIMH to modify the existing interview to incorporate DSM-III criteria and to allow for the determination of the recency of the disorders when present.

Although the focus on clinical definitions of disorder is an important feature of the DIS, the instrument is actually a hybrid that incorporates important aspects of earlier surveys and clinical interviews. Previous studies of psychiatric disorder in the community relied primarily on symptom scales, which assessed the existence of specific symptoms. These scales ascertained information about the existence of symptoms during a specified period of time but provided no information about the recency of symptoms. In addition, these instruments did not exclude symptoms that might have had a cause other than a psychiatric disorder.

The key to the utility of the DIS is its ascertainment of the criteria for diagnosis contained in the DSM-III and its probe structure, which allows for the exclusion of symptoms that neither meet a predefined threshold of severity or which were always the result of the use of drugs, alcohol, or physical illness or injury. In addition, the DIS provides information about the onset of symptomatology related to the disorder, recency of this symptomatology, and frequency and duration of episodes of illness for disorders where this information is relevant. Not that the collection of this information is without problems. As Robins et al. (1985) discuss, DSM-III has not resolved all problems in ascertaining diagnostic criteria, onset of disorder, or excluding symptoms as criteria for a disorder because they actually result from another preexisting psychiatric disorder. Indeed, the ongoing discussion concerning revisions of DSM-III suggest that these difficulties are not limited to epidemiologic studies but reflect the problems inherent in establishing the existence of certain psychiatric disorders. Rather than claiming to have solved all problems related to psychiatric nosology, the DIS and the ECA project provide data for understanding the nature and extent of these problems, and the flexibility of the DIS allows for exploring the implication of alternative solutions.

Since the DIS was to be applied in a community setting, it was not possible for all DSM-III disorders to be assessed. Priority was given to those disorders with parallel criteria in Feighner and RDC classifications, that had been well studied, and for which the diagnostic criteria was least ambiguous (Robins et al., 1985). This resulted in the exclusion of the majority of the Axis II disorders, as well as disorders such as schizoaffective disorder where the criteria were not well specified. In addition, since the diagnoses had to be made on the basis of self-reports and in the absence of a medical history of physical examination, disorders such as organic affective syndrome were excluded. Table 5–2 indicates the DSM-III disorders that can be assessed with the DIS.

Because the focus of this volume is on alcohol abuse and dependence, the manner in which the DIS ascertains the existence of these disorders will be described in detail. The DIS section focusing on alcohol abuse and dependence is presented at the end of this volume. According to DSM-III:

the essential feature of Alcohol Abuse is a pattern of pathological use for at least a month that causes impairment in social or occupational functioning. The essential features of Alcohol Dependence are either a pattern of pathological alcohol use or impairment in social or occupational functioning due to alcohol, and either tolerance or withdrawal (APA 1980:169)

Table 5–2 Diagnoses Covered by the DIS

DSM-III	RDC	Feighner
Cognitive impairment	RDC does not provide criteria	Organic Brain Syndromes (criterion A only)
Severe	—	—
Mild	—	—
Affective disorders	—	—
Manic episode	Manic disorder[a]	Mania[a]
with impariment[a]	Hypomanic disorder[a]	—
without impairment[a]	—	
Major depressive episode	Major depressive disorder[a]	Depression[a]
with impairment[a]	—	—
without impairment[a]	—	—
Dysthymia[a]	—	—
Bipolar	—	—
Major depression	—	—
single episode	—	—
recurrent	—	—
Atypical bipolar	—	—
Grief reaction	—	—
Schizophrenic disorders	—	—
Schizophrenia	Schizophrenia[a]	Schizophrenia[a]
problems in current year[a]	Schizoaffective disorder, manic type	—

(continued)

Table 5–2 (Continued)

DSM-III	RDC	Feighner
earlier symptoms only[a]	Schizoaffective disorder, depressed type	—
Substance use disorders	Alcoholism	Alcoholism[b]
Alcohol abuse	—	—
Alcohol dependence	—	—
Barbiturate, hypnotic abuse	Sedatives, hypnotics, tranquilizers abuse	Drug dependence[b]
Barbiturate, hypnotic dependence	Sedatives, hypnotics, tranquilizers dependence	—
Opioid abuse	Narcotics abuse	—
Opioid dependence	Narcotics dependence	—
Amphetamine abuse	Amphetamine-like stimulants abuse	—
Amphetamine dependence	Amphetamine-like stimulants dependence	—
Cocaine abuse	Cocaine abuse	—
Hallucinogen abuse	LSD or other hallucinogens abuse	—
Canabis abuse	Marijuana, hashish, THC abuse	—
Canabis dependence	Marijuana, hashish, THC dependence	—
	Poly-drug abuse	—
	with impairment	—
	without impairment	—
Anxiety disorders	—	—
Obsessive-compulsive[a]	Obsessive-compulsive disorder[a]	Obsessive-compulsive neurosis
Agoraphobia[a]	Agoraphobia[a]	Phobic neurosis
Social phobia[a]	Social phobias[a]	—
Simple phobia[a]	Simple phobias[a]	—
Summary phobia[a]	Mixed phobias[a]	—
Panic	Panic disorder[a,b]	Anxiety neurosis
Agoraphobia with panic[a]	—	—
Agoraphobia without panic[a]	—	—
Somatization disorder	Briquet's disorder[a]	Hysteria
Antisocial personality	Antisocial personality[b]	Antisocial personality disorder
Anorexia nervosa	—	Anorexia nervosa
Disorders not covered in all ECA sites	—	—
Tobacco use disorder	—	—
Psychosexual dysfunction	—	—
Transsexualism	—	Transsexualism[b]
Egodystonic homosexuality	—	Homosexuality[a]
Pathological gambling	—	—

[a]With and without exclusion criteria.

[b]Probable and definite.

Table 5–3 DSM-III Diagnostic Criteria for Alcohol Abuse or Dependence

Diagnostic Criteria for Alcohol Abuse

A. *Pattern of pathological alcohol use*: need for daily use of alcohol for adequate functioning; inability to cut down or stop drinking; repreated efforts to control or reduce excess drinking by "going on the wagon" (periods of temporary abstinence) or restricting drinking to certain times of the day; binges (remaining intoxicated throughout the day for at least two days); occasional consumption of a fifth of spirits (or its equivalent in wine or beer); amnesic periods for events occurring while intoxicated (blackouts); continuation of drinking despite a serious physical disorder that the individual knows is exacerbated by alcohol use; drinking of non-beverage alcohol.

B. *Impairment in social or occupational functioning due to alcohol use*; e.g., violence while intoxicated, absence from work, loss of job, legal difficulties (e.g., arrest for intoxicated behavior, traffic accidents while intoxicated), arguments or difficulties with family or friends because of excessive alcohol use.

C. *Duration of disturbance of at least one month.*

Diagnostic Criteria for Alcohol Dependence

A. *Either a pattern of pathological alcohol use or impairment in social or occupational functioning due to alcohol use*: (Same as above).

   Pattern or pathological alcohol use: (Same as above).

   Impairment in social or occupational functioning due to alcohol use: e.g., violence while intoxicated, absence from work, loss of job, legal difficulties (e.g., arrest for intoxicated behavior, traffic accidents while intoxicated), arguments or difficulties with family or friends because of excessive alcohol use.

B. *Either tolerance or withdrawal:*

   Tolerance: need for markedly increased amounts of alcohol to achieve the desired effect, or markedly diminished effect with regular use of the same amount.

   Withdrawal: development of Alcohol Withdrawal (e.g., morning "shakes" and malaise relieved by drinking (after cessation or reduction in drinking).

APA 1980:169–70.

The specific criteria used making the diagnosis of alcohol abuse or dependence are presented in Table 5–3.

In addition to establishing whether or not a subject ever met criteria for alcohol abuse or dependence, the DIS also establishes the age at which the subject first drank enough to get drunk, the earliest age at which the subject met one of the diagnostic criteria, and the last time that one of the diagnostic criteria was met. Because each of the symptoms is ascertained independent of other responses, it is possible to develop counts of symptoms as well as identify heavy drinkers not meeting criteria for either alcohol abuse or dependence.

Validity of Cross-Cultural Assessments

An important advantage of the DIS is that it allows comparisons among surveys conducted in vastly different communities. However, the fact that the DIS assessments of alcoholism have proved to be reliable and valid when used in the United States does not assure that this instrument would provide comparable results in other countries and in other communities. Although a detailed discussion of cross-cultural assessment is far beyond the space limitations of this chapter, two important points need to be raised.

First, the epidemiologic techniques described in this volume rely on the acceptance of survey procedures that are quite common in the United States. Indeed, these procedures are so common that they are resulting in a generally decreasing rate of response as individuals begin to encounter frequent requests for interviews, often over the telephone. In many cultures or countries, obtaining interviews door-to-door is not an accepted part of the culture. This could result in greater rates of response due to the novelty of being consulted for an opinion. On the other hand, one might perceive all requests for information as threatening and likely to be misused by the recipient, and in this circumstance we might find a decrease in rates of response, or worse, cooperation without the provision of any real information. It should be pointed out that validity studies conducted on clinical populations do not provide information about how the same questions will be received in the context of the survey.

The second issue that needs to be raised in the context of a discussion of study methodologies is the general problem of developing an instrument that has applicability in a range of countries and cultures. Here many of the studies described in this volume are exemplary. Many of these projects involved efforts at translating and testing the translated DIS, and a number of the studies included extensive comparisons between the DIS and clinician assessments. Possibly because the alcoholism diagnoses had some of the highest reliabilities in the original DIS studies, it is not surprising that this component of the DIS did quite well in the clinical comparison studies conducted in other countries. It is important, however, to recognize that other disorders present different problems, and that considerable care needs to be taken when adopting the DIS to a new culture or language.

Summary

For researchers interested in the epidemiology or etiology of psychiatric disorders, the studies presented in this volume offer considerable encouragement. Not only is it possible to conduct comparable research projects in a wide range of countries and cultures, but computer programs and instrumentation are available for obtaining interpretable findings in each of these communities. The possibilities for cross-national and cross-cultural research are quite extensive. It is important that the efforts of Lee Robins and John Helzer be acknowledged, since the results presented in this monograph are a tribute to their insistence that techniques of epidemiologic research have applications far beyond those envisioned by those developing the instruments. The intellectual and technical support provided by Drs. Helzer and Robins and their many colleagues at Washington University in St. Louis represent an important factor that needs to be taken into account by anyone considering multisite collaborations comparable to those described in this volume. Without the technical backup provided by the Washington University researchers, none of the studies described in this volume would have been possible.

References

American Psychiatric Association (1980). *Diagnostic and Statistical Manual of Mental Disorders*. Third Ed. Washington, D.C.: APA.

American Psychiatric Association (1987). Diagnostic and Statistical Manual of Mental Disorders (DSM-III-R). Third Ed. Revised. Washington, D.C.: APA.

Anthony, J. C.; Folstein, M.; Romanoski, A. J.; Von Korff, M. R.; Nestadt, G. R.; Chahal, R.; Merchant, A.; Brown, C. H.; Shapiro, S.; Kramer, M.; and Gruenberg, E. M. (1985). Comparison of the lay Diagnostic Interview Schedule and a standardized psychiatric diagnosis. *Arch. Gen. Psychiatry* 42:667–75.

Cohen, P., and Cohen, J. (1984). The clinician's illusion. *Arch. Gen. Psychiatry* 41:1178–82.

Eaton, W. W., and Kessler, L. G. (1985). *Epidemiologic Methods in Psychiatry: The NIMH Epidemiologic Catchment Area Program*. New York: Academic Press.

Feighner, J. P.; Robins, E.; Guze, S. B., et al. (1972). Diagnostic criteria for use in psychiatric research. *Arch. Gen. Psychiatry* 26:57–63.

Harding, T. W.; De Arango, M. V.; Baltazar, J.; Climent, C. E.; Ibrahim, H. H. A.; Ladrido-Ignacio, L.; Murthy, R. S.; and Wig, N. N. (1980). Mental disorders in primary health care: A study of their frequency and diagnosis in four developing countries. *Psychol. Med.* 10:231–41.

Helzer, J. E.; Robins, L. N.; McEvoy, L. T.; Spitznagel, E. L.; Stoltzman, R. K.; Farmer, A.; and Brockington, I. F. (1985). A comparison of clinical and Diagnostic Interview Schedule diagnoses. *Arch. Gen. Psychiatry* 42:657–66.

Helzer, J.; Robins, L.; and Croughan, J. (1981). Renard Diagnostic Interview: its reliability and procedural validity with physicians and lay interviewers. *Arch. Gen. Psychiatry* 38:393–98.

Holt, D., and Smith, T. M. F. (1979). Poststratification. *J. R. Stat. Soc. Ser. A.* 142:33–46.

Holzer, C. E.; Becker, H.; Spitznagel, E.; Jordan, K.; Timbers, D.; and Kessler, L. (1985). Sampling the household population. In W. W. Eaton and L. G. Kessler (eds.), *Epidemiologic Methods in Psychiatry: The NIMH Epidemiologic Catchment Area Program*. Academic Press, New York.

Kessler, R. C., and McLeod, J. D. (1984). Sex Differences in Vulnerability to Undesirable Life Events. *Am. Socio. Rev.* 49:620–631.

Kish, L. (1965). *Survey Sampling*. New York: Wiley.

Leaf, P. J.; and Bruce, M. L. (1987). Gender differences in the use of mental health related services: A reexamination. *J. Health Soc. Behav.* 28:171–183.

Leaf, P. J.; German, P.; Spitznagel, E.; George, L.; Landsverk, J.; and Bartko, J. (1985). Sampling: The institutional survey. In W. W. Eaton and L. G. Kessler (eds.), *Epidemiologic Methods in Psychiatry: The NIMH Epidemiologic Catchment Area Program*. New York: Academic Press, pp. 49–66.

Leaf, P. J.; Weissman, M. M.; Myers, J. K.; Tischler, G. L.; and Holzer, C. E. (1984). Social risk factors for psychiatric disorders: The Yale Epidemiologic Catchment Area Study. *Soc. Psychiatry*, 19:53–61.

Myers, J. K.; Weissman, M. M.; Tischler, G. L.; Holzer, C. E.; Leaf, P. J.; Orvaschel, H.;

Anthony, J.; Kramer, M.; and Stoltzman, R. (1984). Six-month prevalence of psychiatric disorders in three communities: 1980–1982. *Arch. Gen. Psychiatry* 41:959–67.

Robins, L. N.; Helzer, J. E.; Croughan, J.; and Ratcliff, K. S. (1981). National Institute of Mental Health Diagnostic Interview Schedule: Its history, characteristics, and validity. *Arch. Gen. Psychiatry* 38:381–89.

Robins, L. N.; Helzer, J. E.; Ratcliff, K. S.; and Seyfried, W. (1985). Validity of the Diagnostic Interview Schedule, Version II: DSM-III diagnoses. *Psychol. Med.* 12:855–70.

[II] *North America*

[6] Five Communities in the United States: Results of the Epidemiologic Catchment Area Survey

JOHN E. HELZER, KATHLEEN BUCHOLZ, AND LEE N. ROBINS

We begin this chapter with a brief review of the history of alcohol use in the United States. This will help place the findings from the Epidemiologic Catchment Area survey, presented below, into context.

Historical Overview

Some families excel in the method of brewing beer with strange variety of ingredients. Here we commonly make it with pine chips, pine buds, hemlock for leaves, roasted corn, dried appleskins, sassafras roots and bran. With these, to which we add some hops and a little malt, we compose a sort of beverage which is very pleasant (Hector St. John de Crevecoeur, p. 298).

The resourcefulness of early colonists in producing alcohol attested to the integral role it played in their lives. In addition to using alcohol for nourishment and medicinal purposes, the colonists served alcohol at social gatherings: weddings, funerals, and even the ordination of ministers (Levine, 1978; Ames, 1985; Caddy, 1983). Alcohol in the form of rum had an important economic role as well. Distilled from inexpensive imported molasses, rum became a major trading item for New England merchants. Historians estimate that the region exported as much as 600,000 gallons of rum per year, making huge profits for distillers (Lender & Martin, 1982).

Whether rum, beer, or whiskey, the early nineteenth century penchant for hard liquor distinguished Americans from their European forebears. It has been estimated that per capita consumption of distilled spirits increased from 2.3 gallons of absolute alcohol at the end of the eighteenth century to 4.3 gallons by 1830 (Rorabaugh, 1976). The comparable consumption figure for 1983 was about .96 gallon. Alcohol was consumed instead of tea or coffee at job breaks, both morning and afternoon (Lender & Martin, 1982; Clark, 1976).

Drinking was especially rampant on the frontier. It was not only the adventurers who drank excessively and often, but also the stable populace (pioneer farmers) drank greater amounts more frequently than their Eastern counterparts (Winkler, 1968). As one nineteenth-century visitor to this country wrote:

They say that the English cannot settle anything without a dinner. I am sure that Americans can fix nothing without a drink; if you meet you drink; if you part you drink; if you make an acquaintance you drink. They quarrel in their drink, and they make it up with a drink (Winkler, 1968, p. 413).

During the nineteenth century, the drinking preferences of Americans were altered by the thousands of immigrants to the United States throughout the nineteenth century. The shift in the type of alcohol consumed from the beginning of the nineteenth century, when distilled spirits accounted for 85 percent, to the end of that century, when 58 percent of alcohol consumed was beer, was due less to moderation in drinking habits than to the addition of numerous new Americans who preferred beer (Cahalan & Cisin, 1976).

Furthermore, the upper class began to see the pervasiveness of alcohol consumption in the lower classes as a threat to social stability. The treatises of Benjamin Rush, a noted colonial physician, on the addicting qualities of distilled spirits provided a rational foundation for the philosophy of abstinence, even though there was no organized movement to promote this at the time (Gusfield; 1962; Levine, 1984). By the mid-nineteenth century, this ad hoc temperance ethic advocated by the elite was embraced by the rapidly growing and ambitious middle class, whose values emphasized sobriety and industry as keys to achieving prosperity (Gusfield, 1962; Cahalan & Cisin, 1976). Initially focusing on moderation in drinking, the temperance movement eventually adopted abstinence as its goal.

In the twentieth century, the temperance movement underwent an organizational change, becoming the Anti-Saloon League (ASL), a highly organized congressional lobby. There was also a change in its objectives. As its new name suggested, the need to eradicate the evils of the liquor industry, particularly the saloon, was added to the long-held temperance values of preserving the middle class home, protecting women and children, and reducing crime. Saloons, which were frequented by working classes and immigrants, were also seen as offering a convenient forum for socialists and labor union organizers, who posed yet another threat to the middle class.

The goals of the ASL were supported by corporate executives, in part because they anticipated reaping economic benefits both from sober, more productive workers, and from consumers with the disposable income previously used to buy liquor. In addition, advocating prohibition was a symbol of business' caring about social conditions in America and thus had a moral overtone (Levine, 1984, 1985). The support of the corporate world was instrumental in the passage of a constitutional amendment establishing national prohibition in 1919, marking the peak of the political strength of the temperance movement.

The Prohibition Period

Prohibition had complex effects on alcohol use patterns and production. Per capita alcohol consumption decreased (Kyvig, 1979) and mortality from cirrhosis declined sharply (Terris, 1968). But Prohibition also led to the development of a covert system of making and distributing alcohol. Because they were easier to produce and distribute compared to beer (which required refrigeration), distilled beverages took the dominant share of the market in illicit beverages.

The Prohibition era also saw a variety of social changes, particularly among the middle class. These, in turn, altered the political environment that had fostered prohibition. By the end of the 1920s, there was a new middle class character. Instead of farmers, small businessmen, and independent professionals, the middle class was increasingly composed of white collar workers, managers, and professionals. Drinking became more acceptable among this new middle class (Levine, 1984; Howland and Howland, 1978). Perhaps, Bacon observed, "greater social complexity (resulted) in the need for greater integrative functioning; lessening of tension, uncertainty and suspicion is necessary for this function; alcohol had been found useful in its accomplishment" (Bacon, 1962, p. 88).

The repeal focus began to gather strength, perhaps indicating a public consensus that prohibition was an unsuccessful experiment, even though it did result in decreased alcohol consumption (Kyvig, 1979). In view of the widespread corporate backing of prohibition, it is ironic that the major supporters of repeal included corporate moguls like Pierre DuPont and John D. Rockefeller. They, and others, believed that repeal would lower income taxes by substituting taxes from alcohol sales. The belief that widespread violations of prohibition were leading to disrespect for the law in general also contributed to the repeal movement. Lastly, proponents of repeal argued that reinstating the liquor industry would result in more jobs, more revenue for state and local governments, and bring an end to the Depression (Levine, 1985).

The repeal forces prevailed, and in 1933 alcohol again became legal. But the effects of prohibition were felt until well after the Second World war (Kyvig, 1979). Since then, changes in alcohol use have involved the addition of new groups to the ranks of drinkers (e.g., women and adolescents) and shifts in the type of alcohol used, as discussed below.

Social Functions of Alcohol

The functions of alcohol alluded to earlier—nourishment, medicinal, and religious—have been superseded by its use as an enhancer of social conviviality. In the last 40 years, the frequency of use and types of events at which alcohol is available have increased. Previously in this century, alcohol was typically used to signify special occasions and, because it was largely a prerogative of adults, symbolized entrance into adulthood. Its use was restricted to particular leisure time events. Today, however, alcoholic beverages are also commonplace after work, at sports activities, and at a variety of cultural events. Lowering of the legal drinking age to 18 in many states allowed earlier access to alcohol.

In the 1980s, there has been a backlash to the increasing availability of alcohol, particularly to young people. This has been motivated in part by the high rates of teenage deaths in alcohol-related motor vehicle accidents. Many states have raised the drinking age, and there is a movement to establish a national drinking age of 21. In 1984, national legislation was enacted that allowed the federal government to restrict highway funds to states with drinking ages under 21.

Cisin (1978) has summarized the correlates of alcohol in American society. Alcohol is related to age and sex norms. Alcohol use, particularly heavy use, is more common among men and the young, although the proportion of drinkers among women has been increasing recently. Unlike men, most drinking among women occurs in the company of their spouses. Alcohol is also correlated with social status, with fewer abstainers among those of upper and middle than among lower classes. Drinking is more prevalent in urban than in rural areas, and emphasizes religious and ethnic differences. Subcultures of American society exhibit different drinking patterns, as will be discussed in separate chapters in this volume.

Contemporary Population Data on Consumption

What Is Drunk

Statistics on liters of alcohol consumed per capita rank the United States sixteenth in the world (Brenner, 1982). Figure 6–1 presents per capita consumption of alcoholic and nonalcoholic beverages for 1983.

Within the United States, statistics regarding per capita ethanol consumption by type of beverage from 1950 through 1984 (Figure 6–2) reveal that alcohol consumption increased rather steadily from 1950 to 1981, with a very consistent increase between 1960 and 1970. A slight decrease in overall alcohol consumption beginning in about 1982 has continued through the mid-80s (Williams et al., 1986). (See Appendix 3 for statistics on alcohol consumption from 1850–1983.)

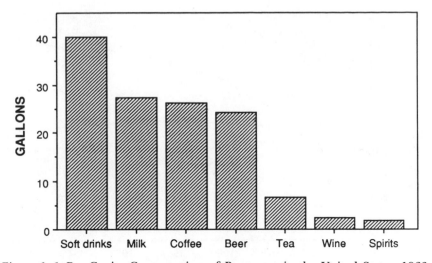

Figure 6–1 Per Capita Consumption of Beverages in the United States, 1963. [*Source: Food consumption, prices and expenditures, 1963–1983*. Statistical Bulletin No. 713. Economic Research Service, U.S. Department of Agriculture, November 1984, p. 34.]

Figure 6–3 shows recent trends for individual beverage types, using 1977 as the base (Williams et al., 1986). These data, from the Alcohol Epidemiologic Data System (AEDS), are based on state sales, taxation,

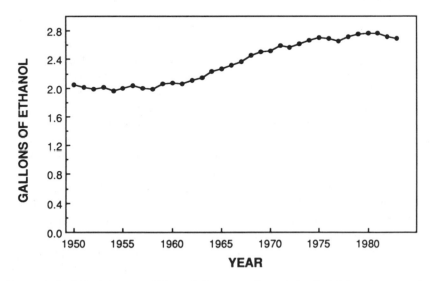

Figure 6–2 U.S. Apparent Ethanol Consumption of the Drinking Age Population. [*Source:* U.S. Alcohol Epidemiologic Data Reference Manual, vol. 1, September 1985. DBF NIAAA]

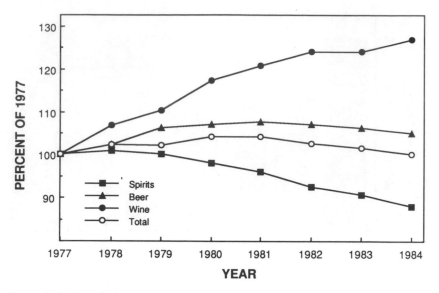

Figure 6–3 Trends in Per Capita Ethanol Consumption as a Percent of 1977 Levels.

and receipt data. Total consumption peaked in 1981 and has declined thereafter to 1977 levels. When broken into component beverage types, wine consumption has increased, while consumption of beer and distilled spirits has declined.

Who Drinks

Data from the supplement on alcohol use included in the 1985 National Health Interview Survey show that 64 percent of the American population aged 18 years or older qualified as drinkers (i.e., consumed at least one alcoholic drink in the past year) with a distinct difference between men (75%) and women (55%) (National Center for Health Statistics, 1986). A larger percentage (72%) of those between the ages of 18 and 44 were drinkers compared to those 45 through 65 (61%) or 65 or older (43%). A drinking index, based on quantity and frequency of drinking during the previous 2 weeks, classified 8% of the population as "heavy," and another 19% as "moderate," drinkers. Heavy drinking differentiated men (13%) from women (3%) but was consistent at 8% across all age groups except for a slight drop to 6% among those 65 or older. Among those 18 through 29, abstention, light, and moderate drinking were equally common drinking patterns. For those 30 through 44, abstention and light drinking were most common, while abstention predominated after age 45.

Trends Over Time

Adding these recent data to a compilation of surveys of alcohol use shows that the proportions of abstainers, light, moderate, and heavy drinkers have remained relatively stable for the total population over the last 15 years (see Appendix 4) (Clark and Midanik, 1982). However, there have been recent changes in particular subgroups. There has been a small shift from the ends of the scale toward light drinking for men. Among women 65 and older, there is a slight upward shift from abstention to lighter drinking. In a separate study, Fillmore (1984) observed that the rate of heavy drinking for unemployed young women remained stable at 2 to 3 percent from 1964 to 1979, while the rate among employed young women rose in the same period from 4 to 10 percent.

In summary, despite methodological and definitional differences, a variety of surveys have established that greater proportions of drinkers and heavy drinkers are found among men and among all those under 45 years of age. There are also suggestive data about the increasing proportion of heavy drinkers among young women, particularly those employed. Problem drinkers are most likely to be males, 18–25 years of age, and not currently married.

The findings from surveys of problem drinking were largely confirmed by one of the first community studies to use standardized diagnostic criteria (Weissman et al., 1980). In a study of a small Northeastern city, they found alcoholism to be more prevalent in men, nonwhites, Protestants, lower social classes, and those not currently married. We now turn to a detailed discussion of a more recent, multisite survey using standardized diagnostic criteria.

The Epidemiologic Catchment Area (ECA) Survey

Composition of the Sample

The ECA is the largest of the surveys presented in this volume. Over 20,000 persons from five geographical areas across the United States were personally interviewed (Figure 6–4). Data from individual sites are weighted to the sampling frame for that site (see Chapter 5). However, for many analyses it would be cumbersome to present separate findings for each of the sites. Since identical assessment methods were used at each site, and since collectively the five sites represent the major regions of the United States, we feel justified in presenting aggregate data for most analyses. The aggregate sample has been weighted so that it is demographically representative of the entire United States as of the 1980 census.

The majority of the sample is between 25 and 64 years of age, the

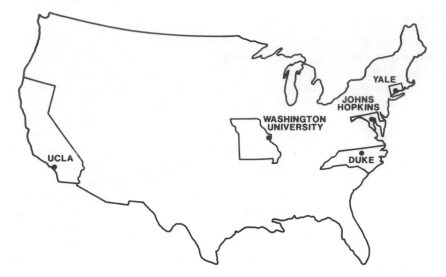

Figure 6–4 ECA Sites in the United States.

mean age is 43 years, and the median is 48 (Table 6–1). The lower age limit of respondents in the ECA was 18 years; there was no upper age limit, and about 5 percent of the respondents were 80 or older. Elderly subjects (65 and older) were oversampled at some of the sites (Baltimore, Durham, and New Haven), as were blacks in St. Louis, and those in long-term institutions at all sites. All oversamples have been weighted back to their true proportion in the sampled areas. Hispanics were oversampled in Los Angeles. The Hispanic sample will not be mentioned further as an independent group in this chapter, but is discussed in detail in Chapter 9.

The mean years of education is 12 (high school completion). In all of the sites, some proportion has obtained an education through equivalence examination. A small minority (9%) had less than 8 years of schooling, and a very few have had no formal education at all.

Most respondents were married and living with their spouse at the time of the interview. The sample is over 90 percent urban; most of the rural residents are from the North Carolina site; and the remainder are from St. Louis, the only other site with a rural component.

We ranked occupations according to their level of prestige in the United States and then trichotomized the prestige scores. Those who were unemployed at the time of interview were assigned the prestige score of their most recent job (Table 6–1). This enabled us to compare occupational status cross-culturally while correcting for the fact that similar occupations may vary in status across cultures.

Table 6–1 Sample Size and Demographic Composition
Combined and Weighted 5-Site ECA Household
and Institutional Samples (Adjusted to National
Demographic Distribution, 1980 Census)

Category	Number or %
Number of subjects interviewed	20,862 76%[a]
Overall response rate	
Age	
18–24	19%
25–44	38%
45–64	27%
65+	16%
Sample mean	49.7 years
Sex (weighted % female)	52%
Race	
Black	11%
White	80%
Other	9%
Years of education	
Mean years	11.8
Proportions with:	
<8 years	9%
8–11 years	24%
12 years	29%
13+ years	38%
Number of marriages	
0	24%
1	63%
2 or more	13%
Residence at time of interview	
Urban	91%
Rural	9%
Occupational status	
Prestige score in	
Upper ⅓	31%
Middle ⅓	38%
Lower ⅓	31%

[a] This percentage is unweighted; all others are weighted (see text).

The Symptoms of Alcoholism

Appendix 1 shows the alcohol section as it actually appears in version III of the DIS. Those items used for the DSM-III (American Psychiatric Association, 1980) diagnoses of alcohol abuse and dependence are asterisked in the right margin. The alcohol symptoms most frequently reported by the total interviewed population were those having to do with excessive consumption. Sixteen percent of the total sample reported drinking heavily, either on a daily (Question 153) or on a weekly (Question 154) basis, at some time in their lives. Fourteen percent said that they had drunk a fifth or more of liquor in one day at least once in their lives. This is a substantial amount of alcohol and we were surprised this symptom was so common. Family objections to the respondent's excessive drinking (11%) and the respondent's own feeling that he was an excessive drinker (10%) are the next two most common symptoms. Only three percent of the sample have ever told a physician about a drinking problem, evidence that treatment seeking in this sample comes well after recognition of problems by family and friends, and even by the drinker himself.

At the other end of the frequency spectrum were work-related symptoms. Losing a job was the least commonly reported symptom, and being unable to work well without having had something to drink was next. These two items were reported by only about 1 percent of the total population. Medical complications of excessive drinking and continuing to drink in the face of an illness that might be made worse by drinking were also rare.

Symptoms that are frequent or rare in the total population occupy roughly that same relative position among those with alcohol abuse and/or dependence, and Table 6–2 shows the proportions of those with an alcohol disorder who responded positively to the alcohol symptoms we asked about. Again, symptoms of heavy alcohol intake are more common and indicators of job or health problems are relatively rare. Relative symptom frequency might be different among alcoholics coming to treatment, but in this general population sample, the correlation for symptom ranking between alcoholics and nonalcoholics is 0.81.

Having widely separated geographical sites in the ECA survey gives us the opportunity to assess the similarities in the expression of alcoholism between various sections of the United States. As it turns out, the intersite correlations of symptom frequencies among alcoholics are also very high. The intersite correlations are all .90 or above (ranging up to .98) except for that between New Haven and Los Angeles, where it is .83.

Drinking Patterns

There is also considerable intersite similarity in drinking patterns between the five ECA sites, but there are some distinct differences as well. For example, total lifetime abstention is relatively rare in all of the sites (Table 6-3), except in Durham. This is the one ECA site that lies in a section of the country known as the "Bible Belt," in which abstaining religious groups are common. Because the abstention rate there is so

Table 6–2 Individual Symptom Frequencies Among Those with Alcohol Disorders Combined and Weighted 5-Site ECA Household and Institutional Samples (Adjusted to National Demographic Distribution, 1980 Census)

DIS Item Number[a]	Symptom	Proportion of Those with Alcohol Abuse and/or Dependence Who Endorsed This Item	
		%	(Rank)
150	Family objected to respondent's drinking	62	(3)
151	Respondent thought himself an excessive drinker	59	(4)
152	Fifth of liquor in one day	70	(2)
153/154	Daily or weekly heavy drinking	80	(1)
155	Told physician about drinking problem	22	(12.5)
156	Friends or professionals said drinking too much	39	(7)
157	Wanted to stop drinking but couldn't	21	(14.5)
158	Efforts to control drinking	19	(16)
159	Morning drinking	21	(14.5)
160	Job troubles due to drinking	15	(17)
161	Lost job	7	(20)
162	Trouble driving	35	(8)
163	Arrested while drinking	31	(9)
164	Physical fights while drinking	50	(6)
165	Two or more binges	29	(10)
166	Blackouts while drinking	57	(5)
167	Any withdrawal symptom	28	(11)
168	Any medical complication	22	(12.5)
169	Continued to drink with serious illness	14	(18)
170	Couldn't do ordinary work without drinking	12	(19)

[a]See Appendix 1 for Alcohol section of DIS-III.

high, Durham is the only site at which social (nonheavy/nonproblem) drinking is not the drinking pattern of the majority.

Heavy/nonproblem drinkers are rare at every site. These are drinkers who have had a period of several months when they regularly consumed seven or more drinks at least one evening a week but have never had any social, legal, or medical problems related to alcohol or any withdrawal symptoms. Most who consume that much alcohol are destined to have at least some problems from it.

Problem drinkers are those who have had at least one alcohol-related problem in their lives, but who have not had enough to qualify for a DSM-III diagnosis of alcoholism. Many of these may be sporadic drinkers. Some may not have been drinking long enough to develop symptoms, although across the five sites the mean age of this group is 38 years, compared to 35 years for those with alcohol abuse. The mean age of all those who are alcohol dependent is 41 years.

Although in DSM-III, alcohol abuse was intended to be the less severe form of the alcohol disorders, in every one of the ECA sites it is less

Table 6–3 Lifetime Rates of Various Drinking Categories Combined and Weighted 5-Site ECA Household and Institutional Samples (Adjusted to National Demographic Distribution, 1980 Census)

Drinking Category	ECA Site					
	New Haven (%)	Baltimore (%)	St. Louis (%)	Durham (%)	Los Angles (%)	All Sites (%)
Abstention	5.2	7.5	9.0	28.0	10.7	10.4
Nonheavy/nonproblem (social) drinkers	72.8	61.9	59.0	47.4	56.9	61.3
Heavy/nonproblem drinkers	2.5	3.4	3.7	1.7	2.3	2.9
Problem drinkers (not alcoholic)	8.3	11.9	12.5	11.2	14.8	11.7
Alcohol abuse only	4.9	5.1	7.1	4.6	5.7	5.8
Dependence with or without abuse	6.4	10.1	8.8	6.1	9.5	7.9
Six-month prevalence of alcoholism (abuse and/or dependence)	4.4	6.0	4.7	3.6	5.1	4.7

prevalent than is alcohol dependence. This probably is an artifact of the DSM-III definition (Helzer et al., 1991). In any event, the proportion with a DSM-III-defined alcohol disorder is the sum of these two lifetime prevalences and is about 11 percent for New Haven and Durham and over 15 percent in each of the other three sites.

The Course of Alcoholism

A majority of the sample (71%) reported having been intoxicated with alcohol at some time in their lives. Since 11 percent of the overall sample reported they were lifelong abstainers, this leaves 18 percent who claim to have used alcohol without ever becoming intoxicated. The mean age of first intoxication is lower in alcoholics than in nonalcoholics, but only by 3 years (Table 6–4). Men also have a lower mean age than women, but only by 2 years. While intoxication first occurs in the late teens, the mean onset of alcohol disorders (the age of the first alcohol-related symptom) is in the early 20s, an average of 24 years for the total sample. It is about 8 years from first intoxication to the onset of alcoholism for both sexes. The mean number of lifetime symptoms is similar in male and female alcoholics—between 5 and 6. The findings in Table 6–4 are for the aggregate 5-site ECA sample, but there is considerable similarity among the five sites.

We define remission from alcoholism as having had no alcohol symptoms for at least one year prior to the interview; 51 percent of those with

Table 6–4 *Onset, Severity, and Course of Alcoholism Combined and Weighted 5-Site ECA Household and Institutional Samples (Adjusted to National Demographic Distribution, 1980 Census)*

	Men	Women	Total
Mean age first intoxicated (if ever)			
Total sample	17	19	18
Alcoholics only	15	17	16
Nonalcoholics	18	20	19
Mean value among alcoholics			
Age of onset of alcoholism	23	25	23
Number of years from first intoxication			
to first alcohol symptom	7.5	7.8	7.6
Mean number of lifetime symptoms	5.6	5.1	5.5
Mean values among alcoholics in remission[a]			
Age last symptom	33	32	33
Duration of alcoholism in years	9.5	6.2	8.9
Lifetime symptoms	5.5	5.6	5.6

[a]Remitted alcoholic = no alcohol symptoms for at least one year prior to interview (proportion = 51% of those with a lifetime diagnosis of alcohol abuse and/or dependence).

a lifetime diagnosis of alcohol abuse or dependence met this definition. The mean age of remission is in the early 30s. The average number of lifetime symptoms is virtually identical among those who are in remission compared to those who are still alcoholic, 5.5 lifetime symptoms compared to 5.6, respectively. There is only a slightly greater differential in symptom count based on the duration of alcoholism. Those who have been alcoholic for more than 10 years at the time of the interview report an average of 6.6 symptoms; alcoholics of a shorter duration report an average of 5.4, not a striking difference. Comparable figures for remitted alcoholics are 6.6 lifetime symptoms for those who had been alcoholic for more than 10 years, and 5.1 symptoms among those who had a shorter duration. Thus, these four groups are similar in terms of the severity of their alcohol disorders as measured by lifetime symptom count.

The average duration of alcoholism among those who have remitted is 9 years, and is longer for men than for women, since women and men remit about the same age, but women begin their problems later. The range of duration is broad, from less than 1 to 64 years, but most have a relatively short duration (Figure 6–5). For many who have remitted, the duration of alcoholism was less than a year, and for over half, the duration was 5 years or less. Only about one-quarter of the remitted cases had been alcoholic for 12 years or more. The high remission rates and lesser durations are very different from those seen in treated samples of alcoholics who typically come to treatment only after many years of alcohol problems. These findings may help to explain why so few persons with alcohol problems in the general population seek care. Many appear to be able to reduce their drinking sufficiently to terminate their difficulties, at

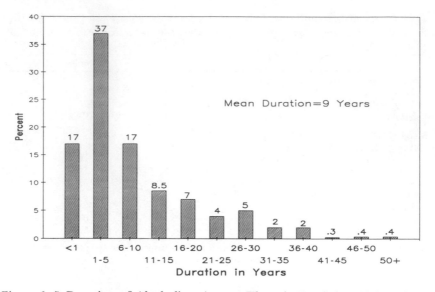

Figure 6–5 Duration of Alcoholism Among Those in Remission 12 Months or More (Combined 5-Site ECA Data Adjusted to National Demographic Distribution).

least for 1 year, quite early in the course of their disorder. It is those who try and fail who appear for treatment.

Risk Factors and Correlates of Alcoholism

Risk factors are variables that are associated with an increased rate of disorder, but are clearly antecedent, such as race and sex. Correlates are associated variables that are not necessarily antecedent, such as other psychiatric diagnoses and education. Sex is clearly an important risk factor for alcoholism. At every age, prevalence rates for men are substantially higher than those for women (Figure 6–6). However, there is evidence of convergence in the rates between sexes in the younger age groups. Male to female ratios are generally lower in younger than in older aged cohorts. Thus there is evidence not only of an age cohort effect, with alcoholism being more prevalent in younger age groups, but also of a sex effect with alcoholism becoming differentially more prevalent in younger women.

The age-specific lifetime rates of alcoholism show strikingly different patterns in blacks and whites (Figure 6–6). Among the youngest men (18–29-year-olds), the lifetime prevalence rate of alcoholism in whites is over twice that in blacks. In the next age group, the rates are more equal, with a slight predominance in blacks. The predominance in black men becomes more apparent with age, so that in the oldest group (65 and

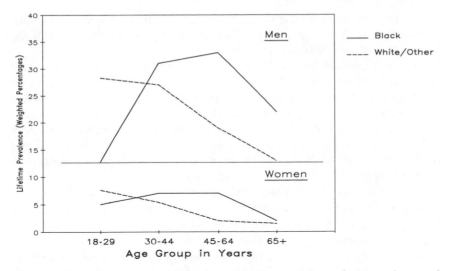

Figure 6–6 Alcohol Abuse and/or Dependence Prevalence by Age, Sex, and Ethnicity (Combined 5-Site ECA Data Adjusted to National Demographic Distribution).

over), the prevalence rates have about reversed, that is, nearly twice as high in blacks compared to whites. The pattern for black and white women is similar to that for men.

Rates by age show an unexpected pattern. At any age, lifetime prevalence is the cumulative rate over all previous ages; thus we would expect lifetime rates to be highest in the older age groups, since they have had more years at risk. As can also be seen from Figure 6–6, this is not the case. Among men, prevalence peaks in the 25–44-year age group and falls thereafter. Among women, there is a consistent downward progression in prevalence from young to old. This seemingly counterintuitive result could be an artifact of recall; older respondents may forget symptoms which occurred earlier in their lives, and thus their lifetime prevalence only appears low because they fail to report past symptoms. While this may be occurring to some extent, it does not appear to be the entire explanation, since the pattern is not as strong among blacks. There is no reason to assume that blacks have better recall for early symptoms than whites.

Another possible explanation for the fall in prevalence in older age groups is differential mortality among alcoholics. As we have seen, the mean onset of alcoholism is in the 20s. As the population ages, the rate of new onsets fall, but alcoholics have an elevated mortality rate relative to the rest of the population so that a higher proportion will be lost to follow-up through early death. Lifetime prevalence estimates based on personal interviews with survivors will miss those who have already died of the disease, thus giving the picture we see here of a lower lifetime prevalence in older age groups. But again, this probably does not explain sex and race differentials.

The explanation with the most serious social implications is that this is not an artifact, but a cohort effect with alcoholism becoming more prevalent in younger age groups, especially for particular subsamples. Such an interpretation is consistent with the rise in per capita consumption shown in Figure 6–2. Other studies are inconsistent on this point. One recent longitudinal cohort analysis of problem drinking did not find evidence of higher rates of alcohol problems among young men (21–29) compared to a cohort of men of the same age 12 years earlier; however, they did have a slightly higher rate of social problems (Fillmore, 1987). Other recent work has suggested that heavy drinking may be increasing among older men (Malin et al., 1986). But it is unclear to what extent these cases represent late onset alcoholism versus relapses.

Other possible correlates and risk factors for alcoholism, based on observations in clinical samples, are considered in Table 6–5. We examine these in the first column of the table as predictors of heavy drinking among all drinkers (lifetime abstainers are excluded from this analysis), and in the second column as predictors of alcoholism among those who are heavy drinkers. The total proportions at the top of the table show that about one-third (32%) of all drinkers have at one time been heavy drinkers, and about half (49%) of all heavy drinkers meet the DSM-III criteria for alcohol abuse and/or dependence.

Drinkers who have been married only once are somewhat less likely to be heavy drinkers compared to those who are single or married more than once. Multiple marriage is also associated with alcoholism among those who have drunk heavily. Education shows a consistent relationship with both outcome variables. Those with the lowest levels of education have the highest rates of heavy drinking and, within heavy drinkers, of alcoholism. There is a consistent fall in these percentages as educational level rises. Occupational status appears to have little impact, perhaps because it reflects job prestige and not job performance or current employment. Region of residence at the time of the interview also shows little association with either heavy drinking or progression to alcoholism.

The last three variables in Table 6–5 show strong associations with both outcome variables. Two of these, number of childhood conduct disorder symptoms and first intoxication before age 15, are clearly antecedent to the development of both heavy drinking and alcoholism, i.e., risk factors. Drug abuse, on the other hand, is a correlate, as it may or may not precede drinking. All three are highly associated with both heavy drinking and alcoholism among heavy drinkers.

Another interesting set of variables to examine in relation to alcoholism is other psychiatric disorders ascertained by the DIS. These are presented in Table 6–6, which shows, in the first column, the lifetime

Table 6–5 Risk Factors and Correlates for Heavy Drinking and Alcoholism Combined and Weighted 5-Site ECA Household and Institutional Samples (Adjusted to National Demographic Distribution, 1980 Census)

	Proportion of All Drinkers Who Are Heavy Drinkers (%)	Proportion of Heavy Drinkers Who Are Alcoholic (%)
Total nonabstaining sample (*N* = 16,441)	32	49
Risk Factor or Correlate		
Sex		
Men	48	53
Women	16	35
Number of marriages		
0	40	46
1	27	48
2+	36	57
Years of education		
<8 years	37	57
8–11 years	34	53
12 years	31	48
13+ years	30	43
Occupational status		
Upper ⅓	33	50
Middle ⅓	34	50
Lower ⅓	29	46
Residence at time of interview		
Urban	31	49
Rural	35	47
Childhood conduct groups positive		
None	20	37
1 or 2	40	46
3 or more	67	67
Intoxicated before age 15		
No	27	43
Yes	66	66
Any drug disorder		
No	29	45
Yes	72	67

prevalence rates for each of the core DIS/DSM-III diagnoses ascertained in the initial ECA surveys. The diagnoses have been listed in order of lifetime prevalence. Alcoholism is the most prevalent diagnosis and, given the severe consequences of this disorder to individuals and to society, the public health implications of this high rate are profound.

Column 2 of Table 6–6 shows the lifetime prevalence of each of these disorders among those who also meet DSM-III criteria for alcohol abuse and/or dependence on a lifetime basis. For every diagnosis shown, there is a higher prevalence among alcoholics than in the total population.

Table 6–6 Lifetime Prevalence Rates of Core Diagnoses and Risk Ratios among Alcoholics Combined and Weighted 5-Site ECA Household and Institutional Samples (Adjusted to National Demographic Distribution, 1980 Census)

Diagnosis in Order of Lifetime Prevalence	Lifetime Prevalence in Total ECA Sample (Weighted %)	Lifetime Prevalence in ECA Alcoholics (Weighted %)	Risk Ratio (Prevalence in Alcoholics/ Prevalence in Nonalcoholics)
Alcoholism	13.7	—	—
Phobic disorder (any)	12.6	16.5	1.4
Drug abuse and/or dependence (any)	6.2	21.4	5.7
Major depression	6.4	9.4	1.6
Cognitive impairment (mild or severe)	4.7	5.1	1.1
Dysthymic disorder	3.2	5.0	1.7
Antisocial personality disorder	2.6	14.3	19.5
Obsessive compulsive disorder	2.6	4.5	2.0
Panic disorder	1.6	3.3	2.6
Schizophrenia	1.3	3.4	3.4
Mania	0.8	2.8	5.4
Somatization disorder	0.1	0.2	1.8
Anorexia nervosa	0.1	0.1	1.1
Any core DIS diagnosis	27.8	48.0	2.0

Run used: job 648,270CT881.

(For anorexia, however, the difference is too slight to be seen.) Column 3 shows the risk ratios of other disorders in alcoholics, that is, the prevalence of each disorder in alcoholics divided by its prevalence in nonalcoholics. Again, the risk ratios are greater than 1 for every diagnosis (indicating higher prevalence in alcoholics), but it is interesting to examine the magnitude of the differences. The diagnosis for which the relative risk is largest is antisocial personality disorder—alcoholics are almost 20 times more likely to have this diagnosis than nonalcoholics. This association has been well recognized in previous studies of both alcoholic (Lewis, 1983; Virkkunen, 1979) and antisocial (Robins, 1966) samples. Although it is questionable whether there is a genetic relationship between these two disorders (Cadoret et al., 1985), it appears that antisocial behavior is a risk factor for alcoholism in this sample, and not just a behavioral correlate. The evidence for this is the strong relationship between the number of conduct disorder symptoms, precursors of adult antisocial behavior occurring in childhood, and both heavy drinking and the development of alcoholism among heavy drinkers. Overall, those with alcoholism are five times more likely to have had three or more conduct disorder symptoms by the age of 15 than are nonalcoholics.

Antisocial personality clearly stands out as the disorder that is most strongly associated with alcoholism. Drug abuse and/or dependence is next, but a distant second. This is true even among younger age groups, in which drug abuse is more common. In fact, although drug disorders are rare in the older ages, they are more highly associated with alcoholism in older than in younger age groups.

After antisocial and drug disorders, mania is next most strongly associated with alcoholism. Mania is a relatively rare diagnosis in the general population—only 94 persons met the DSM-III criteria on a lifetime basis—but the association with alcoholism is high. In fact, it is even stronger than the association between alcoholism and depression.

Based on experience with clinical samples, it may seem surprising that the risk ratio for depression is so low. Alcoholics seen in clinical settings often report multiple depressive symptoms, and patients who seek care for depression often use alcohol, perhaps for symptomatic relief. We thus tend to think of these two disorders as highly associated. In fact, it has been suggested that they might be genetically related (Winokur et al., 1970). From the population data here, it would appear that neither major depression nor dysthymic disorder co-occur very strongly with alcoholism, a finding that is consistent with other recent data (Schuckit, 1986). It may be that alcoholics who are depressed or depressives who drink heavily are more likely to seek or be brought to treatment, thus giving a false impression of general comorbidity. On the other hand, the clinical impression of a strong association between alcoholism and mania is borne out in this population survey. Numbers are relatively small here since mania is a rare diagnosis, but comorbidity is frequent. Schizophrenia, which is not as rare as mania in the population and of which we have 254 diagnosed cases in the total sample, also shows a relatively strong association with alcoholism.

Overall, those with alcoholism are about twice as likely as nonalcoholics to have some other core psychiatric diagnosis. This is consistent with a previous report that those with any diagnosis are more likely to also have some other diagnosis (Boyd et al., 1984).

Conclusions

In this chapter, we have reviewed the history of alcohol use in American society and have examined recent trends in alcohol consumption in order to provide a context for the detailed cross-sectional examination undertaken in the ECA survey.

Although the ECA is not a nationwide probability sample, the results depict some of the diversity of the United States. The five samples reported here represent only portions of some of the communities from which they were drawn, but the communities themselves are widely distributed across the continent; the North, East, Midwest, South, and West are all represented. The ECA is the largest psychiatric epidemiologic survey ever done in this country and is one of the few in which the interview instrument was based directly on specific diagnostic criteria.

The sample includes respondents from households as well as a variety of institutions, and so is comprehensive. Since group quarters are included in the sampling frame, only those persons who are not attached to any type of domicile, such as vagrants, would be absent from the survey.

Our review of the history of its use suggests that alcohol, particularly in the form of beer and spirits, has always occupied a prominent role in the United States. The results of the ECA survey tend to support this by indicating that most Americans drink and that alcoholism, as defined by the DSM-III criteria, is a highly prevalent disorder in American society. Of all the psychiatric disorders we assessed, alcohol abuse and dependence are among the most prevalent. Only phobic disorder has a similarly high prevalence, and the public health implications of the latter are much different. Phobic disorder is typically fairly circumscribed and, while there may be social inconvenience associated with avoiding the feared object(s) or situation(s), it is rarely incapacitating. Furthermore, phobic disorder does not have the serious physical complications nor the extreme social consequences that alcoholism engenders for the alcoholic, his family, and society at large. Thus, of the psychiatric disorders assessed in the ECA survey, alcoholism is particularly important—it is both a prevalent and a serious disorder.

It is well known from multiple studies of clinical samples that sex is a major risk factor for alcoholism. It is clear from Figure 6–6, that the strong association between sex and alcoholism found in many previous studies is present in this general population sample as well. Taken all together, men are about five times more likely to have a lifetime diagnosis of alcoholism than women and, even in the youngest groups, men clearly predominate. But there is also evidence that alcoholism is becoming more common among women; for both races, there is a consistent and dramatic fall in the male:female ratio from about 7:1 in the oldest age group to around 3:1 in the 18–24-year-olds. This finding is particularly unlikely to be either a recall artifact (such as an explanation would have to presuppose that men are considerably better historians than women) or a manifestation of differential mortality (since that would require that alcohol-related mortality in women greatly exceeds that in men). Assuming this finding is not artifactual, it raises concern that there are increasing numbers of female alcoholics in this country.

The strong sex effect can also be seen in Table 6–5. Two reasons suggested for a higher prevalence of alcoholism in men are the social stigma attached to drinking by women and the fact that women are less physically tolerant of alcohol, that is, that many women cannot consume enough alcohol to become dependent on it. Our analysis of risk factors has shown that men are three times more likely than women to be heavy drinkers. However, we might expect the sex ratio for alcoholism to decrease when only heavy drinkers are included, since heavy drinking women have overcome both of the obstacles noted above. Indeed, the risk differential is reduced, but heavy drinking men are still 1.5 times more likely to be alcoholic than their female counterparts.

Although alcoholism has a high prevalence rate overall, we found differences in the prevalence rates across the five study sites (Table 6–3). Durham, North Carolina, which is located in a region of the country with a strong religious influence, had the lowest rates of both alcohol abuse and dependence and a very high lifetime abstention rate. This suggestion of a religious influence on drinking patterns is consistent with the finding by Caetano and Herd (1984) of high rates of both abstention and light drinking among religious fundalmentalists in California.

Although not located in a Bible Belt region, New Haven has an equally low lifetime prevalence of alcoholism. However, the abstention rate is lowest in New Haven. All categories of excessive alcohol intake are low in the New Haven sample, with the difference made up in the relatively high rate of nonproblem social drinking. As we noted, the educational level in New Haven is higher than the other sites, and this may be an important factor in the high rate of social drinking. Years of education showed a consistent inverse relationship with both rates of heavy drinking and, among those who were heavy drinkers, rates of alcohol abuse and dependence (Table 6–5).

In contrast to the prevalence of alcoholism, where we see some regional differences, the expression of alcoholism as manifested by relative lifetime frequency of specific symptoms, age of onset, lifetime symptom count, and duration is similar across the sites. For example, there is little variation in the relative prevalence of the alcohol-related symptoms we asked about, and the intersite correlations range up to nearly unity.

As expected, excessive drinking is a common symptom, but we were surprised at the frequency of positive reports of drinking as much as a fifth of liquor in one day. This was the second most common symptom among the alcoholics. The third most common symptom is family objections to the respondent's drinking. Not surprisingly, this source of complaints is quite a bit more common than friends or professionals telling the respondent he drinks too much. Alcoholism tends to disrupt the home before it disrupts outside relationships, and the threshold for tolerance is reached first in the former setting. Support for this is seen in Table 6–5, where those with multiple marriages are more likely both to be heavy drinkers and to progress to alcoholism compared to those who have been married only once.

Apart from the burden borne by the families, the costs of drinking seem to fall more frequently on society at large than on the drinker himself. These costs are in the form of trouble driving (a significant risk factor for those the alcoholic encounters on the highway), arrests, and violence. Personal health consequences are less frequently endorsed than social complications, although reports of job-related difficulties by the alcoholic are rare. It is also interesting to note that, in this general population sample, high occupational status appears to offer no protection against either heavy consumption or, among heavy drinkers, against alcoholism (Table 6–5).

The results from this study also provide clues about the future prevalence of alcoholism in the United States. Our finding that the ratio of male to female alcoholics is decreasing in younger age cohorts suggests that there will be an increase in female alcoholics. In addition, if early age of first intoxication is an important precursor of alcoholism, as seems to be the case in our data, the increasingly early exposure of adolescents to alcohol may presage an increase in the rates of alcoholism as these young people enter adulthood, although as Babor points out (Chapter 4), this probably depends on the nature of the exposure. Introduction to alcohol in family or ritualistic settings that are sanctioned by society may have very different implications than an introduction in peer group settings. One recent longitudinal cohort analysis of problem drinking, however, did not find evidence of higher rates of alcohol problems among young (21–29-year-old) men compared to men of the same age 12 years earlier, although they did have a slightly higher rate of social problems (Fillmore, 1987). This is an important issue that needs further investigation.

Although not a principal objective of this chapter, we close with some comments about the discouraging picture our data present for the identification of alcoholics by treatment services. Only 20 percent of alcoholics reported ever discussing drinking problems with a doctor. While a positive response to this question cannot be considered synonymous with treatment, it is an indication of how rarely alcoholics seek care for alcohol problems. This is especially disturbing in light of our findings suggesting that families and society bear a major share of the effects of alcoholism. Aside from consumption, the most common symptoms were those that impinged on personal (family objecting) and societal (physical fights, trouble driving, and arrests) domains.

This picture of a minority of alcoholics coming to treatment contrasts very sharply with the view obtained from examining treatment facility statistics. A sharp (65%) increase in alcoholism treatment units was recorded in the United States between 1982 and 1984 (Noble, 1986). Furthermore, the character of ownership of these facilities is shifting, with government (local, state, and federal) reducing its role, and for-profit companies and not-for-profit entities becoming more prominent. The appearance of investor-owned companies in particular suggests that this area is seen as a highly lucrative one. There is some evidence from ECA data that alcoholics can be influenced to seek treatment by the urgings of others even when the individual himself sees no such need (McEvoy et al., submitted). But it remains to be seen whether the greater availability and intense marketing of these facilities will substantially affect the treatment statistics for alcoholism.

Despite the increased availability of facilities, the process by which alcoholics come to treatment is not well understood. Recommendations that focus on employee assistance plans, while well motivated, overlook evidence presented here and elsewhere (Cahalan & Room, 1970) that work performance is among the last aspect of the alcoholic's life to be affected. Because alcoholism remains hidden from employers and co-workers until it is well advanced, employers may have to be more aggressive in identifying cases if such programs are to have an impact on bringing alcoholics to early treatment.

Prevention is another little-understood area. Our data did not uncover any factors that prevented the progression from heavy drinking to alcoholism. This would suggest that prevention strategies that focus on stopping the progression from light to heavy drinking might be a gainful approach. Targeting certain high risk groups (such as children with three or more symptoms of conduct disorder) for special education on alcohol abuse might be an effective preventive strategy. The enormous societal and personal costs of alcoholism, including family anguish, loss of productivity, early illness, and high mortality and morbidity, call for greater activity in the recognition and prevention of this highly prevalent, highly disruptive disorder.

References

American Psychiatric Association, Committee on Nomenclature and Statistics (1980). *Diagnostic and Statistical Manual of Mental Disorders—Edition 3 (DSM-III)*. Washington, D.C.: American Psychiatric Association.

Ames, G. M. (1985). American beliefs about alcoholism: Historical perspectives on the medical-moral controversy. In L. A. Bennett and G. N. Ames (eds)., *The American Experience with Alcohol: Contrasting Cultural Perspectives*. New York: Plenum Press, pp. 23–39.

Bacon, S. D. (1962). Alcohol and complex society. In D. J. Pittman and C. R. Snyder (eds.), *Society, Culture and Drinking*. New York: John Wiley & Sons, pp. 78–93.

Boyd, J. H.; Burke, J. D.; Gruenberg, E.; Holzer, C. E.; Rae, D. S.; George, L. K.; Karno, M.; Stoltzman, R.; McEvoy, L.; and Nestadt, G. (1984). Exclusion criteria of DSM-III: A study of co-occurrence of hierarchy-free syndromes. *Arch. Gen. Psychiatry* 41:983–89.

Brenner, M. H. (1982). International trends in alcohol consumption and related pathologies. In *Alcohol Consumption and Related Problems*. Alcohol and Health Monograph No. 1. Washington, D.C.: National Institute on Alcohol Abuse and Alcoholism (NIAAA), Alcohol, Drug Abuse, and Mental Health Administration (ADAMHA), United States Public Health Service, pp. 157–76.

Caddy, G. R. (1983). Alcohol use and abuse: Historical perspective and present trends. In B. Tabakoff, P. Sutker, and C. Randall (eds.), *Medical and Social Aspects of Alcohol Abuse*. New York: Plenum Press, pp. 1–30.

Cadoret, R. J.; O'Gorman, T. W.; Troughton, E.; and Heywood, E. (1985). Alcoholism and antisocial personality: Interrelationships, generic and environmental factors. *Arch. Gen. Psychiatry* 42:161–67.

Caetano, R., and Herd, D. (1984). Black drinking practices in northern California. *Am. J. Drug Alcohol Abuse* 10:571–87.

Cahalan, D., and Cisin, I. H. (1976). Drinking behavior and drinking problems in the U.S. In B. Kissin and H. Begleiter (eds.), *The Biology of Alcoholism, Volume 4. Social Aspects of Alcoholism.* New York: Plenum Press, pp. 77–115.

Cahalan, D., and Room, R. (1974). *Problem Drinking Among American Man* (Monograph No. 7). New Brunswick, N.J.: Rutgers Center for Alcohol Studies.

Cisin, I. G. (1978). Formal and informal social controls over drinking. In B. Rouse and J. Ewing (eds.), *Drinking: Alcohol in American Society: Issues and Current Research.* Chicago: Nelson Hall, pp. 145–58.

Clark, N. H. (1976). *Deliver Us from Evil: An Interpretation of American Prohibition.* New York: W. W. Norton.

Clark, W. B., and Midanik, L. (1982). Alcohol use and alcohol problems among U.S. adults: Results of the 1979 Survey. *Alcohol Consumption and Related Problems* (Alcohol and Health Monograph No. 1), U.S. Government Printing Office, Washington, D.C.: DHHS Pub. No. (ADM) 82-1190, pp. 3–52.

de Crevecoeur, H. S. J. (1963). *Letters from an American Farmer and Sketches of Eighteenth Century America.* New York: New American Library of World Classics.

Fillmore, K. M. (1984). When angels fall: Women's drinking as cultural preoccupation and as reality. In S. Wilsnack and L. Beckman (eds.), *Alcohol Problems in Women: Antecedents, Consequences and Intervention.* New York: Guilford Press, pp. 7–36.

Fillmore, K. M. (1987). Prevalence, incidence and chronicity of drinking patterns and problems among men as a function of age: A longitudinal and cohort analysis. *Br. J. Addict.* 82:77–83.

Gusfield, J. R. (1962). Status conflicts and the changing ideologies of the American temperance movement. In D. J. Pittman and C. R. Snyder (eds.), *Society, Culture and Drinking Patterns.* New York: John Wiley & Sons, pp. 101–20.

Helzer, J. E., Burnam, A., McEvoy, L. T. (1991). Alcohol abuse and dependence. In L. N. Robins and D. A. Regier (eds.), *Psychiatric Disorders in America.* New York: The Free Press.

Howland, R. W., and Howland, J. W. (1978). Two hundred years of drinking in the United States: Evolution of the disease concept. In B. A. Rouse and J. A. Ewing (eds.), *Drinking Alcohol in American Society: Issues and Current Research.* Chicago: Nelson Hall, pp. 39–60.

Kyvig, D. E. (1979). *Repealing National Prohibition.* Chicago: University of Chicago Press.

Lender, M. E., and Martin, J. K. (1982). *Drinking in America: A History.* New York: Free Press.

Levine, H. G. (1978). The discovery of addiction: Changing conceptions of habitual drunkenness in America. *J. Stud. Alcohol.* 39:143–74.

Levine, H. G. (1984). The alcohol problem in America: From temperance to alcoholism. *Br. J. Addict.* 79:109–19.

Levine, H. G. (1985). The birth of American alcohol control: Prohibition, the power elite, and the problem of lawlessness. *Contemporary Drug Problems* 12, 63–115.

Lewis, C. R.; Rice, J.; and Helzer, J. E. (1983). Diagnostic interactions: Alcoholism and antisocial personality. *J. Nerv. Ment. Dis.* 171, 105–13.

Malin, H.; Wilson, R.; Williams, G.; and Aitken, S. (1986). 1983 Alcohol/Health Practices Supplement. *Alcohol Health and Research World* 10, 48–50.

McEvoy, L., Robins, L. H., Helzer, J. E., and Spitznagel, E. L. (submitted for publication). Alcoholism and mental health services: Who comes to treatment?

National Center for Health Statistics; Thornberry, O. T.; Wilson, R. W.; and Golden, P. M. (1986). *Advance Data from Vital and Health Statistics.* No. 1265, DHHS Publication No. (PHS) 86-1250. Myatteville, Maryland: Public Health Service.

Noble, J. (1986). Mental health services: Who comes to treatment? Presented at the ADPA, West Palm Beach, Florida, February. (Submitted for publication.)

Regier, D. A.; Myers, J. K.; Kramer, M.; Robins, L. N.; Blazer, D. G.; Hough, R. L.; Eaton, W. W.; and Locke, B. Z. (1984). The NIMH Epidemiologic Catchment Area program: Historical context, major objectives, and study population characteristics. *Arch. Gen. Psychiatry* 41:934–41.

Robins, L. N. (1966). *Deviant Children Grown Up: A Sociological and Psychiatric Study of Sociopathic Personality.* Baltimore: Williams and Wilkins.

Robins, L. N., Helzer, J. E., Croughan, J., and Ratcliff, K. S. (1981). National Institute of Mental Health Diagnostic Interview Schedule: Its history, characteristics, and validity. *Arch. Gen. Psychiatry* 38:381–89.

Rorabaugh, W. J. (1976). Estimated U.S. alcoholic beverage consumption, 1790–1860. *J. Stud. Alcohol* 37:357.

Schuckit, M. A. (1986). Genetic and clinical implications of alcoholism and affective disorder. *Am. J. Psychiatry* 143:140–47.

Terris, M. A. (1968). A social policy for health. *Am. J. Public Health* 58:5–12.

United States Department of Agriculture, Economic Research Service (1984). *Food Consumption, Prices and Expenditures, 1963–1983.* Statistical Bulletin No. 713. Washington, D.C.: U.S. Department of Agriculture, November.

Virkkunen, J. (1979). Alcoholism and antisocial personality. *Acta Psychiatr. Scand.* 59:493–501.

Weissman, M. M.; Myers, M. K.; and Harding; P. S. (1980). Prevalence and psychiatric heterogeneity of alcoholism in a U.S. urban community. *J. Stud. Alcohol* 41:672–81.

Williams, G. E.; Doernberg, D. G.; Stinson, F.; and Noble, J. (1986). State, regional, and national trends in apparent per capita consumption. *Alcohol, Health and Research World* 10:60.

Winkler, A. M. (1968). Drinking on the American frontier. *Quart. J. Stud. Alcohol* 29:413.

Winokur, G.; Reich, T.; and Rimmer, J. (1970). Alcoholism III: Diagnosis and familial psychiatric illness in 259 alcoholic probands. *Arch. Gen. Psychiatry* 23:104–11.

[7] Alcohol Abuse and Dependence in Edmonton, Canada

Roger C. Bland, Stephen C. Newman, and Helene Orn

Alberta, the westernmost of Canada's three prairie provinces, became a province in 1905. It is bounded on the north by the Northwest Territories, and on the south, at the 49th parallel, by the state of Montana. The province is landlocked, the eastern boundary is with Saskatchewan, and the western with British Columbia, at the Rocky Mountains. The area is 661,185 sq.km., with a north–south dimension of 1221 km. and an east–west dimension of 650 km. In the 1981 national census the population was 2.2 million. Edmonton, the capital city of the province, is situated centrally and has a population of over half a million. Following the Second World War and with the discovery of oil and gas deposits, the provincial economy expanded rapidly, but agriculture is still significant to Alberta. From the early 1970s to 1982, oil and gas developments increased rapidly and there was a 37.5 percent growth in the provincial population from 1971 to 1981. Since 1982, there has been a marked downturn in the economy, particularly the natural resource sector, but also in agriculture, and the unemployment rate has gone from less than 3 percent in the late 1970s to about 12 percent currently.

History of Alcohol Legislation

In 1906, 1 year after the province of Alberta came into being, the Liquor License Ordinance was placed on the Alberta Statutes (ALCB, 1975). This legislation provided for the issuing of licenses and the sale of alcohol at both wholesale and retail levels. About this time a number of

This study was supported by the Alberta Mental Health Advisory Council and Alberta Mental Health Services. Vipin Sharma of Mental Health Services assisted in preparation of background material.

"clubs," specially incorporated by provincial legislation, also came into being. Most were nothing more than liquor-selling outlets, and the subsequent abuse of government-granted privileges led to an outcry by prohibitionists who in 1915 forced a referendum. The campaigns by the "Wets" and the "Drys" were vigorous, but in the end the polls were three to two in favour of prohibition. The following year a new Liquor Act was proclaimed which abolished the clubs and put an end to the availability of wholesale liquor licenses. The sale of alcohol was restricted to specially appointed vendors; however, physicians and druggists (on receipt of a prescription) could also sell liquor. Interestingly, the new legislation allowed liquor to be obtained from outside the province, and this resulted in a flourishing mail order business in alcoholic beverages. Following World War I the mood in the province changed with steadily mounting pressure against prohibition. In 1924 the Government Liquor Control act was passed with broad public support. It gave the provincial government complete control over the retail and wholesale selling of alcoholic beverages, including the issuing of licenses and permits, the setting of prices, deciding where retail outlets could be established, their hours of operation, and the brands that could be imported. The administration of the legislation became the responsibility of the newly created Liquor Control Board. Over the years the legislation governing liquor in Alberta has undergone many changes, and with it changes in the powers of the Board, a body that functions to this day. The 1960s in particular brought innovations. In 1965 the regulations surrounding advertising were relaxed so that producers of alcoholic beverages could advertise their product in the media. In 1969 the first self-service liquor retail outlet was opened. Despite the relaxation of certain regulations, virtually complete control over the sale of alcoholic beverages in the province remains under government control. Legislation regarding the legal age of drinking has also changed. In 1971 the limit was lowered from age 21 to its current level of 18.

Alcohol Consumption

Based on retail liquor sales during 1973–1983, it has been estimated that on average an Albertan aged 18 or over consumed the equivalent of approximately 12 liters of absolute alcohol in 1973, 15 liters in 1981 (a maximum for the period) and 13 liters in 1983 (AADAC, 1985). In 1983 consumption was mostly in the form of spirits (45%), followed closely by beer (42%), with the remainder consumed as wine (13%). Since 1981 there have been major increases in the price of alcohol when taken as a percentage of disposable income. This has been followed by a corresponding decrease in per capita consumption. About three percent of the disposable income of an Albertan aged 18 or over was spent on alcohol in 1983. Alcohol consumption is closely paralleled by a number of health and social indicators. In 1983 the death rate for alcohol-related liver disease was approximately 9 deaths per 100,000 Albertans aged 18 or over. This represents two-thirds of the death rate due to all liver disease. Also in 1983 almost 5 percent of divorces in Alberta that were granted on the grounds of marriage breakdown were directly attributed to alcohol addiction. In that same year over one-quarter of motor vehicle fatalities involved alcohol-impaired drivers. An additional 15 percent of non-fatal collisions involved drinking and driving.

Attitudes

A survey of 1,400 Albertans selected from all walks of life was conducted in 1974 with the aim of determining attitudes and beliefs toward alcohol and alcoholism (DMI, 1974). Personal experience with alcohol had by far the most significant influence on the respondent's feelings towards alcohol, followed by television, religious institutions, and the printed media. About half of those interviewed regarded alcoholism as a serious societal problem when compared to such concerns as inflation and pollution. Twenty percent of respondents felt that alcohol abuse could be attributed to family and marital difficulties, with an additional twenty percent believing emotional instability and various mental disorders to be the root cause. About three-quarters of those interviewed held the opinion that difficult social conditions like poverty and the stresses of modern society result in people drinking too much. Although 90 percent felt that alcoholism is a treatable disorder, just under half of those voicing this opinion said that an alcoholic is cured only when drinking ceases completely. When asked about advertising and alcohol, almost one-third of those surveyed wanted such advertising banned altogether, and an additional 17 percent wanted it reduced. Opposition to advertising was greatest in the older age groups and in those with less education. The emotional response to someone drinking while driving was anger in about half of the respondents, followed by fear in a further third.

Adolescents and Alcohol

In 1980, a survey of 261 junior and senior high school students (ages 12–18 years) was conducted in Alberta with the aim of determining alcohol-related attitudes and habits (AADAC, 1980). Only one-fifth of the respondents indicated that they never drank. Sixty percent believed that most people drink in order to "have a good time." Half said that getting drunk was "O.K. once in a while." One-third of the students felt that their friends would think they were "O.K." if they did not drink, but one-quarter said they would be considered a "goody goody." Most of the students tended to look to adults to teach them the responsible use of alcohol, while only a few suggested that television was important in forming their attitudes. Group discussions with the students revealed that at the younger ages drinking is motivated by curiosity and social approval. At this stage alcohol consumption is infrequent but in relatively large amounts with a small group of friends. This is the time when individuals learn how much alcohol they can tolerate. Later, drinking becomes more of a social challenge, taking place in large gatherings and more frequently. When the legal drinking age is reached, alcohol becomes less of a challenge.

Methods

The results in this chapter are based on the first 3,258 interviews conducted in a community survey of Edmonton, the capital city of the province of Alberta, Canada. Data collection took place between January 1983 and May 1986. The sampling frame was restricted to the city proper, and so outlying suburban and rural areas were excluded. The survey has recently been extended to include an institutional sample, but the interviews considered below were obtained only from private residences. The population of Edmonton aged 18 years or over was just under 398,000 in the 1981 national census, with an age distribution somewhat younger than that in Canada as a whole.

Subjects were sampled using a two-stage design. First, addresses were selected in systematic samples from a 1982 computerized list of residences. A minimum of four, and as many as eight, attempts were made to contact someone at each address. At the second stage, a household member was chosen using the method of Kish (1949). To be eligible the subject had to be a "usual" occupant of the household and at least 18 years of age. If the index subject refused to be interviewed, no data was collected from that household. No substitution or interview by proxy was allowed. Version III of the DIS was used in all the interviews.

All interviewers were selected and trained by one of us (HO), who attended a training session in the use of the DIS at Washington University in St. Louis. Data were checked for completeness and consistency prior to being double-entered into the computer. Printouts of raw data underwent additional checks and credits, and a sample of questionnaires was further verified by triple-entering. Survey weights were constructed according to the method described by Kessler et al. (1985), with post-stratification to the 1981 age-sex distribution of Edmonton. Most of the data analysis was performed using the same program as that employed by the St. Louis group (see Chapter 2), according to which diagnoses are made hierarchy-free. Standard errors were computed using SESUDAAN (Shah, 1981).

Results

The Composition of the Sample

The Edmonton survey was conducted entirely in the City of Edmonton, and includes 3,258 interviewed respondents. Table 7–1 shows the demographic composition of the sample. All results except the response rate have been weighted to the 1981 census population of Edmonton unless stated otherwise.

The response rate (71.6%) is the proportion of eligible addresses at which an interview was obtained. Nonresponse was due to refusal (17.3%), contact not being made at an address (8.8%), and language barriers (2.3%). Addresses that were vacant and where security systems

Table 7–1 Sample Size and Demographic Composition, Edmonton Household Sample (Weighted Except Where Indicated)

Category	Number or %	
Number of subjects interviewed	3,258	
Overall response rate[a]	72%	
Age	Unweighted	Weighted
18–24	17.7%	25.5%
25–44	49.0%	42.0%
45–64	22.3%	22.8%
65+	11.0%	9.8%
Sex		
Weighted % female	50.1%	
Unweighted	59.2%	
Number of marriages		
0	31.2%	
1	60.0%	
2 or more	8.8%	
Residence at time of interview		
Urban	100.0%	
Rural	0.0%	
Employment		
Employed	53.0%	
Unemployed	11.0%	
Not in labor force	36.0%	

[a]This percentage is unweighted; all others are weighted (see text).

precluded contact were considered ineligible and excluded from the calculations.

The interviewed sample shows an excess of females. Whereas women made up 50 percent of the total Edmonton population aged 18 or over at the 1981 census, they constituted 59 percent of the survey sample. This excess may be because women usually spend more time in the home and are therefore more readily available for interview. There is also an overrepresentation of respondents in the 25–44 age group, with a corresponding deficit for the 18–24-year-olds. These findings demonstrate the necessity of weighting the survey data in order to obtain a valid picture of psychiatric disorders in Edmonton.

No data were collected on race. The predominant racial group in Edmonton is white, with small numbers of North American Indians, blacks (of American, Caribbean or African origin), and Asians (from various countries). The latter two groups include new immigrants—first generation Canadians—as well as those who have been in the country for decades. Since the sample was drawn from the whole of the city there seems little likelihood of a racial bias, as would be the case if only selected subdivisions had been sampled.

As mentioned earlier, the entire sample was selected from an urban population. Most respondents were married once, and most were living with their spouse. Occupational data shows 11 percent to be unemployed, defined as having been out of work more than twelve months in the last 5 years and actively seeking a job. Just over half (53.0%) of the sample were employed, with the remainder (36.0%) not in the labor force.

The Symptoms of Alcoholism

The alcohol section of the DIS is shown in Appendix 1, with items used for the DSM-III diagnoses of alcohol abuse and dependence asterisked in the right margin. The most frequently reported alcohol symptoms were related to excessive consumption. Twenty-one percent of the entire sample reported drinking heavily on either a daily (Question 153) or weekly (Question 154) basis at some time in their life. Eighteen percent reported drinking a fifth of liquor or more in one day at least once in their life (Question 152). The respondent thinking he was an excessive drinker (Question 151) (6.6%) and family objections to the respondent's excessive drinking (Question 150) (12.4%) were the next most common symptoms in the overall sample.

Work-related symptoms were relatively infrequent. Losing a job was reported by 2.0 percent (Question 161) and being unable to work well without having had something to drink by 2.2 percent (Question 170).

Medical complications of excessive drinking were also quite unusual, being reported by only 3.9 percent of respondents (Question 168); only

2.1 percent (Question 169) reported that they continued to drink in the face of an illness that may be made worse by drinking.

Relative frequencies of alcohol symptoms in the total population were similar to frequencies in those meeting criteria for alcohol abuse or dependence. Quantity-related symptoms (Questions 152–54) were the most frequently reported among both alcoholics and the total population, while employment-related symptoms were the least. Table 7–2 shows the (weighted) proportions of those who gave a positive response to each of the alcohol symptoms enquired about. This detail allows comparison with the other sites, although weighting of results must be considered. The correlation for the ranking of symptom frequencies between alcoholics and nonalcoholics is 0.78.

Drinking Patterns

In Table 7–3 lifetime prevalence rates are given for various categories of drinking. Since the lifetime rates for the different categories are mutually exclusive, these figures are additive. The current (six-month) prevalence rate for alcohol abuse and/or dependence is also shown.

Lifetime abstention from alcohol is uncommon, with only 4.1 percent of the population in this category. Over half the population (62.0%)

Table 7–2 Individual Symptom Frequencies among Those with Alcohol Disorders Edmonton (Weighted Percentages)

DIS Item Number[a]	Symptom	Proportion of Those with Alcohol Abuse and/or Dependence Who Endorsed This Item %
150	Family objected to respondent's drinking	53
151	Respondent thought himself an excessive drinker	61
152	Fifth of liquor in one day	71
153/54	Daily or weekly heavy drinking	82
155	Told physician about drinking problem	19
156	Friends or professionals said drinking too much	39
157	Wanted to stop drinking but couldn't	15
158	Efforts to control drinking	16
159	Morning drinking	21
160	Job troubles due to drinking	20
161	Lost job	12
162	Trouble driving	38
163	Arrested while drinking	37
164	Physical fights while drinking	54
165	Two or more binges	46
166	Blackouts while drinking	56
167	Any withdrawal symptom	35
168	Any medical complication	23
169	Continued to drink with serious illness	13
170	Couldn't do ordinary work without drinking	13

Table 7–3 Lifetime Rates of Various Drinking Categories (Weighted Percentages)

Drinking Category		Edmonton %
Total abstention		4.1
Nonheavy/nonproblem (social) drinkers		62.0
Heavy/nonproblem drinkers		3.1
Problem drinkers (not alcoholic)		12.8
Alcohol abuse only		7.1
Dependence with or without abuse		10.9
Six-month prevalence of alcoholism (abuse and/or dependence)		
	Total	5.4
	Men	9.2
	Women	1.6

are classified as social (nonheavy/nonproblem) drinkers. Heavy/nonproblem drinkers are rare (3.1%). These are persons who have had a period when they regularly consumed seven or more drinks at least one evening per week, but never had any social, legal, or medical problems related to alcohol, and never had withdrawal symptoms. Since few people are in this category it seems likely that most of those consuming this amount of alcohol suffer further problems.

Problem drinkers have had at least one alcohol-related problem in their lives, but not enough to qualify for a DSM-III diagnosis of alcoholism. While it is possible that some problem drinkers had not been drinking long enough to develop symptoms, the weighted mean age of this group was 34, compared to 33 for those with alcohol abuse, and 36 for those who are alcohol dependent. The weighted mean age of abstainers was 44.

Although alcohol abuse was intended in DSM-III to be the less severe form of alcohol disorder, it is actually less prevalent than alcohol dependence (7.1% compared to 10.9%). The total lifetime prevalence for alcoholism is the sum of these two figures, namely 18.0 percent.

Lifetime prevalence includes anyone accumulating the required number of alcohol symptoms regardless of the concurrence of other disorders. The 6-month prevalence includes those who met the diagnostic criteria on a lifetime basis, and who had one or more symptoms in the 6 months preceding the interview. At 5.4 percent (9.2% for men, 1.6% for women), this is the highest 6-month prevalence for any individual disorder detected by the DIS. Lifetime prevalence, with an overall rate of 18 percent (29.3% for men and 6.7% for women), is also the commonest individual lifetime disorder.

Table 7–4 Onset, Severity, and Course of Alcoholism
Edmonton Sample (Weighted Estimates)

	Men	Women	Total
Mean age first intoxicated (if ever)			
Total sample	17	18	17
Alcoholics only	15	16	15
Nonalcoholics	17	19	18
Mean value among lifetime alcoholics			
Age of onset of alcoholism	21	22	21
Number of years from first intoxication			
to first alcohol symptom	6.2	5.8	6.1
Mean number of lifetime symptoms	5.9	5.1	5.8
Mean values among alcoholics in remission[a]			
Age last symptom	30	27	29
Duration of alcoholism in years	9.2	5.9	8.5
Mean number of lifetime symptoms	5.5	4.8	5.3

[a]Remitted alcoholic = no alcohol symptoms for at least one year prior to interview.

The Course of Alcoholism

The onset and course of alcoholism is shown in Table 7–4. Most Edmontonians (77%) have been intoxicated with alcohol at some time in their lives, 4 percent have been lifelong abstainers, leaving only 19 percent who have used alcohol but never been intoxicated.

The mean age of first intoxication (Table 7–4) is lower by 3 years in alcoholics compared to nonalcoholics. Men have a slightly lower mean age at first intoxication than women. Although the age at first intoxication is in the late teens, the mean age at onset of alcohol disorders (the age of the first alcohol-related symptom) is a few years later at age 21, men again being slightly younger at onset than women. The number of years from first intoxication to the onset of alcoholism is about 6 years. Among alcoholics the mean number of lifetime symptoms is between 5 and 6.

Alcoholics in remission are defined as those who, while meeting the lifetime criteria, have had no alcohol symptoms in the year prior to the interview. For those who have remitted, the mean age of remission is the late 20s to 30. The average number of lifetime symptoms of alcoholism is very similar in those who have remitted (5.3) and those who are still alcoholic (5.8). The symptom count varies only slightly with the duration of alcoholism. Those who have been alcoholic for more than 10 years and were not in remission at the time of the interview reported an average of 6.2 symptoms; those with a shorter duration of alcoholism reported 5.5 symptoms. For those in remission the comparable average symptom counts were 6.6 and 5.0, respectively. Thus, measured by lifetime symptom counts, those four groups appear to be quite similar in severity.

The mean duration of alcoholism among those who have remitted is 8.5 years (both sexes), with a differential between the sexes (9.2 years for men and 5.9 years for women). The range of duration is broad, from 0 (where first and last symptoms occurred in the same year) to 46 years, but is highly skewed towards a shorter duration. For 30 percent of those who have remitted, the duration of alcoholism was 2 years or less, and for half of this group the duration was 6 years or less. Only 25 percent of those who remitted had been alcoholic for 10 years or more.

Overall 57 percent of those who met the lifetime criteria for alcoholism were in remission. This suggests that for many individuals alcoholism may be a self-limiting disorder with a quite high remission rate.

Risk Factors and Correlates of Alcoholism

This section examines risk factors. These include characteristics associated with an increased rate of alcoholism but are antecedent, such as age and sex; and correlates—factors that are associated but not necessarily antecedent, such as other psychiatric disorders.

Table 7–5 shows lifetime prevalence rates by age and sex. In all age groups the prevalence for men is considerably higher than for women. In the youngest age group, where the highest rates for women are found, the male to female ratio is 3:1. In the over-65 age group this ratio is 7:1. Overall, men are 4 times more likely to have a diagnosis of alcoholism than women.

The rates of alcoholism by age show an interesting pattern. Lifetime prevalence at any given age is the cumulative rate over all earlier ages. Thus, if the rates of alcoholism are constant in a population; the instrument for detection is similarly reliable across all age groups; and alcoholics are not subject to excessive mortality compared to the remainder of the population, lifetime prevalence should rise with succeeding age groups in proportion to the increased years at risk. Table 7–5 clearly indicates that this is not the case. In men, prevalence is very similar in the two younger age groups (18–44) and decreases thereafter, particularly

Table 7–5 Lifetime Prevalence of Alcoholism by Sex and Age Edmonton Sample (Weighted Percentages)

Age Group	Men %	Women %	Total %
18–24	31	11	21
25–44	33	7	20
45–64	27	4	15
65+	14	2	7
Total	29	7	18

in the over-65 age group. In women, the highest rate is found in the 18–24 age group and progressively decreases thereafter.

Possible reasons for these findings have been given above. Artifacts of recall, while they may occur, do not seem to be a satisfactory explanation. In other surveys employing similar study instruments, rates were found to increase with increasing age (Helzer et al., 1988).

Differentially high mortality among alcoholics is another possible explanation, but mathematical models constructed to test this hypothesis demonstrated that an unrealistically high mortality risk due to alcohol-related diseases would have to be operating to produce the prevalence rates that were found.

The most likely explanation is that alcoholism has been increasing in recent years, particularly among the younger age groups and in women. This is consistent with increased per capita alcohol consumption in Alberta from the 1950s until recently, and with the changing role of women in society.

Some other possible correlates and risk factors that are thought to be associated with alcoholism are shown in Table 7–6. The first column of the table shows these factors as possible predictors of heavy drinking

Table 7–6 Risk Factors and Correlates for Heavy Drinking and Alcoholism Edmonton Sample (Weighted Percentages)

	Proportion of All Drinkers Who Are Heavy Drinkers (%)	Proportion of Heavy Drinkers Who Are Alcoholic (%)
Total sample	35	53
Risk Factor or Correlate		
Number of marriages		
0	47	57
1	28	47
2+	42	67
Childhood conduct groups positive		
0	17	41
1–2	49	46
3+	80	75
Intoxicated before age 15		
No	28	47
Yes	71	66
Any drug disorder		
No	32	49
Yes	82	76
Sex		
Male	54	56
Female	16	44

among all drinkers (abstainers are excluded from this analysis). The second column shows the same factors as possible predictors of alcoholism among those who are heavy drinkers. Figures for the total sample are shown at the top of the table for comparison and show that about one third (35%) of all drinkers are heavy drinkers and just over half (53%) of all heavy drinkers meet DSM-III criteria for alcohol abuse and/or dependence.

Drinkers who have been married once are less likely to be heavy drinkers than those who have never been married or have had more than one marriage. Never having been married, and to a greater extent multiple marriages, are associated with a higher risk of alcoholism even among those who drink heavily.

The last three variables in Table 7–6 show quite striking associations with heavy drinking among all drinkers and alcoholism in heavy drinkers. Childhood conduct disorder and first intoxication before age 15 are risk factors as they are antecedent to the development of heavy drinking or alcoholism. Drug abuse is a correlate; it may or may not be antecedent. All three are strongly associated with heavy drinking and alcoholism after controlling for heavy drinking.

Table 7–7 shows other psychiatric diagnoses ascertained by the DIS in relation to alcoholism. The first column gives the lifetime prevalence rates for each of the core DIS/DSM-III diagnoses found in the Edmon-

Table 7–7 Lifetime Prevalence Rates of Core
Diagnoses and Risk Ratios Among Alcoholics
Edmonton Sample (Weighted Estimates)

Diagnosis	Lifetime Prevalence in Total Sample	Lifetime Prevalence in Alcoholics	Risk Ratio (Prevalence in Alcoholics/ Prevalence in Nonalcoholics)
Alcoholism	18.0		
Phobic disorder (any)	8.9	12.1	1.5
Drug abuse and/or dependence (any)	6.9	23.8	7.5
Cognitive impairment (mild or severe)	1.3	2.1	1.8
Major depression	8.6	14.6	2.0
Dysthymic disorder	3.7	6.2	2.0
Antisocial personality disorder	3.7	17.4	26.4
Obsessive compulsive disorder	3.0	5.9	2.6
Panic disorder	1.3	3.8	5.4
Schizophrenia	0.4	1.3	6.5
Mania	0.6	1.4	3.7
Somatization disorder	0.1	0.3	a
Anorexia nervosa	0.1	0.2	3.1
Any core DIS diagnosis (except alcoholism)	24.4	47.7	2.5

aNo somatization disorder in nonalcoholics.

ton survey. Diagnoses in the Edmonton sample rank in the same order as those in the ECA sample with the exception of cognitive impairment, major depression, and schizophrenia. Cognitive impairment is much less frequent in Edmonton, probably because the Edmonton survey includes only household respondents with no institutional sample, and because the Edmonton population is younger. Major depression with a lifetime prevalence of 8.6 percent is more frequent in Edmonton, and schizophrenia less than in the ECA.

The diagnosis with the highest lifetime prevalence is alcohol abuse/dependence at 18.0 percent. No other disorder reaches even half this rate. The closest are phobic disorder at 8.9 percent and major depression at 8.6 percent. The medical and social consequences of alcoholism far outweigh those of phobias. Major depression obviously has considerable social implications, particularly for the family, but much less potential for a wider range of social consequences and disruption. The next commonest disorder is drug abuse and dependence (6.9%). Other disorders have lower prevalence rates.

The second column of Table 7–7 shows the lifetime prevalence of each of the disorders in those meeting the DSM-III criteria for (lifetime) alcohol abuse and/or dependence. For every diagnosis the prevalence in alcoholics is higher than the prevalence in the total population. This is particularly evident for drug abuse/dependence (diagnosed in 23.8% of alcoholics), antisocial personality (found in 17.4%), and major depression (identified in 14.6%).

The third column in Table 7–7 compares the prevalence for other disorders in alcoholics to that in nonalcoholics. If the prevalence is the same, this indicates that the other disorder is neither positively or negatively associated with alcoholism and the risk ratio will be one. For all diagnoses the risk ratios are greater than one, indicating higher prevalence in alcoholics. By far the greatest relative risk (26.4) is that associated with antisocial personality disorder. It was shown in Table 7–6 that early conduct disorder symptoms (which form part of the DSM-III criteria for antisocial personality disorder) are highly associated with later alcoholism.

The next highest risk ratio is found with drug abuse/dependence (7.5). Although this is a much lower ratio, it is seen from the second column of Table 7.7 that drug abuse/dependence has a higher prevalence in alcoholics than does antisocial personality disorder. This is followed by the risk ratios found with schizophrenia, panic disorder, and mania. Other disorders including, somewhat surprisingly, depression, have lower ratios. It is also worth noting that those disorders with a high risk ratio—antisocial personality and drug abuse/dependence—like alcoholism, show a strong male predominance in the lifetime prevalence figures. Mania and schizophrenia show no sex predominance, and major depression, dysthymia, and panic disorder show a female predominance. Overall, alcoholics were 2.5 times more likely to have another lifetime diagnosis than nonalcoholics.

Discussion and Conclusions

Edmonton is only one city in Canada and is unlikely to be representative of the whole of the country, which has one of the largest land masses in the world. Language, culture, economic factors, and racial patterns differ significantly across Canada and its major regions.

As mentioned above, in recent years alcohol has been relatively inexpensive in Alberta, and per capita consumption rose steadily until the early 1980s. At the same time Alberta had a relatively young population with high levels of disposable income, and a drinking age of 18. Female participation in the labor force also rose markedly during the 1970s, when there was low unemployment. These changes were paralleled by increasing divorce and crime rates, a high proportion of single parent families, and increasing suicide rates. All of these influences bear on the alcohol problem in Alberta.

The general impression is that there are high rates of alcoholism, and this is one of the findings of the study. Also, although lifetime rates for men greatly exceed those for women (29% to 7%), the rates for females are also quite high. Although alcoholism is not restricted to younger age groups, it is here that both the highest lifetime rates and the highest 6-month prevalence rates are found. The proportion of women to men who are alcoholic is also greatest in the age group 18–24, where women constitute one-quarter of all alcoholics.

The most obvious conclusion is that alcoholism has increased in the young to such an extent that they have much higher lifetime rates than the older age groups, especially in the case of younger women. This is consistent with the social changes that have taken place in recent years, and with studies of attitudes toward alcohol.

The finding that 57 percent of alcoholics are in remission, and that their median duration of alcoholism is 6 years, clearly suggests that many alcoholics may have a better prognosis than is usually thought to be the case. This is perhaps even more remarkable when some of the symptoms are examined; only one in five alcoholics told a physician about their drinking problem and only 16 percent claimed to have made efforts to control their drinking. Perhaps efforts to control drinking are denied by the alcoholic, since only 61 percent thought themselves to be excessive drinkers, while at the same time a high proportion had either family objections to their drinking, got into fights, or been arrested while drinking. The lower rate of alcoholism found in older age groups raises methodological issues as discussed above, particularly the ability of an older person to recall alcohol symptoms from many years in the past, a problem that could be exacerbated by a high rate of remission of the disorder. Not all disorders follow the age or sex distribution patterns of alcoholism, and there seems no immediately apparent reason why remembering symptoms associated with alcohol should be differentially subject to recall problems.

A striking feature of the results is the high level of comorbidity found in alcoholics. They have higher to much higher rates of other psychiatric disorders than the remainder of the population. Almost one-quarter of alcoholics have a lifetime history of drug abuse or dependence. Since drug abuse/dependence is also a disorder that is primarily found in younger age groups and in males, this may suggest at least some common underlying factors. Similar comments can be made regarding antisocial personality disorder, which also links with the finding that childhood conduct disorders are more frequent in those who subsequently develop alcoholism, and obviously also in those developing antisocial personality disorder. In total, just less than half of those with a lifetime disorder of alcoholism have another lifetime psychiatric disorder, making them 2.5 times more likely to have another psychiatric illness than those who are not alcoholic. It cannot be determined on the basis of these data whether alcoholism predisposes to other disorders, whether those with other psychiatric disorders are especially vulnerable to alcoholism, or whether there is an underlying predisposition to several disorders. There is evidence to suggest that those with any disorder are more likely to develop another disorder than those with no disorder. Psychiatric disorders do not appear to be randomly distributed in the population (Sturt, 1981 Boyd et al., 1984, Bland et al., 1987).

There can be little doubt that in Edmonton, alcoholism poses a major public health problem since a significant proportion of the population, particularly young adults, with increasing numbers of young women, are affected. The impact on social behavior, such as arrests, drinking and driving, getting into fights, employment problems, and involvement in spouse and child abuse, is possibly more serious than the medical complications (Bland and Orn, 1986). It is hoped that recent measures such as increases in the price of alcohol will have the effect of reducing rates of alcoholism.

References

Alberta Liquor Control Board (1975). *Fifty Years.* Edmonton, Alberta: Alberta Liquor Control Board.

Alberta Alcohol and Drug Abuse Commission (1985). *Alcohol Use in Alberta.* Edmonton, Alberta: Alberta Alcohol and Drug Abuse Commission.

Alberta Alcohol and Drug Abuse Commission (1980). *Alcohol and Youth.* Edmonton, Alberta: Alberta Alcohol and Drug Abuse Commission.

Bland, R. C.; Newman, S. C.; and Orn, H. (1987). Schizophrenia: Lifetime comorbidity in a community sample. *Acta Psychiatr. Scand.* 75:383–91.

Bland, R. C., and Orn, H. (1986). Family violence and psychiatric disorder. *Can. J. Psychiatry* 31:129–37.

Bland, R. C., and Orn, H. (1986). Psychiatric disorders, spouse abuse and child abuse. *Acta Psychiatr. Belg.* 86:444–49.

Boyd, J. H.; Burke, J. D.; Gruenberg, E.; Holzer, C. E.; Rae, D. S.; George, L. K.; Karno, M.; Stoltzman, R.; McEvoy, L.; and Nestadt, G. (1984). Exclusion criteria of DSM-III. *Arch. Gen. Psychiatry* 41:983–89.

Decision Making Information (1974). *Public Perceptions of Alcoholism in Alberta.* Edmonton, Alberta: Decision Making Information.

Helzer, J. E.; Canino, G. J.; Yeh, E-K.; Bland, R. C.; Lee, C. Y.; Hwu, H-G.; and Newman, S. (1988). Alcoholism—North America—Asia. In R. M. Rose and J. Barrett (eds.), *Alcoholism: A Medical Disorder.* New York: Raven Press.

Kessler, L. G.; Folsom, R.; Royall, R.; Forsythe, A.; McEvoy, L.; Holzer, C. E.; Rae, D. S.; and Woodbury, M. (1985). Parameter and variance estimation. In W. W. Eaton and L. G. Kessler (eds.), *Epidemiologic Field Methods in Psychiatry.* Orlando: Academic Press.

Kish, L. (1949). A procedure for objective respondent selection within the household. *J. Am. Stat. Assoc.* 94:380–398.

Shah, B. V. (1981). SESUDAAN: Standard Errors Program for Computing Standardized Rates from Sample Survey Data. Research Triangle Park, N.C.: Research Triangle Institute.

Sturt, E. (1981). Hierarchical patterns in the distribution of psychiatric symptoms. *Psychol. Med.* II:783–94.

[8] Alcohol Abuse and Dependence Among American Indians

SPERO M. MANSON, JAMES H. SHORE,
ANNA E. BARON, LYNN ACKERSON,
AND GORDON NELIGH

Current, community-based epidemiologic studies of alcohol abuse and dependence among American Indians are nonexistent. Indeed, state-of-the-art diagnostic techniques only recently have been applied in this special population (Manson et al., 1987; Walker, Walker, & Kivlahan, 1988; Westermeyer & Neider, 1984, 1985). Reasons for this delay include long-standing concerns about the cultural factors that affect reliable measurement and diagnosis (Levy & Kunitz, 1974; Manson, Walker, & Kivlahan, 1987; Walker & Kivlahan, 1984). Difficulties in sampling and resulting limits to meaningful generalization have also slowed the advance of scientific inquiry. Our work inevitably reflects these circumstances and has addressed itself to the first order problem. Specifically, we are attempting to improve the assessment process by combining local explanatory models for dysfunction with psychiatric diagnostic criteria (Manson & Shore, 1981; Manson, Shore, & Bloom, 1985). The DIS has played a central role in this endeavor.

Given our interest in assessment, the focus of the present chapter is slightly different than others in this volume. The case control design and sampling plan used in our study do not permit estimates of prevalence. However, we are able to report on the DIS's performance with several American Indian tribes and to describe patterns of alcohol abuse/dependence among select segments of their populations.

Demographic, Socioeconomic, and Health Characteristics

American Indians constitute a dispersed, mobile, young, and rapidly growing group. The 1980 census indicates that the Indian population numbers approximately 1.37 million, nearly double the 1970 count (U.S. Bureau of the Census, 1984a). Although more than half (63%) of the Indian population lives in cities and urban areas, much attention has

113

been given to those who live in rural areas on 278 reservations. American Indian communities are culturally heterogenous, having been classified into as many as seventeen distinct regions in terms of language, social organization, religious practice, and ecological relationships. At present there are well over 300 federally recognized tribes.

This population is markedly young. Their median age (22.9 years) is much lower than that of the general U.S. population (30.0 years), due mainly to a higher fertility rate in past decades. By and large American Indians are economically impoverished. The mean income for Indian families ($13,678) is considerably lower than the national average ($19,917). It is not surprising, then, that unemployment is extremely high (at least 2 times the national average) and is well over 60 percent on some reservations (U.S. Bureau of Census, 1984a, 1984b). Lastly, when measured by college experience, the educational attainment of American Indians is far below the national average (Brod & McQuiston, 1983). Among individuals 25 years of age and older, twice as many members of the general population (16%) than Indians (8%) have completed four years of college.

Rates of infant mortality and death from infectious disease among American Indians have declined dramatically in recent years, but remain much higher than those for the national population (Indian Health Service, 1978). Chronic physical illnesses such as diabetes, rheumatoid arthritis, biliary dysfunction, and cardiac disease are of increasing concern and, in some instances, affect unparalleled proportions of Indian communities. Recent estimates place the excess death rate of American Indians under age 45 at 43 percent, which is significantly higher than Blacks (39%) and other U.S. ethnic minority groups (U.S. Department of Health and Human Services, 1985).

Extent of Alcohol Abuse and Dependence

Alcohol use varies considerably from one tribe to another. Indeed, some tribes have proportionately fewer drinking adults than the U.S. population as a whole (30 percent compared to 67 percent). However, other tribes have many more drinkers (69 to 80 percent), with a correspondingly higher prevalence of alcohol-related problems (Jessor et al., 1969; Longclaws, Barnes, Grieve, & Dumoff, 1980; May, 1986; Whittaker, 1962).

Three psychiatric epidemiological studies of adult American Indians have been conducted, all more than a decade and a half ago (Shore, Kinzie, Hampson, & Pattison, 1973; Roy, Chaudri, & Irvine, 1970; Sampath, 1974). While each study focused on a single, small tribe or native village, the results suggest alarmingly high rates of alcohol abuse and dependence in this population. For example, Shore et al. (1973) interviewed half of the adult members of a Pacific Northwest reservation community and reported that 27 percent of the total population qualified for diagnoses of alcoholism.

In the absence of current epidemiological data, estimates of the extent to which alcohol abuse and dependence affect the lives of American Indians typically rely upon inferences from measures of mortality and morbidity. These measures indicate that alcohol abuse is a major factor in five of the ten leading causes of death among most tribes. The age-adjusted mortality rates among U.S. Indians for alcohol-related causes of death are higher than those for the nation. Specifically, their mortality rate is 5.5 times higher for motor vehicle accidents, 3.8 times higher for alcoholism, 4.5 times higher for cirrhosis of the liver, 2.3 times higher for suicide, and 2.8 times higher for homicide (May, 1986). Unintentional injuries account for an estimated 21 percent of all deaths in Indian communities and are the leading cause of mortality. Available estimates suggest that 75 percent of all accidental deaths among Indians are alcohol-related (National Institute on Alcohol Abuse and Alcoholism, 1980). Suicide accounts for 2.9 percent of all Indian deaths, eighty percent of which are believed to be alcohol-related. The tenth-ranked cause of death in Indian communities is homicide, which is responsible for two percent of total deaths. At least 90 percent of homicides committed in Indian communities involve alcohol.

Alcohol abuse also is an important contributor to morbidity. Indian Health Service data on inpatient and outpatient care indicate that alcohol-related trauma and disease are frequent reasons for health care problems and disability among many tribes (Indian Health Service, 1978; May & Broudy, 1980). In 1981, hospital discharge rates for Indian males and females with alcohol-related diagnoses (e.g., alcoholic psychosis, alcohol abuse/dependence, and liver disease) were three times higher than the United States as a whole and twice the rates for other nonwhites (Walker et al., 1988).

Study Method

Design

We conducted a multistage study, partially described here, to assess the performance of a modified version of the NIMH Diagnostic Interview Schedule (DIS) and of the Schedule for Affective Disorders and Schizophrenia-Lifetime Version (SADS-L) (Endicott & Spitzer, 1978). Our investigation proceeded within a known cases/noncases matched control design that involved adult tribal members of three reservation communities. The long-range objectives of this effort included developing culturally sensitive diagnostic instruments to be used in community-based psychiatric epidemiologic studies with these special populations.

The study began by eliciting cultural conceptualizations of serious psychological dysfunction and/or major mental disorder from three different reservation communities representing the Pueblo, Plains, and Plateau culture areas in North America. These indigenous categories of illness and culturally meaningful symptoms were incorporated within an interview schedule that included select sections of the DIS that had been modified through extensive reviews by local health professionals and paraprofessionals. The resulting protocol, hereafter referred to as the Indian Depression Schedule (IDS), was patterned after the DIS in terms of its logic of inquiry and response format. The SADS-L subsequently was employed to identify a clinically depressed index group (CIG) of tribal members from each reservation community. Individuals who, in the opinion of local health professionals, exhibited significant signs of depression were interviewed by one of four research psychiatrists using the SADS-L. Respondents diagnosed as depressed were assigned to the index group that serves as a criterion referent. The IDS then was administered to the CIG and to a community sample (MCS), the members of which were matched to subjects in the CIG on a two-to-one basis according to relative age and sex. Previous clinical experience suggested that response patterns might vary along these demographic parameters. The matched community samples from two reservations, specifically the Pueblo and Plains sites, were drawn from general outpatient medical clinics and screened for prior histories of mental health and/or alcohol problems. The MCS at the Plateau site was derived from a random sampling of tribal rolls. All interviews were conducted by local mental health paraprofessionals who received extensive training in the protocol.

The overall design of the study and some findings from the Pueblo site have been described (Manson, Shore, & Bloom, 1985). Other reports detail the nature and pattern of depression (Shore et al., 1987) and alcoholism (Manson et al., 1987) as reflected in the SADS-L interviews conducted among clinic index group members across the three study sites.

Instrumentation

The central diagnostic instruments in this study are the IDS, adapted from the DIS, and the SADS-L. The IDS is comprised of five sections: 1) an extensive set of sociodemographic questions; 2) a series of linked, recurring questions about one's knowledge and personal experience of indigenously defined illness; and 3) those portions of the DIS pertaining to depression, alcohol abuse/dependence, and somatization. Sociodemographic items covered age, sex, marital status, family size, recent deaths, residential pattern, religious affiliation, education, occupation, employment, and a brief medical history. Questions specific to community life addressed such matters as tribal and clan membership, blood quantum, languages spoken, fluency, participation in ceremonial activities, special stresses, and recent deaths of loved ones.

The second section asked whether the respondent was familiar with any of the indigenous categories of illness, about their meaning, whether the respondent had ever felt these ways and, if so, frequency of occurrence, duration, and cause. Other questions in this section focused on the nature of assistance sought and rendered, compliance, and effectiveness of treatment(s).

The remaining three sections were adopted directly from the DIS and need no elaboration other than to note that, based upon systematic review by local community members, the wording of certain items was altered slightly to render them more intelligible to these respondents.

No inter-rater reliability study was conducted of the IDS in part because only one interviewer administered the instrument at each of the respective study sites. Given that the study required SADS-L assessments by multiple interviewers across different sites, an inter-rater reliability test was conducted involving four research psychiatrists (Shore, Bloom, Keepers, and Neligh). This process is described in detail elsewhere (Manson et al., 1987). In summary, the degree of agreement was examined through a variety of comparisons employing the kappa statistic. The overall kappa coefficients for alcoholism (1.0) and major depressive disorder (.89) were excellent.

Study Sites

As previously noted, the study was designed to permit intertribal comparisons of the diagnostic instrumentation for certain psychiatric disorders. Hence, three reservation communities were chosen to represent several of the major culture areas that characterize the diverse social, religious, political, and linguistic aspects of the American Indian life experience. For the purposes of the present discussion, these three communities are referred to as the Pueblo, Plateau, and Plains study sites.[1] The Pueblo study site is situated in the Southwest. A relatively small reservation, especially in comparison to its Plateau and Plains counterparts, this site is well above sea-level, semi-arid, and dominated by large mesas. Over 80 percent of the 10,000 tribal members live on the reservation. A large on-reservation IHS hospital and outpatient clinic provide a wide spectrum of primary and mental health care. Part-time satellite clinics offer limited services to residents living 30 or more miles from the hospital. The tribe that occupies this reservation is among the most traditional of Indian communities. It has long resisted social and cultural change, though residents are concerned about the increase of nontribal marriages, off-reservation migration, and the decline in native language ability. Traditional healing is a strong and deeply engrained practice, as is the ceremonial life of tribal members.

The Plateau study site is located in the Pacific Northwest and encompasses a large tract of land that extends from the foothills of the mountains to the arroyos of a semi-arid plateau. Tribal membership numbers approximately 3,800 and is comprised of several confederated tribes. Health and mental health facilities on the reservation include a wide range of outpatient services. Most of these are tribally operated, though primary care remains an IHS responsibility. The nearest hospital, to which the IHS physicians and tribal mental health professionals have admitting privileges, is located off-reservation in a small rural town. The tribes living at the Plateau study site have been subjected to a long history of acculturative pressure, but much of the traditional ceremonial life has remained intact, and is undergoing active revitalization.

The Plains study site is situated in the northern Midwest and covers a large land mass consisting mainly of high, rolling prairies interrupted by numerous rivers, creeks, lakes, buttes, and hills. About 6,200 tribal members and slightly more than half this number of non-Indians live on the reservation. The bulk of the health and mental health services are delivered through an IHS hospital and clinic located in the agency town. Like the Pueblo study site, a series of part-time satellite clinics offer care to outlying areas. The reservation is occupied by a single tribe with several bands. Here, too, social and cultural change have eroded traditional subsistence patterns, language, and religion. However, indigenous healing practices and such ceremonies as the Sun Dance quietly continue.

Results

In order to maximize the relevance of this study to the theme of the present volume, the data are considered without reference to the original case control design. Hence, the results are reported in an aggregate form, combining the CIG and MCS samples.

Table 8–1 presents the demographic characteristics of the individuals who were administered the IDS interview. Approximately 53 percent ($n = 106$) were under 40 years of age at the time of the interview. The majority are female (73%) and 54 percent ($n = 107$) were married or cohabiting. Seventy-two percent of the respondents are three- to four-quarters American Indian. Thirty-one percent have at least some college education, and 45 percent were unemployed at the time of the study. Church membership and ceremonial participation characterize 63 and 79 percent of the study subjects, respectively. Ninety-five percent of the subjects have lived on their reservations for more than 10 years.

Table 8–1 Demographic Characteristics of the Study Sample

Variable	Category	Number	%
Age	<20 years	9	4.6
	20–29	50	25.4
	30–39	47	23.8
	40–49	54	27.4
	50–59	22	11.2
	60+	15	6.6
Sex	Female	144	73.1
	Male	53	26.9
Marital Status	Married	99	50.2
	Cohabitation	8	4.1
	Widowed	15	7.6
	Separated	15	7.6
	Divorced	27	13.7
	Never married	32	16.2
Blood Quantum	$<1/4$	3	1.5
	$1/4–1/2$	26	13.2
	$1/2–3/4$	24	12.2
	$3/4–4/4$	142	72.1
Education Level	< High school	62	31.0
	High school	75	38.1
	Some college	47	23.9
	College degree+	14	7.1
Occupation	Unemployed	89	45.2
	Unskilled	4	2.0
	Skilled	24	12.2
	Clerical/technical	27	13.7
	Administrative/ professional	50	25.4
Church Member	No	73	37.1
	Yes	124	62.9
Ceremonial Participation	No	41	20.8
	Yes	156	79.2
Number of years on reservation	<10 yrs.	10	5.1
	10–19	28	14.2
	20–29	47	23.9
	30–39	40	20.3
	40–49	43	21.8
	50+	29	14.7

Table 8–2 illustrates the relationships among demographic characteristics and alcohol-related diagnoses according to DSM-III criteria as specified by the DIS. Women exhibit much lower rates of both alcohol abuse and dependence than men ($p < .01$). Younger age is highly associated with both alcohol abuse and dependence ($p < .01$). Married and widowed respondents exhibit significantly lower levels of both abuse and

Table 8–2 DIS Alcohol Diagnoses and Demographic Characteristics

Demographic Variable	Negative N	Negative (%)	Abuse Only N	Abuse Only (%)	Dependence N	Dependence (%)	Insufficient information N	Insufficient information (%)	Total
Total	93	(47)	41	(21)	60	(30)	3	(2)	197
Sex									
Male	10	(19)	16	(30)	27	(51)	0		53
Female	83	(58)	25	(17)	33	(23)	3	(2)	144
Age									
<29	21	(36)	22	(37)	16	(27)	0		59
30–39	21	(45)	9	(19)	17	(36)	0		47
40–49	26	(48)	5	(9)	21	(39)	2	(4)	54
50–59	13	(59)	5	(23)	3	(14)	1	(4)	22
60+	12	(80)	2	(13)	1	(7)	0		15
Marital status									
Married/cohabitation	57	(53)	18	(17)	31	(29)	1	(1)	107
Widowed	10	(67)	3	(20)	1	(7)	1	(7)	15
Separated/divorced	16	(38)	7	(17)	18	(43)	1	(2)	42
Never married	10	(31)	12	(38)	10	(31)	0		32
Blood Quantum									
<1/4	0		1	(33)	1	(33)	1	(33)	3
1/4–1/2	9	(35)	12	(46)	5	(19)	0		26
1/2–3/4	8	(33)	6	(25)	10	(42)	0		24
3/4–4/4	75	(53)	21	(15)	44	(31)	2	(1)	142
Education level									
< High school	10	(46)	3	(14)	8	(36)	1	(4)	22
High school	51	(45)	28	(25)	33	(29)	2	(1)	114
College +	32	(52)	10	(16)	19	(31)	0		61
Church member									
No	40	(55)	11	(15)	22	(30)	0		73
Yes	53	(43)	30	(24)	38	(31)	3	(2)	124
Ceremonial participation									
No	22	(54)	10	(24)	9	(22)	0		41
Yes	71	(45)	31	(20)	51	(33)	3	(2)	156
Deaths									
No	35	(59)	13	(22)	10	(17)	1	(2)	59
Yes	57	(42)	28	(20)	50	(36)	2	(2)	137
Stress									
No	38	(51)	23	(31)	14	(18)	0		75
Yes	51	(44)	18	(15)	45	(39)	2	(2)	116
DIS depression diagnosis									
Negative	74	(47)	35	(22)	45	(29)	3	(2)	157
Lacks severity/bereavement	3	(50)	3	(50)	0		0		6
Positive	16	(47)	3	(9)	15	(44)	0		34
Years on reservation									
<20	11	(29)	13	(34)	14	(37)	0		38
20–39	35	(40)	19	(22)	32	(37)	1	(1)	87
40+	47	(65)	9	(13)	14	(19)	2	(3)	72

dependence than the never married or divorced. Neither education level, membership in a church, nor ceremonial participation are related to alcohol diagnosis. Among those with recent losses or deaths in family or of friends, alcohol dependence is approximately twice as common as among those with no recent losses or deaths, but the difference is not statistically significant. For those experiencing a special stress compared to those who have not, dependence is twice as prevalent and abuse half as prevalent compared to the group not experiencing special stress. A DIS/DSM-III diagnosis of depression is equally associated with alcohol abuse and dependence. Those who have lived on a reservation for 40 years or more show significantly lower levels of abuse and dependence than those living there for a shorter period of time, but this association is attenuated when we control for age, which is highly confounded with years on the reservation.

Table 8–3 shows the percentages of those endorsing the individual items on the DIS alcohol section. At the Pueblo site, where the study began, it became apparent that some respondents had never consumed alcohol, were offended by being asked the question that introduces this section: "Have you ever been drunk?", and were perplexed, even angered by other questions about alcohol abuse. Consequently, this section

Table 8–3 Response Frequencies on DIS Alcohol Questions

	Total Sample						Those with Alcohol Abuse/ Dependence	
	No		Yes		Below critical		Yes	
Response	N	(%)	N	(%)	N	(%)	N	(%)
Question								
Ever been drunk	47	(25)	143	(75)	0		97	(97)
Family objects to drinking	109	(56)	77	(39)	9	(5)	73	(72)
You think you drink too much	103	(54)	89	(46)	0		82	(81)
Drink a fifth in one day	136	(70)	53	(27)	5	(3)	52	(52)
Excessive drinking, >2 weeks	153	(78)	41	(21)	1	(1)	42	(42)
Excessive drinking, >2 months	131	(69)	58	(30)	1	(1)	56	(56)
Told a doctor	165	(85)	29	(15)	0		29	(29)
Others commented on drinking	145	(75)	49	(25)	0		48	(48)
Wanted to stop but couldn't	141	(73)	52	(26)	1	(1)	48	(48)
Ever promised to stop drinking	152	(78)	41	(21)	1	(1)	37	(37)
Drink before breakfast	171	(88)	23	(12)	0		23	(23)
Job troubles due to drinking	149	(77)	44	(22)	1	(1)	43	(43)
Loss of job due to drinking	172	(89)	22	(11)	0		21	(21)
Drunk driving or car accident	139	(72)	54	(28)	0		51	(51)
Arrested due to drinking	137	(71)	56	(29)	0		53	(53)
Physical fights due to drinking	115	(60)	77	(40)	0		67	(67)
Binges	89	(59)	61	(41)	0		62	(64)
Blackouts	84	(56)	66	(44)	0		64	(66)
Shakes, DTs, seizures, voices, visions	108	(74)	38	(26)	0		38	(40)
Health problems	118	(79)	31	(21)	0		31	(32)
Continued drinking when ill	129	(88)	18	(22)	0		19	(20)
Couldn't do daily work without drinking	132	(90)	15	(10)	0		15	(16)

Table 8–4 Risk Factors and Correlates for Heavy Drinking and Alcoholism

	Proportion of All Drinkers Who Are Heavy Drinkers	Proportion of Heavy Drinkers Who Are Alcoholic
	% (n =)	% (n =)
Total Sample	46 (72)	70 (52)
Risk Factor or Correlate		
Sex		
Men	65 (32)	76 (25)
Women	38 (40)	66 (27)
Years of education		
<8 years	82 (9)	80 (8)
8–11 years	62 (20)	90 (18)
12 years	34 (20)	48 (10)
13+ years	43 (23)	70 (16)
Occupational status		
Upper ⅓	42 (18)	56 (10)
Middle ⅓	33 (13)	79 (11)
Lower ⅓	57 (40)	73 (30)
Intoxicated before age 15		
No	39 (45)	67 (30)
Yes	77 (27)	78 (21)

was modified to begin with the question: "Do you drink or have you ever drunk alcohol?". Those responding "no" were not asked the remaining alcohol questions, but were presumed to have a negative answer for all of them.

Table 8–4 summarizes the risk factors and correlates for heavy drinking and alcohol that, in this study, approximate some of those discussed for other studies reported in the present volume. Almost half of the respondents who drink are heavy drinkers; nearly three-quarters of the heavy drinkers are alcoholic. Significantly greater proportions of male than female drinkers are heavy drinkers; yet, the male to female ratio of heavy drinkers who are alcoholic is approximately equal (1.15:1). Years of formal education and occupational status reflected the expected patterns. Drinkers with less formal schooling are more likely to drink heavily and to be alcoholic than their better educated counterparts. Drinkers of lower occupational status are more likely to drink heavily and to be alcoholic than those who are employed in more prestigious positions. Finally, the proportion of drinkers to heavy drinkers is almost twice as great for individuals who became intoxicated before 15 years of age than those who did not.

Table 8–5 shows the agreement of the SADS lifetime diagnosis for alcoholism with respect to that obtained by the DIS for the subset of individuals in the study who were administered both interviews. The kappa statistic for these data, combining the abuse and dependence

Table 8–5 Agreement of SADS and DIS on Alcohol Diagnoses

		DIS Alcohol Diagnosis									
		Negative		Abuse		Dependence		Insufficient information		Total	
		N	(%)	N	(%)	N	(%)	N	(%)	N	(%)
SADS	NO	25	(58)	9	(21)	7	(16)	2	(5)	43	(65)
Alcohol diagnosis	YES	2	(9)	4	(17)	17	(74)	0		23	(35)

categories as positive for the DIS diagnosis, and excluding the insufficient information category, is .46; the SADS did not assign a diagnosis of alcoholism to 16 of those individuals who were DIS positive.

Table 8–6 depicts agreement for each DIS alcohol-related question and its SADS counterpart. The kappa statistics ranged from .24 to .77 for these comparisons.

Discussion

Before considering the implications of the above findings, the limits to their interpretation and generalization must be clearly understood. First, the nature of the sample precludes extrapolation to the broader communities in which these individuals live. Second, the determination of risk factors for alcohol abuse/dependence is confounded by the criteria for inclusion in the study. Hence, our discussion of these results is framed primarily in terms of within sample and interscale comparisons. We attempt, however, to place these observations in the context of other findings specific to this special population.

Let us begin by considering the relationships between certain demographic characteristics of the respondents and DIS alcohol-related diagnoses. The observed sex and age differences in rates of alcohol abuse

Table 8–6 Inter-Scale Agreement Between the DIS and SADS by Item

Question	Kappa
You think you drink too much	.66
Excessive drinking, > 1 month	.51
Others commented on drinking	.59
Wanted to stop but couldn't	.27
Drink before breakfast	.52
Job troubles due to drinking	.59
Loss of job due to drinking	.49
Drunk driving or car accident	.77
Arrested due to drinking	.51
Physical fights due to drinking	.64
Binges	.49
Blackouts	.63
Shakes, DTs, seizures, voices, visions	.46
Health problems	.24

and dependence are consistent with clinical experience and with the available literature. Twice as many male (81%) as female (40%) respondents in this study met criteria for alcohol abuse/dependence. The number of drinkers among Indian women is said to be increasing rapidly with each subsequent generation, and many now consume alcohol, as do their male counterparts, in communal settings, as a part of everyday social intercourse (Medicine, 1982; Whittaker, 1962). However, Indian women apparently still tend to drink less in a single sitting than men (Weisner, Weibel-Orlando, & Long, 1984; Whittaker, 1962) and to decrease or stop drinking as they assume parental responsibilities. Indeed, given the high prevalence of abusive and dependent drinking among the men, the burdens of child rearing and even income production often fall exclusively on these women.

In a study of a small Pacific Northwest Indian community, Shore et al. (1973) also found that women had a lower prevalence of alcoholism than men, but had a significantly greater prevalence of depression, anxiety, and psychophysiologic syndromes, visited local health clinics with higher frequency, and used far more prescribed medications. Some investigators have suggested that alcohol abuse and dependence may serve as a cultural mask of depression among Indian men (Shore & Manson, 1981). Two previous papers based upon the present study (Manson, Shore, et al., 1987; Shore, Manson, et al., 1987) reported a close association between these two disorders among male respondents within the clinic index group and underscored the diagnostic problems involved.

In the present study, the proportion of respondents determined to have abused or been dependent upon alcohol at some point in their lives decreases fairly steadily with age, from a high of 64 percent among those under 30, to 20 percent among those 60 years or older. Though various factors may be at work, notably sample bias and mortality influenced selection, these findings reflect several general trends. Lifetime prevalence rates of substance use—particularly alcohol, marijuana, and inhalants—have risen dramatically among Indian youth over the last decade. Fifty-three percent of Indian, compared with 35 percent of non-Indian youth, are now considered to be "at risk" for serious drug involvement (Beauvais, Oetting, & Edwards, 1985). Alcohol remains the drug of choice and of most frequent abuse (Oetting & Beauvais, 1987). Adolescent socialization to drinking begins in familial contexts (Medicine, 1982) and is reinforced through peer clusters (Oetting & Beauvais, 1987); thus, patterns of drinking among Indian youth mirror those of adults. Probable causes for continued, pathological drinking include unemployment, prejudice, poverty, lack of optimism about the future, and alienation (Beauvais et al., 1985; Binion et al., 1988; Holmgren, Fitzgerald, & Carman, 1983).

The high frequency of death and other stresses in American Indian communities may place members of this population at elevated risk for psychiatric disorder, including alcohol abuse and dependence (Walker et al., 1988). Such experiences were common to those participating in the present study. Seventy percent of the respondents reported the loss of a family member or friend within 2 years of interview; 60 percent acknowledged suffering special stresses at the time of interview. We found that alcohol abuse/dependence did in fact occur with disproportionately greater frequency among these individuals. However, at present it is difficult to draw any causal inferences from this intriguing association.

It is generally presumed that such factors as social support, religious involvement, and cultural affiliation serve a protective role in terms of vulnerability to alcohol abuse and dependence among American Indians (Dozier, 1966; Jilek & Todd, 1974; Westermeyer & Peake, 1983; Westermeyer & Neider, 1985). The significant difference in the observed frequency of alcohol abuse/dependence among the married and widowed, compared to the never married and divorced, is similar to Shore et al.'s (1973) earlier finding and is congruent with prevailing assumptions. However, the same relationship did not obtain between church membership or ceremonial participation and diagnosis.

Responses to the DIS symptoms provide several interesting insights into the pattern of alcohol abuse/dependence in this population. Given what is already known about the population in general and the construction of this sample in particular, it is not surprising that 75 percent reported having been drunk, almost half admitted they drink too much, and 39 percent reported that family members object to their drinking. Blackouts, binges, and physical fights are the most common symptoms and correspond to those frequently described in clinical studies of Indian alcoholics (Westermeyer & Neider, 1984, 1985; Westermeyer & Peake, 1983). The relatively low endorsement of items associated with work-related activities may be due to several factors. For example, social norms in these communities may be such that there is higher tolerance for alcohol-impaired behavior. Alternatively, job troubles may be less common because of the high unemployment rates in Indian communities. It is also striking that although 46 percent of the sample believed that they drink too much, only one-third of them had mentioned their possible drinking problem to a physician. One would expect this among Indian men, who are much less likely than women to utilize local health services. Yet, among respondents assigned a DIS diagnosis of alcohol abuse or dependence, men and women differed on only two symptoms. Being arrested for drunkenness and getting into fights while drinking were more common in men.

Like the marked variation among Indian communities in the prevalence of alcohol use reported earlier, the range of "heavy use" is also considerable. For the U.S. in general, between 9 percent (National Institute of Alcohol Abuse and Alcoholism, 1981) and 18 percent (Cahalan & Cisin, 1968) of the population uses alcohol heavily. By comparison, among American Indians, heavy use has been reported at between 9–24 percent of the Standing Rock Sioux (Whittaker, 1962), 14 percent of the Navajo (Levy & Kunitz, 1974), 26 percent of the Ute (Jessor et al., 1969), and 42 percent of the Ojibwa (Longclaws et al., 1980). Thus, the literature suggests that heavy alcohol use is common among American Indians, perhaps more so than in other populations. The present study bears out certain aspects of this, although the overall patterns in terms of risk factors and correlates for heavy drinking and alcoholism appear similar. For example, the proportion of males who drink heavily as opposed to those who drink more moderately is almost twice that of females. Likewise, there is a fairly clear relationship between fewer years of formal education, lower occupational status, early age of first intoxication, and a higher preponderance of heavy drinkers. Yet, as Helzer et al. point out in Table 8–5, Chapter 3 of this volume, controlling for heavy drinking—and therefore the effects of potentially different social factors on drinking styles—reduces the ratio of alcoholics to non-alcoholics along these dimensions. Nonetheless, for the American Indian respondents in this study, the percentage of heavy drinkers who are alcoholic is remarkably high.

Turning now to the degree of agreement between the DIS and SADS-L, a kappa of .46 was observed in the classification of respondents for an alcohol disorder. As noted above, 16 respondents were DIS positive for alcohol abuse/dependence, but did not receive a SADS-L lifetime diagnosis of alcoholism. The individuals in question were predominantly from the Plains ($n = 10$) and Pueblo ($n = 5$) tribes, with equal representation of both sexes. According to the DIS criteria, nine respondents were assigned diagnoses of alcohol abuse, and the remaining seven were determined to be alcohol dependent. Without exception, each of these respondents indicated experiencing periods of heavy drinking that lasted at least 2 weeks, but none met the one month criteria of the SADS-L. Eleven of the sixteen cases exhibited large numbers of SADS-L symptoms of alcoholism (mean = 6.7). Clearly, the different duration criterion constituting "period of heavy drinking" largely is responsible for the lack of concordance between the DIS and SADS-L on this dimension. The difference in this regard, of course, stems from the fact that the DIS diagnoses are generated on the basis of DSM-III criteria, whereas the SADS-L employs RDC criteria[2]. This finding underscores the role of a well-defined cultural pattern of binge or episodic heavy drinking in Indian communities (Hill, 1980; Levy & Kunitz, 1974; Weisner, et al., 1984). Such patterns of consumption may last 2 weeks, but typically not an entire month, and often are related to a variety of community events.

An examination of the concordance between these two protocols on individual questions indicates that only one item "drunk driving/traffic difficulties due to drinking," achieved excellent agreement. Two items, "could not stop drinking" and "having been told by a doctor that physical health problems were due to alcoholism," exhibited poor agreement.

Conclusion

We view this study as the first in a series of steps that are necessary to launching a large scale, community-based epidemiological investigation of alcohol abuse and dependence among American Indians. The emergence of diagnostic tools such as the DIS are causes for considerable excitement. Highly structured protocols of this type reduce the criterion and information variance that have contributed to the unreliability of previously available procedures. We are encouraged by its emphasis on a descriptive rather than etiological approach to diagnosis, on clear standards for severity of symptoms, and on determining the extent to which physical illness, medical experiences, and drug/alcohol use may explain symptoms. To date, our experience with the DIS has underscored these strengths.

Our use of the DIS in this study has enabled us to move beyond the limits of past studies of alcohol abuse and dependence among American Indians, which have emphasized drinking styles and patterns of consumption. We have some sense for its discriminant validity and can now consider questions of clinically meaningful "cases" and subtypes thereof.

In our opinion, however, much work remains to be done before one should feel confident in promoting the application of the DIS, and the DSM-III criteria, across all American Indian communities. Certain diagnostic criteria, particularly those pertaining to symptom duration, severity, and functional impairment, demand closer scrutiny to be certain they are appropriate for this population. Given drinking styles common to this population (e.g., passing a bottle), the use of standard drink equivalents (e.g., seven glasses) as an index of consumption deserves further consideration. This protocol's performance characteristics, especially with respect to response biases, need to be better understood. Lastly, local knowledge of and explanatory models for alcohol abuse and dependence may contribute in important ways to population appropriate adjustments in such instrumentation, yielding even more reliable and valid means for assessing these phenomena.

Notes

The research reported herein originally was conducted through the Department of Psychiatry at the Oregon Health Sciences University. The preparation of this chapter was supported in part by grants from the National Institute of Mental Health (R01-MH33280 and R01-MH4247) and the National Institute of Alcohol Abuse and Alcoholism (R01-AA04401). The authors wish to acknowledge the important contributions of Dr.

Joseph D. Bloom, Dr. George Keepers, and the mental health personal, as well as Indian Health Service programs at the three Indian reservation communities.

1. This convention has been adopted to avoid stigmatizing the communities in question, which, by virtue of their small size, might be singled out inappropriately as examples of widespread psychiatric problems in this special population.

2. A study by Hasin and Grant (1987) found that the DIS assessed the DSM-III and RDC criteria very similarly across all forms of substance abuse and dependence.

References

Beauvais, F.; Oetting, E. R.; and Edwards, R. W. (1985). Trends in drug use of Indian adolescents living on reservations: 1575–1983. *A. J. Drug Alcohol Abuse* 11(3 and 4):209–29.

Binion, A.; Miller, C. D.; Beauvais, F.; and Oetting, E. R. (1988). Rationales for the use of alcohol, marijuana, and other drugs by Indian youth. *Int. J. Addict.* 23:47–64.

Brod, R. L., and McQuiston, J. M. (1983). American Indian adult education and literacy: the first national survey. *J. Am. Indian Educ.* 1:1–16.

Broudy, D. W., and May, P. A. (1983). Demographic and epidemiologic transition among the Navajo Indians. *Soc. Biol.* 30:1–16.

Cahalan, D., and Cisin, H. (1968). American drinking practices. *Q. J. Stud. Alcohol*, 29, 130–51.

Cohen, J. (1960). A coefficient of agreement for nominal scales. *Educational Psychology Measurement* 20:37–46.

Dozier, E. P. (1966). Problem drinking among American Indians: The role of sociocultural deprivation. *Q. J. Stud. Alcohol* 27:72–87.

Endicott, J., and Spitzer, R. L. (1978). A diagnostic interview: The Schedule for Affective Disorders and Schizophrenia. *Arch. Gen. Psychiatry* 35:837–44.

Fleiss, J. L. (1981). *Statistical Methods for Rates and Proportions.* New York: John Wiley & Sons.

Hasin, D. S., and Grant, B. F. (1987). Psychiatric diagnosis of patients with substance abuse problems: A comparison of two procedures, the DIS and the SADS-L. *J. Psychiatr. Res.* 21(1):7–22.

Hill, T. W. (1980). Life styles and drinking patterns of urban Indians. *J. Drug Issues* 10:257–72.

Holmgren, C.; Fitzgerald, B. J.; and Carman, R. S. (1983). Alienation and alcohol use by American Indian and Caucasian high school students. *J. Sch. Psychol.* 120:139–40.

Indian Health Service (1978). *Indian Health Trends and Services, 1978. Department of Health, Education, and Welfare Publication No. (HSA) 78-12009. Washington, D.C.: U.S. Government Printing Office.*

Jessor, R.; Grave, T.; Hanson, R.; and Jessor, S. (1969). *Society, Personality and Deviant Behavior: A Study of a Tri-ethnic Community.* New York: Holt, Rinehart & Winston.

Jilek, W. W. G., and Todd, N. (1974). Witchdoctors succeed where doctors fail: Psychotherapy among Coast Salish Indians. *Can. Psychiatr. Assoc. J.* 19:351–56.

Levy, J. E., and Kunitz, S. (1974). *Indian Drinking.* New York: Wiley Interscience.

Longclaws, L.; Barnes, G.; Grieve, L.; and Dumoff, R. (1980). Alcohol and drug use among the Brokenhead Ojibwa. *J. Stud. Alcohol* 41:21–36.

Manson, S. M., and Shore, J. H. (1981). Psychiatric epidemiology among American Indians: Methodological issues. *White Cloud J.* 2(2):48–56.

Manson, S. M.; Shore, J. H.; and Bloom, J. D. (1985). The depressive experience in American Indian communities: a challenge for psychiatric theory and diagnosis. In A. Kleinman and B. Good (eds.), *Culture and Depression.* Berkeley, Calif: University of California Press.

Manson, S. M.; Walker, R. D.; and Kivlahan, D. R. (1987). Psychiatric assessment and treatment of American Indians and Alaska Natives. *Hosp. Community Psychiatry* 38(2):165–73.

Manson, S. M.; Shore, J. H.; Bloom, J. D.; Keepers, G.; and Neligh, G. (1987). Alcohol abuse and major affective disorders: Advances in epidemiologic research among American Indians. In D. L. Spiegler, D. A. Tate, S. S. Aitken, and C. M. Christian (eds.), *Alcohol Use Among U.S. Ethnic Minorities*. NIAAA Research Monograph No. 18. Department of Health and Human Services Publication No. (ADM) 87-1435. Washington, D.C.: U.S. Government Printing Office.

May, P. A. (1986). Alcohol and drug misuse prevention programs for American Indians: Needs and opportunities. *J. Stud. Alcohol* 47(3):187–95.

May, P. A., and Broudy, D. W. (1980). *Health Problems of the Navajo and Suggested Interventions*. Window Rock, Ariz.: Navajo Health Authority.

Medicine, B. (1982). New roads to coping—Siouan sobriety. In S. M. Manson (ed.), *New Directions in Prevention Among American Indian and Alaska Native Communities*. Portland, Ore: Oregon Health Sciences University, pp. 189–212.

National Institute on Alcohol Abuse and Alcoholism (1980). *Facts in Brief: Alcohol and American Indians*. Rockville, Md: National Clearinghouse for Alcohol Information.

National Institute on Alcohol Abuse and Alcoholism (1981). *Fourth Special Report to the U.S. Congress on Alcohol and Health* (DHHS Publication No. ADM 81-1080). Washington, D.C.: U.S. Government Printing Office.

Oetting, E. R., and Beauvais, F. (1987). Epidemiology and correlates of alcohol use among Indian adolescents living on reservations. In D. L. Spiegler, D. A. Tate, S. S. Aitken, and C. M. Christian (eds.), *Alcohol Use Among U.S. Ethnic Minorities*. NIAAA Research Monograph No. 18. Department of Health and Human Services Publication No. (ADM) 87-1435. Washington, D.C.: U.S. Government Printing Office.

Roy, C., Chaudhri, A.; and Irvine, D. (1970). The prevalence of mental disorders among Saskatchewan Indians. *J. Cross-Cultural Psychol.* 1(4):383–92.

Sampath, B. M. (1974). Prevalence of psychiatric disorders in a southern Baffin Island Eskimo settlement. *Can. Psychiatr. Assoc. J.* 19:303–367.

Shore, J. H.; Kinzie, J. D.; Hampson, D.; and Pattison, M. (1973). Psychiatric epidemiology of an Indian village. *Psychiatry* 36:70–81.

Shore, J. H., and Manson, S. M. (1981). Cross-cultural studies of depression among American Indians and Alaska Natives. *White Cloud J.* 2:5–12.

Shore, J. H.; Manson, S. M.; Bloom, J. D.; Keepers, G.; and Neligh, G. (1987). A pilot study of depression among American Indians. *American Indian and Alaska Native Mental Health Research* 1(2):4–15.

U.S. Bureau of the Census (1984a). *U.S. Census of Population, 1980: American Indian Areas and Alaska Native Villages*. (PC80-S1-B). Supplementary report. Washington, D.C.: U.S. Government Printing Office.

U.S. Bureau of the Census. (1984b). *U.S. Census of Population, 1980: American Indian Areas and Alaska Native Villages*. (PC80-S1-13). Supplementary report. Washington, D.C.: U.S. Government Printing Office.

U.S. Department of Health and Human Services. (1985). *Report of the Secretary's Task Force on Black and Minority Health*. Washington, D.C.: U.S. Government Printing Office.

Walker, R. D., and Kivalhan, D. R. (1984). Definitions, models, and methods in research on sociocultural factors in American Indian alcohol use. *Substance and Alcohol Actions/Misuse*, 5:9–19.

Walker, P. S.; Walker, R. D.; and Kivlahan, D. R. (1988). Alcoholism, alcohol abuse and health. In S. M. Manson and N. G. Dinges (eds.), *Health and Behavior: A Research Agenda for American Indians and Alaska Natives*. Denver, Col.: National Center for American Indian and Alaska Native Mental Health Research.

Weisner, T. S.; Weibel-Orlando, J. C.; and Long, J. (1984). "Serious drinking," "White man's drinking," and "teetotaling": drinking levels and styles in an urban American Indian population. *J. Stud. Alcohol* 45:237–50.

Westermeyer, J., and Neider, J. (1984). Depressive symptoms among Native American alcoholics at the time of a 10-year follow-up. *Alcohol. Clin. Exp. Res.* 8(5):429–34.

Westermeyer, J., and Neider, J. (1985). Cultural affiliation among American Indian alcoholics: Correlations and change over a ten year period. *J. Operational Psychiatry* 16(2):17–23.

Westermeyer, J., and Peake, E. (1983). A ten-year follow-up of alcoholic Native Americans in Minnesota. *Am. J. Psychiatry* 140(2):189–94.

Whittaker, J. O. (1962). Alcohol and the Standing Rock Sioux I: The pattern of drinking. *Q. J. Stud. Alcohol* 24:80–92.

[9] The Prevalence of Alcohol Abuse and/or Dependence in Two Hispanic Communities

Glorisa J. Canino, Audrey Burnam,
and Raul Caetano

The main purpose of this chapter is to compare the prevalence rates and correlates of alcohol abuse and/or dependence between Mexican Americans and Puerto Ricans. We will briefly review results from prior research with Hispanics in the U.S. and Puerto Ricans in Puerto Rico. This will provide a context against which the new data presented here can be considered.

It is difficult to imagine a single ethnic label that would adequately represent the diversity of cultural and social experiences existing among U.S. Hispanics. Currently, the most common of these labels is the term Hispanic, which although convenient has not been uniformly accepted as a valid identifier of Hispanic ethnicity. Comprising now approximately 6 percent of the U.S. population (U.S. Bureau of the Census, 1985), Hispanics come from all the countries of Latin America, brining to the U.S. a very diverse cultural heritage.

They also migrate to the United States for diverse reasons. The majority are unskilled or semiskilled workers who come from rural areas of Latin America in search of economic betterment. But there are also many professionals seeking better opportunities for career development, and people fleeing political persecution in their countries of birth. Upon arrival they are incorporated into different Hispanic ethnic groups, in urban or rural areas, having differing life experiences, and develop differing levels of acculturation to the U.S. Altogether, variations in cultural heritage, immigration experience, and life in the new

This investigation was supported by grant IRl-MH36230 from the Division of Biometry and Epidemiology of the National Institute of Mental Health. We would like to acknowledge Maritza Rubio-Stipec, M.A., Miligros, Bravo, Ph.D., and Hector Bird, M.D.—coinvestigators of this study—and José Martinez, M.A.—data analyst—for their invaluable collaboration with this investigation.

131

country come together to create an extremely diverse and culturally rich ethnic mosaic.

Alcohol Use in Latin America

The diversity of the cultural experiences of Latin American nations is reflected in a wide variation in alcohol use. Latin American countries can be characterized not only by their political systems or level of economic development but also by national drinking patterns, beverage preference, attitudes toward alcohol consumption, and attention given to alcohol problems. There are wine-producing and wine-drinking countries such as Argentina and Chile; there are countries, such as Puerto Rico, where distilled spirits are preferred; and there are beer drinking countries like Mexico. Some of these differences in alcohol use arise from demographic factors, such as the presence of a large indigenous population, which may have contributed since colonial times to the development and survival of certain patterns of drinking in the non-European population. A possible example of this is the pattern of infrequent drinking with high consumption per occasion observed in Mexico, which may have emerged from ritual drinking among the natives in precolonial times (Heath, 1982 and Taylor, 1979).

Puerto Rico, a country with close ties with the U.S. and a large representation in the U.S. Hispanic population, had a per capita consumption in liters of absolute alcohol of 8.4 in 1982–1983 (Canino et al., 1987), close to the 9.7 per capita consumption of liters in the U.S. in the same period. In Mexico, another country with a very intense flow of migration to the U.S., this figure was 5.4 liters (in 1984) (Rosovsky, 1985). Data on alcohol-related indicators such as cirrhosis mortality, traffic accidents involving alcohol, suicides, and admissions to psychiatric hospitals show great variation across Latin American countries (Caetano, 1984a), suggesting differences in alcohol use and in the pattern of responses to alcohol-related problems.

But if there is a wide variation in alcohol use among the different nations of Latin America from which U.S. Hispanics come, there is also some uniformity. Alcohol is closely associated with everyday life in Latin America. No Latin American country has a history of Prohibition. Drinking is frequently associated with cultural activities such as baptisms, funerals, religious ceremonies, and so on. It is therefore not unusual for people to drink early in the morning, during weekdays, and weekends. Drinking and drunkenness by men and the young is more accepted than by women and the elderly (Caetano, 1984a). A comparison between Mexico and the United States showed that in the latter country norms regulating alcohol use are more egalitarian, and access to alcohol by gender and age group is not as different as it seems to be in Mexico (Roizen et al., 1983).

Following these normative prescriptions, drinking in Latin America is predominantly a male activity, something that men do when they get together after work, during sports activities, or when socializing. Excessive drinking is also a male problem, the great majority of women being either abstainers or very light drinkers. Thus, most of the people in treatment for alcohol problems are men. Data on drinking patterns, attitudes and norms toward alcohol consumption, and alcohol problems among Hispanics in the United States and island Puerto Ricans reflect these patterns found in Latin American countries (Alcocer, 1982; Caetano, 1984b; Gilbert & Cervantes, 1986; Garcia, 1976).

Alcohol Use in Puerto Rico

The age adjusted death rate per 100,000 population for cirrhosis in Puerto Rico is almost three times higher than in the United States (36.5 versus 13.4, respectively). In 1987 liver cirrhosis was among the first five causes of death for ages 40 to 44 in the general population of Puerto Rico (Department of Health Vital Statistics, 1987).

There have been few studies of drinking patterns in the Puerto Rican general population. Garcia (1976) reported results from a national survey based on a multistage area probability sample of households (N = 782). The study classified drinkers as occasional, social, heavy, and alcoholics, the difference between the latter and the others being the presence of loss of control. Unfortunately definitions were vague, and drinkers' classification was not by self-report: In each household the person interviewed was asked to classify all the drinkers in the family. The proportion of individuals who were drinkers in the population 13 years of age and older (29%) was low when compared to other Latin American surveys and the United States. The proportion of individuals who drank and had some kind of alcohol-related problem ranged from 1.5 percent in the Northeast District to 5 percent in the South District. The estimated prevalence of those who drank and had problems in the total Puerto Rican population was 2.5 percent.

A second survey of the Puerto Rican general population was conducted by Gonzalez (1983). He defined heavy, moderate, and occasional drinking based on self-reported quantity of drinks consumed. Results showed that about 48 percent of the population 15 years of age and older were drinkers. Among heavy drinkers, who comprised 30 percent of all drinkers, the proportion of men and women was 89 and 11 percent, respectively. However, young women had lower rates of abstention than older women, and about 80 percent of the women who drank were in the 15 to 39 year-old-group. Among the 12 percent of the drinkers who reported loss of control, 84 percent were men and 16 percent were women. The differences observed in the rate of abstention among men and women in Puerto Rico seem to reflect the drinking norms in the country. Aviles Roig (1973) suggested that norms are more liberal for men than for women, and that drinking by men is associated with independence and "machismo."

Alcohol use among U.S. Hispanics

Reports from several community surveys have assessed levels of drinking or problems from alcohol use among Hispanic samples of differing regional and cultural backgrounds (Haberman & Sheinberg, 1967; Maril & Zaveleta, 1979; Cahalan & Room, 1974; Caetano, 1984; Holck et al., 1984). However, the Hispanic samples in many of these studies are small or have not included comparative population groups. In order to examine drinking patterns and alcohol problems in a national sample of U.S. Hispanics, the Alcohol Research Group conducted in 1984 a national study of this ethnic group. A total of 1,453 individuals who identified themselves as Hispanics were interviewed in this survey (Caetano, 1989). Data from this survey showed that the rate of abstention was twice as common among women as among men. Frequent heavy drinking among men was most common in the 30–39 age group. Comparable research in the U.S. general population shows heavy drinking among men as most common in the 20–29 age range, that is, a decade younger (Cahalan & Room, 1974; Clark & Midanik, 1981; Hilton).

The results of this national survey also showed that drinking predominated among the young, the better educated, and those with higher incomes. Among women, those who were 40 years of age and older, who were married, who had a job, who were born in the United States of U.S. born parents, and who were highly acculturated had a particularly high rate of drinking once a week or more often, and drinking five or more drinks at a sitting at least once a week. When the relationship between heavy drinking and sociodemographic characteristics was examined with multivariate analysis (logistic regression), women who were highly acculturated were 9 times more likely to be heavy drinkers than women in the low acculturation group (Caetano, 1986d).

Among women who identified themselves as Mexican American, acculturation was strongly related to being born in the United States (Caetano & Medina Mora, 1986). Thus, the rate of abstention among women born in Mexico was 61 percent and did not decline with number of years of life in the United States; very few of these women were highly acculturated to the United States. Almost all of those born in the U.S.

were in the high acculturation group and the abstention rate was comparatively low (32% versus 61% for foreign born women). For Mexican men the change in drinking patterns occurred very early, within 5 years of their arrival in the United States. At this point drinking patterns were already very similar to those found among men born in the United States. There was a shift from infrequent drinking of high amounts to a more frequent and heavier drinking as compared to drinking in Mexico (Caetano & Medina Mora, 1986).

Acculturation was also associated with attitudes toward drinking in various social settings. Hispanics who were high in acculturation were more liberal regarding drinking, especially drinking by women and by older people. Attitudes toward what is appropriate drinking across gender and age groups was more egalitarian among acculturated than nonacculturated Hispanics (Caetano, 1986e).

Finally, this national survey collected data on the frequency of a number of alcohol-related social, medical, and psychiatric problems among Hispanics. Among men the most prevalent problems were salience of drink seeking behavior (7% of the sample), impaired control over drinking (6%), problems with spouse (6%), problems with other people (7%), and health problems (6%). Among women the most prevalent problems were salience of drink seeking behavior (3% of the sample), belligerence (3%), health problems (3%), and problems with people other than the spouse (3%). Given the fact that men drank more than women and that attitudinal and consumption norms were more liberal for men than for women, the higher rate of problems among men should not come as a surprise. Whether this relationship between men and women will change as the demographics of the Hispanic population in the United States change, that is, as more women enter the workforce and as acculturation and the consequent liberalization of norms increase, remains to be seen.

Conclusions

There are some commonalities between island Puerto Ricans and U.S. Hispanics, especially Mexican Americans. Both groups admit to permissive attitudes toward drinking and drunkenness. For men, drinking is associated with family reunions and festivities, and excessive drinking in women is curtailed. Similarities in attitudes toward alcohol consumption seem to be greater between island Puerto Ricans and nonacculturated Mexican Americans as compared to Mexican Americans acculturated to the United States. Furthermore, lifetime prevalence rates of alcohol abuse and dependence have been reported as different for these two groups of Mexican Americans (Burnam et al., 1987). Because of this, the analyses presented in this chapter will make the distinction between the Mexican Americans born in the United States and those born in Mexico.

The statistics for both U.S. Hispanics and island Puerto Ricans show elevated death rates due to cirrhosis of the liver, and a great number of accidents while driving under the influence of alcohol. These statistics, coupled with permissive cultural attitudes toward drunkenness, would suggest a high prevalence of alcoholism for these two Hispanic groups. Yet no previous studies were identified that assessed the prevalence rates of alcohol abuse or dependence for either island Puerto Ricans or Mexican Americans.

Data on alcohol abuse/dependence among Mexican Americans were collected in Los Angeles as part of the Epidemiologic Catchment Area study (Regier et al., 1984). The data from Puerto Rico were obtained from the Epidemiologic Study of Mental Disorders in Puerto Rico (Canino et al., 1987a). Both studies were designed to provide estimates of the prevalence of major psychiatric disorder in the general population as assessed by the DIS based on the diagnostic criteria of the American Psychiatric Association (DSM-III).

The comparison between Puerto Ricans and Mexican Americans is of great interest because it will permit an examination of cultural similarities and differences between these two Hispanic groups in the prevalence and correlates of alcohol abuse and/or dependence. The data from Los Angeles are shown for all Mexican Americans in the study, and are also presented separately for two subgroups; those born in the United States (natives) and those born in Mexico (immigrants). The comparisons of these two Mexican American groups to island Puerto Ricans is useful for determining the influence that acculturation to the United States may have on the prevalence and correlates of the disorder.

Method

Sampling Design

The design and methodology of the ECA program surveys and of the Puerto Rican survey are presented in Chapter 5. Detailed methods for the two surveys may be found in Eaton et al. (1984) and Canino et al. (1987b) and will only be briefly reviewed here.

The sample designs for the two studies are similar since both are probability household samples. Both studies employed postratification weights to adjust the age and sex distributions of the respective samples to the 1980 Census. The Los Angeles investigators also adjusted their samples for ethnic origin (Hispanic versus non-Hispanic) as well as age and sex. Although the Los Angeles (LA) study included an over-sample of adults who were institutionalized (prisons, psychiatric hospitals, homes for the elderly), the present analysis is restricted to the household sample. The LA study design was longitudinal, with follow-up interviews 6 months and 1 year later. However, the data presented here are from the index interview only, for the purpose of cross-sectional comparisons of the Los Angeles and Puerto Rico samples.

The major difference between the surveys is that the Puerto Rico sample is representative of the entire island of Puerto Rico, while the LA sample is representative of the populations of two mental health catchment areas in metropolitan Los Angeles.

LOS ANGELES SAMPLE   Los Angeles respondents were selected in 1983 and 1984 from a catchment area in East Los Angeles, which was 83 percent Hispanic American (by 1980 U.S. Census data), and one in Calver City (West Los Angeles), the population of which was principally (63%) non-Hispanic white. The Hispanic Americans in each of these catchment areas were largely of Mexican origin.

The sample was a two stage area probability sample stratified by catchment area. The primary sampling units (PSU) were census blocks aggregated or disaggregated to maintain a relatively uniform PSU size; and secondary sampling units were households. Using a modified Kish method (Kish, 1965), one adult age 18 or older from each sampled household was randomly selected for the study. A total of 3,132 adults were interviewed in the sample, with an overall completion rate of 68 percent.

THE PUERTO RICO SAMPLE   The study population was defined as all persons 17–64 years of age living in a household in Puerto Rico, including those household members temporarily away and those in institutions with families in the community. As in Los Angeles, a two-stage probability sample design was used to select 2,036 households. The primary sampling units were census blocks and the secondary sampling units were households. Individuals within a household were selected using a modified Kish procedure (Kish, 1965). Eighty-four percent (1,701 out of 2,036) of the households contained at least one eligible respondent. Among the 1,701 respondents selected, 1,551 were successfully interviewed during the spring and fall of 1984, yielding a completion rate of 91 percent. The demographic characteristics of the unweighted sample are similar to those of the Puerto Rican population and are described in detail elsewhere (Canino et al., 1987a).

In order to make the sample comparable with L.A., the 17-year-olds were excluded from the Puerto Rico sample.

DIS Adaptation to Puerto Ricans and Mexican Americans

In both the Puerto Rico and Los Angeles studies, the Spanish translation of the DIS developed by Karno et al. (1983) was used. However, this translation was adapted to the Puerto Rico population and is reported elsewhere (Bravo et al., 1987).

The reliability and validity of the DIS for use in Mexican American and Puerto Rican populations has been reported elsewhere (Burnam et al., 1983; Canino et al., 1987b). However, it is relevant to note here that the DIS demonstrated high levels of test-retest reliability and equivalence to the English version for most diagnoses, including the alcohol abuse and or dependence schedule (Burnam et al., 1983). The procedural validity (test-retest reliability comparing lay and psychiatric interviewers) of the alcohol abuse and dependence schedule of the instrument was reported as excellent in the Puerto Rico study (Canino et al., 1987b). Agreement was similarly high ($K = .73$) when the DIS administered by a lay interviewer was compared to the clinical judgment of two highly qualified native Puerto Rican psychiatrists, and when the DIS administered by a lay interviewer was compared to the clinical judgment of masters level psychologists and social workers from Los Angeles ($K = .62$).

Results

Composition of the Samples

Table 9–1 shows the size and demographic composition of the Los Angeles and Puerto Rican samples. Except for the response rate which is unweighted, all the percentage figures in this and subsequent tables are weighted to the population to which they refer (See Chapter 2).

The sample composition by age and sex is very similar in the Los Angeles and Puerto Rican samples. However, there are considerable subsample differences in years of education. The majority of the Mexican American immigrants have less than 8 years of education and only a small percentage have completed high school or have some college. The reverse is true of the native Mexican Americans. In Puerto Rico, although slightly more than half of the sample has completed high school or have some college, about one-quarter has less than 8 years of schooling.

Number of marriages, area of residence, and occupational status are also shown in Table 9–1. The number of marriages was not determined in the Puerto Rican study. Rural residence is not relevant to the Los Angeles sample, since the whole sample was drawn from an urban setting. In Puerto Rico 64 percent of the sample is urban, and 36 percent is rural.

The majority of Mexican Americans have had only one marriage,

Table 9–1 Sample Size and Demographic Composition of Los Angeles Mexican American Household Samples (Weighted Percentages and Means)

Category	Puerto Ricans	Mexican Americans		
		Total[a]	Immigrants	Natives
Total number interviewed	1,513	1,244	706	538
Overall response rate	91%	68%	—	—
Age				
18–24	23%	21%	18%	25%
25–44	48%	46%	53%	36%
45–64	29%	24%	18%	32%
65 or more	—	9%	11%	7%
Sex (weighted % female)	53%	51%	49%	55%
Years of education				
Mean years	10.5	8.8	6.9	11.4
8 years	24%	39%	61%	9%
8–11 years	20%	25%	20%	31%
12 years	26%	20%	12%	30%
13+ years	30%	16%	6%	30%
Number of marriages[b]				
0	—	29%	25%	34%
1	—	62%	68%	53%
2+	—	9%	6%	13%
Occupational status prestige score in				
Upper ⅓	—	12%	7%	19%
Middle ⅓	—	35%	29%	43%
Lower ⅓	—	52%	63%	38%

[a]Total Mexican Americans refers to the sum of the immigrant and Native Mexican Americans.

[b]This information was not ascertained by the Puerto Rico survey, since it is part of the schedule of antisocial personality, which was not included as part of the study.

regardless of their country of birth. On the other hand, there are intergroup differences in occupational status. Immigrants are overrepresented in the lower prestige occupations and underrepresented in prestige occupations compared to the native Mexican Americans. This is expected, since most Mexican American immigrants are unskilled workers. However, it is important to note that even though the natives do have higher prestige occupations than immigrant Mexican Americans, a large percentage of both Mexican American groups have low prestige occupations.

The Symptoms of Alcoholism

The overall evidence regarding patterning of symptoms among those who have met criteria for a DIS/DSM-III diagnosis of alcohol abuse and

Table 9–2 *Individual Symptom Frequencies Among Those with Alcohol Disorders for Puerto Rican and Mexican American Samples*

DIS Item No.	Puerto Rico	% with Alcohol Abuse/Dependence Who Endorsed this Item Total Mexican Americans[a]	Immigrants	Natives
150	76	73	71	74
151	50	62	72	55
152	83	65	67	63
153/54	83	70	68	57
155	17	13	7	17
156	50	38	35	40
157	28	27	28	26
158	23	20	20	20
159	19	23	27	20
160	15	15	16	15
161	7	7	10	4
162	21	42	41	43
163	13	29	32	27
164	39	38	32	43
165	30	31	33	30
166	59	57	52	60
167	29	21	22	21
168	[b]	19	15	22
169	24	12	12	11
170	13	8	8	8

[a]Total Mexican Americans refers to the sum of imigrants and native Mexican Americans.

[b]Was not included in the Puerto Rico study; only DSM-III criteria items were included.

or dependence (also referred to as alcoholism in this chapter) suggests no substantial difference between the Puerto Rican and Los Angeles samples, or by country of birth in Los Angeles. The most frequently reported symptoms by both Puerto Ricans and Mexican Americans were those having to do with family objections to drinking, excessive consumption, and "blackouts." Compared to U.S. anglos, (See chapter 6 of this book), a high proportion of all Hispanics endorse these items (DIS items 166, 150, 154) (see Table 9–2).

Of great importance is the fact that as compared to other ethnic or national groups reported in this book (e.g., U.S., Taiwan, etc.), a very large percentage of Puerto Rican alcoholics (83%) and Mexican American alcoholics (70%) admit to drinking heavily either on a daily or on a weekly basis at some time in their lives. On the other hand, losing a job or having problems at work are among the least commonly reported symptoms in the Hispanic samples.

The few differences observed between the two samples are related to problems (Question 162) or arrests (Question 163) while driving under the influence of alcohol. In Puerto Rico, the percentage of alcoholics endorsing these items was considerably smaller than in Los Angeles.

Table 9–3 Lifetime Rate of Various Drinking Categories for Puerto Rican and Mexican American Samples (Weighted Percentages)

	Puerto Rico	Total Mexican Americans	Immigrants	Natives
Total abstention	20.2	16	23	7
Males	7.2	2.5	2.8	2.1
Females	31.7	29.5	44.2	11.9
Nonheavy/nonproblem (social) drinkers	69.1	47	44	52
Heavy/nonproblem drinkers	7.0	2	1	3
Problem/drinkers (not alcoholic)	10.2	17	19	14
Alcohol abuse only	4.4	8	5	10
Dependence with or without abuse	8.2	10	8	13
Six-month prevalence of alcoholism (abuse and/or dependence)	4.9	6	4	8

Patterns of Drinking

Table 9–3 shows lifetime prevalence rates for various levels of drinking and current (6-month) prevalence rates for alcohol abuse and/or dependence for the two Hispanic samples. The lifetime categories are mutually exclusive (and thus additive).

Approximately one-fourth of Puerto Ricans, Mexican Americans, and immigrants are abstainers. Native Mexican Americans reported a considerably lower abstention rate. Abstention rates by sex in Puerto Rico reveal that 4 times as many women abstain from drinking as men. An even larger sex difference is observed in immigrant Mexican Americans where women abstain from drinking 15 times more often than men. On the other hand, the pattern of abstention by sex for the Native Mexican American is very different. In this group, women abstain from drinking only 6 times more frequently than men.

Social drinking (nonheavy/nonproblem) is the most frequent pattern of drinking for all four Hispanic groups, with Puerto Rico having a higher percentage of social drinkers. Conversely, heavy/nonproblem drinking is the least frequent pattern observed in all groups. However, the percentage of heavy/nonproblem drinkers among Puerto Ricans is considerably higher than among Mexican Americans. This may be related to the permissive attitudes toward drinking and drunkenness exhibited by the majority of Puerto Ricans. While similar attitudes toward drinking exist in Mexican American groups, the fact that they live in the

U.S. where the attitudes toward drunkenness are not as liberal probably increases the probability of having problems when they do drink heavily.

Problem drinkers are those who have had at least one alcohol-related problem in their lives, but who have not had enough to qualify for a DSM-III diagnosis of alcoholism. Puerto Rico has fewer problem drinkers than any other Hispanic group (10%) and considerably fewer than Mexican American immigrants (19%).

In all three Hispanic groups, alcohol abuse is less prevalent than alcohol dependence. As discussed in Chapter 2, this result may be an artifact of the DSM-III definition of alcoholism. However, it is of interest to note that Puerto Ricans and Mexican American immigrants have very similar lifetime rates of both alcohol abuse/and dependence. Consequently, the proportion of Puerto Rican and Mexican American immigrants with any DSM-III alcohol disorder is identical (13%). On the other hand, native Mexican Americans have nearly 2 times this rate (23%). The same pattern is observed for the 6-month prevalence of alcohol disorders. However, in spite of these differences, alcoholism is the most prevalent of the major psychiatric disorders in all of these Hispanic samples.

The Course of Alcoholism

The course of alcoholism can be examined retrospectively in Table 9–4. Because so few Hispanic women are alcoholic (see Table 9–5), the retrospective course of alcoholism is described only for Hispanic males, and the combined sample of male and female alcoholics.

The mean age of first intoxication is lower in male alcoholics compared to nonalcoholics for both immigrant and native Mexican Americans. (The age of first intoxication was not ascertained in Puerto Rico). First intoxication typically occurs in the early teens, and the mean age of the first alcohol symptom is in the early 20s. Therefore, the number of years from first intoxication to the onset of alcoholism is around 7 years for the Mexican American males.

The mean age of first alcohol symptom in Puerto Rico is in the late 20s (27) as compared to the early 20s for the two Mexican American groups (22–23). Similarly, the mean age of the most recent symptom among alcoholics in remission is higher in the Puerto Rican sample (37 years) compared to 34 years in the Mexican American natives, and only 29 years among immigrants.

The duration of alcoholism in years among those who have remitted is similar for Puerto Ricans and Mexican American natives, but the Mexican American immigrant group has a slightly lower duration of the disorder. The mean number of lifetime alcohol symptoms is the same for both Mexican American groups (5) and slightly higher for Puerto Rico (6).

Table 9–4 Onset, Severity and Course of Alcoholism for Puerto Rican and Mexican American Samples

	Men				Women				Total			
	Puerto Rico	Total Mexican Americans	Immigrants	Natives	Puerto Rico	Total Mexican Americans	Immigrants	Natives	Puerto Rico	Total Mexican Americans	Immigrants	Natives
Mean age first intoxicated[a]												
Total sample		17	17	16	***	21	21	20		18	18	18
Alcoholics		15	15	14		***	***	***		15	15	15
Nonalcoholics		17	18	17		21	21	21		19	19	19
Mean value among alcoholics												
Age of onset	27	22	23	22	***	***	***	***	27	23	23	23
Number of years first intoxicated to first alcohol symptom		7	7	7		***	***	***		8	7	8
Mean No. lifetime symptoms	6.2	5	5	5	***	***	***	***	6.1	5	5	5
Mean values among alcoholics in remission[b]												
Age last symptom	37	32	29	34	***	***	***	***	37	32	29	34
Duration of alcoholism in years	10.3	10	8	11	***	***	***	***	9.2	9	8	10

***Denominator less than 30.

[a]Was not included in the Puerto Rico study; only DSM-III items were included.

[b]Remitted alcoholic = No alcoho. symptoms for at least 1 year prior to interview.

Table 9–5 Lifetime Prevalence of Alcoholism by Sex and Age:
Puerto Rican and Mexican American Samples
(Weighted Percentages)

Total Mexican Americans	N Unweighted	Men (%)	Women (%)	Total (%)
Age				
18–24		27	8	18
25–44		36	4	20
45–64		30	4	16
65 or more		21	1	9
Total		31	5	18
Immigrants				
Age				
18–24		21	2	12
25–44		30	0	16
45–64		20	0	10
65 or more		12	0	5
Total		25	0	13
Natives				
Age				
18–24		33	13	23
25–44		50	12	29
45–64		38	7	20
65 or more		41	2	18
Total		41	10	24
Puerto Ricans				
Age Group				
18–24	295	10.7	0.9	5.6
25–44	768	26.7	2.2	13.3
45–64	450	32.3	2.6	17.2
Total	1,513	24.6	2.0	12.6

Risk Factors and Correlates of Alcoholism

Table 9–5 examines the lifetime prevalence rates of alcoholism by age and sex. At every age, and for both Puerto Ricans and Mexican Americans, the rates for men are considerably higher than those for women. This pattern is accentuated in the 25–64 age group. However, the male/female ratio is much higher among immigrant Mexican Americans (25:0) as compared to native Mexican Americans who have a male/female ratio of 4:1. Puerto Ricans have a sex ratio intermediate to the two Mexican American groups (12:1).

Rates by age show a different pattern for Puerto Ricans as compared to Mexican Americans. In Puerto Rico, the lifetime prevalence of alcoholism increases with age. This is what would be intuitively expected, since the lifetime prevalence of any disorder is the cumulative rate over all previous ages. However, this pattern was not observed for the Mexican American groups. In these two groups, the pattern observed is a relatively high prevalence rate in the 18–25 age range, followed by an increase of this rate in the 25–45 age range, and thereafter a decline for the older age groups.

Various hypotheses have been proposed by Robins et al. (1984) as explanations for the decline with age after 45 years of age found not only in the Los Angeles Mexican American sample, but in all ECA samples. Possible reasons include faulty recall in the older group, selective mortality (i.e., alcoholics die younger), and a true cohort effect (i.e., that there is a true increase in the condition in the younger age groups). It would be reasonable to assume that the effects of the first two factors should have also prevailed in Puerto Rico. Resolving this issue requires further analysis. However, one may postulate several alternatives that could explain the differences observed between the Los Angeles sample and Puerto Rico: First, drinking patterns among alcoholics in Puerto Rico may be less deleterious to physical health and more individuals survive to an older age, thus increasing lifetime prevalence. Second, alcoholics in Puerto Rico may begin having problems at a later age, and thus it is not possible to see the full effects of selective mortality in the oldest age group studied in Puerto Rico (45–65). In fact, the mean age of the first alcohol symptom in Puerto Rico is higher (27 years) than in the three LA groups, which is 23 years for all groups. The third possible explanation for the differences observed between Puerto Rico and Los Angeles is that a true cohort effect may exist—that is, younger cohorts of Americans generally, including Mexican Americans, are more prone to suffer from alcoholism than cohorts born in the first three decades of the century, while the same would not be true of Puerto Rico.

Table 9–6 depicts a number of other possible correlates and risk factors associated with alcoholism. The first column of the table shows the predictors of heavy drinking among all drinkers, and the second column the predictors of alcoholism among heavy drinkers. Data for Puerto Rico is available only for the items on occupation and education. The remaining variables were not ascertained in this study. The base percent for the total samples of all Hispanic groups are shown at the top of Table 9–6. These show that more than a third (43%) of all Hispanic drinkers are heavy drinkers, and that for all groups except immigrants (39%), half or more of all heavy drinkers meet DSM-III criteria for alcoholism.

Table 9–6 also shows that among those who are heavy drinkers, educational level is not a consistent predictor of alcohol disorder. Occupational status as measured by job prestige does not appear to show a consistent relationship to alcoholism among heavy drinkers. However, belonging to the upper one-third of prestige occupations seems to be related to a lower prevalence of heavy drinking in all Hispanic groups.

The last three variables in Table 9–6 show a very clear association with both heavy drinking among all drinkers and with alcoholism among heavy drinkers. Childhood conduct disorder and first intoxication be-

Table 9–6 Risk Factors and Correlates for Heavy Drinking and Alcoholism for Puerto Rican and Mexican American Samples (Weighted Percentages)

	% of Drinkers Who Are Heavy Drinkers				% of Heavy Drinkers Who Are Alcoholic			
	Puerto Rico	Total Mexican Americans	Immigrants	Natives	Puerto Rico	Total Mexican Americans	Immigrants	Natives
Total sample	31	43	43	44	51	49	39	59
No. of marriages								
0	a	47	48	47		49	36	60
1		41	41	41		47	39	57
2+		44	43	45		50	***	***
Years of education								
6	37	43	42	46	54	41	36	***
8–11	41	44	43	46	57	54	43	61
12	27	47	49	46	58	53	51	54
13+	23	39	37	39	41	50	***	57
Occupational status								
Lower 1/3		44	44	44		47	35	68
Middle 1/3		48	51	46		52	49	55
Upper 1/3		38	29	42		51	***	54
Childhood conduct groups positive								
0	a	31	35	25		34	31	41
1–2		48	43	53		50	38	59
3		75	75	75		67	58	76
Intoxicated before age 15								
No	a	37	39	36		39	33	46
Yes		70	65	75		72	57	84
Any drug disorder								
No	a	41	42	39		45	38	55
Yes		89	***	96		77	***	77

***Denomination size less than 30.

a The Puerto Rico study did not include antisocial personality or drug abuse/or dependence DIS items.

146

fore age 15 are clearly risk factors of heavy drinking or alcoholism for the Mexican American sample. The presence of any drug abuse diagnosis is a correlate (i.e., may or may not be antecedent) of heavy drinking or alcoholism. Thus, for these three variables, Mexican Americans appear to be very similar to other ethnic groups.

Table 9–7 shows the relationship of alcoholism to other psychiatric diagnoses. The first column shows the lifetime prevalence rates for all diagnoses ascertained in both the Los Angeles and Puerto Rico sites. For all groups, alcoholism is the more prevalent disorder, but as previously discussed, it is almost twice as high in the native Mexican American group as in Puerto Ricans and immigrant Mexican Americans. The lifetime prevalence of cognitive impairment for both the Puerto Rican and immigrant Mexican American groups is inordinately high. However, this is probably an artifact of the low educational level of a great part of the Puerto Rican and Mexican American immigrant population. Recent research has demonstrated that the Minimental State Examination, the cognitive test used in the DIS, is highly sensitive to language, ethnicity, and low educational level (Escobar et al., 1986; Anthony et al., 1982; Folstein, et al., 1983; Bird et al., 1987).

The second column in Table 9–7 shows the lifetime prevalence of all disorders among those who also meet DIS/DSM-III criteria for alcohol abuse and/or dependence. For most diagnoses shown in this column, and for both Puerto Ricans and Mexican Americans, there is a higher prevalence of disorders among alcoholics as compared to the general population.

The third column shows the prevalence of each disorder in alcoholics divided by the prevalence in nonalcoholics, that is, risk ratios for psychiatric disorders among alcoholics relative to nonalcoholics. For Mexican Americans, the diagnoses for which the relative risks for alcoholics are larger are antisocial personality and mania, followed by drug abuse and/or dependence. The relationship of alcoholism to antisocial personality is not surprising. As was previously discussed, conduct disorder symptoms that are part of the DSM-III definition of antisocial personality were highly associated with later alcoholism.

No strong association was observed between depression and alcoholism for any of the Hispanic groups. This finding is not surprising in the light of recent evidence, which suggests that affective disorder uncommonly produces secondary alcoholism (Schuckit, 1981). Family studies have led to the conclusion that depression and alcoholism are not manifestations of the same underlying disorder (e.g., Merikangas et al., 1985).

No cases of somatization were found in the Mexican American groups, so an association with alcoholism could not be tested. It is of great interest, however, that in Puerto Rico a strong association was observed between alcoholism and somatization disorder. At present, we

Table 9–7 Lifetime Prevalence Rates of Core Diagnoses and Risk Ratios Among Total Sample and Alcoholics for Puerto Rican and Mexican American Samples

	Prevalence in All Persons				Prevalence in Alcoholics				Risk Ratio			
	Puerto Rico	Total Mexican Americans	Immigrants	Natives	Puerto Rico	Total Mexican Americans	Immigrants	Natives	Puerto Rico	Total Mexican Americans	Immigrants	Natives
Alcoholism	12.6	17.6	13.0	23.9	20.0	15.0	7.8	20.3	1.6	0.9	0.6	0.8
Phobic disorder	12.2	13.4	10.3	17.6	16.3	16.1	12.3	21.2	1.3	1.2	1.2	1.2
Drug abuse and/or dependence (any)	a	4.2	1.6	7.7		16.4	6.0	24.0		3.9	3.8	3.1
Cognitive impairment	13.46	8.9	12.7	3.7	16.3	5.2	8.3	3.0	1.2	0.6	0.7	0.8
Major depression	4.6	4.6	3.1	6.5	7.5	8.6	2.8	13.0	1.8	1.9	0.9	2.0
Dysthymic disorder	5.0	4.7	3.4	6.5	5.7	6.6	1.7	10.2	1.2	1.4	0.5	1.6
Antisocial personality	a	3.7	2.8	4.9		14.8	13.3	15.9		4.0	4.8	3.3
Obsessive-compulsive	3.2	1.7	1.5	2.0	6.6	2.6	1.6	3.2	2.4	1.5	1.1	1.6
Panic disorder	1.7	1.1	1.1	1.3	2.4	0.5	0.7	0.3	1.5	0.4	0.6	0.2
Schizophrenia	1.6	0.3	0.4	0.3	3.0	0.0	0.0	0.0	2.2	0.0	0.0	0.0
Mania	.51	0.1	0.0	0.3	.00	0.8	0.0	1.3	.0	5.9		4.2
Somatization	0.8	0.0	0.0	0.0	2.3	0.0	0.0	0.0	4.7			
Anorexia nervosa	a	0.0	0.0	0.0		0.0	0.0	0.0				
Any core DIS dx	18.7	30.1	28.0	33.0	28.6	44.0	32.0	52.9	1.7	1.5	1.1	1.6

aThe Puerto Rico study did not include the DIS schedules of antisocial personality, anorexia nervosa, or drug abuse and/or dependence.

148

have no clear explanation for this finding, but our prior analyses have shown that somatization disorder was more prevalent in Puerto Rico than in the five U.S. communities represented in the ECA (Canino et al., 1987a). We are presently in the process of comparing the prevalence and correlates of somatic complaints in the Los Angeles and Puerto Rican samples. Our preliminary findings suggest that the prevalence of somatic complaints among Puerto Ricans is two times that of any Hispanic or Anglo Los Angeles group. This finding persists even after standardizing the Los Angeles sample to the Puerto Rican sample by sex, education, and age.

Discussion

One of the advantages of cross-cultural research is that it permits us to better describe the way in which sociocultural factors may influence the course, content, and manifestations of a particular disorder (Sartorious, 1979). The veracity of this premise becomes obvious after examining the data from the Hispanic groups represented here, island Puerto Ricans and Mexican Americans living in the United States. Our data in general confirm what has been described in previous surveys of alcohol use and alcohol problems among Mexican Americans and Puerto Ricans. In all the samples, there were high rates of heavy drinking even among those who did not meet the DSM-III criteria for alcoholism. Excessive drinking and the problems associated with it were predominantly male activities. In fact, the characteristics of alcoholism in women could not be described for either the Puerto Rican or Mexican American samples because the number of women who met criteria for the disorder was so low. The pattern of heavy drinking among Hispanic males, and the low prevalence of the disorder in women, has been explained as resulting from culturally defined permissive attitudes toward drinking and drunkenness in men, coupled with strong social disapproval of alcohol use by women (García, 1976; Caetano, 1983; Schaefer, 1982; White, 1982; Alcocer, 1982; and Gomberg, 1982).

The high prevalence of social drinking found in the two Hispanic samples is also consistent with what has been described previously. Alcohol consumption in Hispanic cultures is typically seen in relation to sports events, as well as other socialization activities such as baptisms and festivities. The acceptance of alcohol as a normal part of such routine socializing coupled with a permissive attitude toward drinking and drunkenness may be related to the high prevalence of social drinking found in these Hispanic samples.

These cultural attitudes toward drinking, especially toward female drinking, have been described as changing with increased acculturation among Mexican Americans. Caetano (1986c) found that acculturated Mexican Americans had a more liberal attitude toward drinking by women and older people than nonacculturated Mexican Americans. Furthermore, acculturated women themselves more often endorsed drinking five or more drinks at a sitting, and were less likely to be abstainers. Our data seem to confirm these findings.

Burnam (1989) found that whatever protection Mexican American women have from developing an alcohol disorder seems to diminish with increased exposure to the Anglo American culture. Consistent with that, we found that overall prevalence of alcoholism was identical for both the Puerto Rican and immigrant samples (13%), and considerably higher for the native Mexican American group (23%). One possible explanation for this difference in rates is that native Mexican Americans, as compared to immigrants, have been exposed to a longer period of discrimination, social alienation, and frustration, for which alcohol abuse becomes a commonly used means of escape (Burnam, 1989). Immigrants who are newly arrived to the United States are still able to guard against the long term effects of discrimination, and would tend to bring the drinking habits of their home culture with them. Island Puerto Ricans, of course, are not subjected to discrimination, since they constitute a majority in their own country. In fact, this may be the more plausible explanation for the higher rate of alcoholism among Mexican Americans as compared to non-Hispanic Los Angeles males reported by Burnam (1989).

Although they may certainly influence the patterns of drinking, the liberal attitudes toward drinking and drunkenness typical of Hispanic cultures does not seem to affect the prevalence of alcoholism. Neither the Puerto Rican nor the immigrant sample had higher rates of alcohol abuse and/or dependence than did the non-Hispanic ECA community samples in the United States. However, these two Hispanic groups exhibited very high rates of heavy drinking and intoxication among nonalcoholics.

Puerto Ricans and Mexican American immigrants thus exhibited not only similarities in the overall prevalence rates of alcoholism, but also similarities in rates of abstention and heavy drinking. The native Mexican Americans differed from the other two Hispanic groups regarding these variables, possibly due to their higher exposure to the U.S. culture, which, in turn, may have changed their attitudes and beliefs toward drinking practices.

There are a number of variables that do not seem to be influenced by cultural background. Although the male:female ratio varies between Puerto Ricans and immigrant and native Mexican Americans, alcoholism is a predominantly male disorder in all the Hispanic groups studied. Similarly, the presence of childhood conduct disorder and first intoxication before age 15 seem to be strong risk factors independent of culture. Drug addiction, mania, and antisocial personality were strongly associated with alcoholism in both the U.S. and Mexican American samples. Conversely, no strong association was found between alcoholism and depression for any of the samples studied. Similar results are reported in the chapter on the U.S. sample, and are corroborated by recent longitudinal research (Vaillant & Milofsky, 1982; Schuckit, 1983) on the association between affective disorders and alcoholism.

Puerto Ricans and Mexican Americans (whether natives or immigrants) differed on a number of variables associated with alcoholism. The mean age of onset of the first and last symptoms in Puerto Rico, as well as social drinking, was higher on the island as compared to the Mexican American sample. Similarly, there were fewer problem drinkers and fewer alcohol-related traffic offenses among the island Puerto Ricans as compared to Mexican Americans. One essential difference between island Puerto Ricans and Mexican Americans is that the former live in their country of origin and consequently are less exposed to the societal restrictions associated with alcohol use and drunkenness in the Anglo American culture.

Lower educational level was associated with a higher prevalence of heavy drinking among nonalcoholics and alcoholics in both the Puerto Rican and native Mexican American samples. This pattern was not observed in the immigrant sample. On the contrary, a higher educational level was associated with heavy drinking in this latter group. The association between lower educational level and higher prevalence of alcoholism as well as of heavy drinking has been established for different cultural groups such as Orientals, Anglo Americans, Canadians, and Mexican Americans (Robins et al., 1984; Helzer et al., 1989; Cahalan et al., 1969; Cahalan, 1970). One possible explanation for the increased rates of alcoholism with higher education among the immigrants is that higher educational level in this group is positively correlated with higher acculturation and consequently with a more liberal attitude toward drinking. Another possibility is that low education in immigrants is associated with income levels that are so low they inhibit alcohol consumption.

The comparison of two distinct Hispanic groups, one living in its country of origin and the other living in an Anglo culture, has allowed us to compare risk factors and correlates of alcoholism associated with Hispanic culture. We have found that sex, age of first intoxication, and childhood conduct disorder are risk factors that do not seem to vary across subcultural groups. Antisocial personality disorder as well as drug addiction and mania also appear to be strongly associated to alcoholism independent of the group studied. On the other hand, age of onset of the disorder, patterns of drinking, and symptoms associated to the social consequences of the disorder, as well as sex differences in risk for alcoholism, seem to vary across groups.

References

Alcocer, A. M. (1982). Alcohol use and abuse among the Hispanic American population. In U.S. National Institute on Alcohol Abuse and Alcoholism, *Alcohol and Health Monograph 4: Special Population Issues*. Rockville, Md.: Department of Health and Human Services, pp. 361–82.

Anthony, J. C.; LeResche, L.; Niaz, U.; et al. (1982). Limits of the Minimental State as a screening test for dementia and delirium among hospital patients. *Psychol. Med.* 12:397–408.

Aviles-Roig, C. A. (1973). Aspectos socioculturales del alcoholismo en Puerto Rico. In E. Tongue, R. T. Lambo, and B. Blair (eds.), *Proceedings of the International Conference on Alcoholism and Drug Abuse*. San Juan, Puerto Rico: ICAA Publication, pp. 78–85.

Barba, J., and Arana, M. Utilización y limitaciones de los indicadores para el estudio del alcoholismo en México. In U. M. Piñeiro, L. A. Berruecos, L. S. Medal (eds.), *El Alcoholismo en México: II. Aspectos Sociales, Culturales y Económicos*. México, D.F.: Fundación de Investigaciones Sociales, A.C., pp. 277–96.

Bird, H.; Canino, G.; Rubio-Stipec, M.; and Shrout, P. E. (1987). The use of the Minimental State Examination in a probability sample of a Hispanic population. *J. Nerv. Ment. Dis.* 175(12):731–737.

Bravo, M.; Canino, G.; and Bird, H. (1987). El DIS en español. *Acta Psiquiátr. Psicol. Am. Lat.* 33:27–42.

Burnam, A. (1989). Prevalence of alcohol abuse and dependence among Mexican-Americans and Nonhispanic whites in the community. In Spiegler, D. L.; Tate, D. A.; Aitken, S. S.; and Christian, C. M. (eds.), *Alcohol use Among U.S. Ethnic Minorities*. NIAAA Research Monograph No. 18; DHHS Publication No. (ADM) 88–1435. Washington, D.C.: U.S. Government Printing Office.

Burnam, M. A.; Karno, M.; Hough, R. L.; Escobar, J. I.; and Forsythe, A. B. (1983). The Spanish Diagnostic Interview Schedule: Reliability and comparison with clinical diagnoses. *Arch. Gen. Psychiatry* 40:1189–96.

Burnam, A. M.; Hough, R.; Karno, M.; Escobar, J.; and Telles, C. (1987). Acculturation and lifetime prevalence of psychiatric disorders among Mexican Americans in Los Angeles. *J. Health Soc. Behav.* 28:89–102.

Caetano, R. (1983). Drinking patterns and alcohol problems among Hispanics in the U.S.: A Review. *Drug Alcohol Depend.* 12:37–59.

Caetano, R. (1984). Ethnicity and drinking in northern California: A comparison among Whites, Blacks, and Hispanics. *Alcohol & Alcoholism* 19:31–44.

Caetano, R. (1984a). Manifestations of alcohol-related problems in Latin America: A Review. *Bull. Pan Am. Health Organ.* 8:258–80.

Caetano, R. (1984b). Hispanic drinking practices in Northern California. *Hispanic J. Behav. Sci.* 6:345–64.

Caetano, R. (1986b). Patterns and Problems of Drinking Among U.S. Hispanics. In *Report of the Secretary's Task Force on Black and Minority Health, Vol. VII: Chemical Dependency and Diabetes*. Washington, D.C.: U.S. Department of Health and Human Services pp. 143–86.

Caetano, R. (1986c). Drinking patterns and alcohol problems in a national sample of U.S. Hispanics. Forthcoming in U.S. National Institute on Alcohol Abuse and Alcoholism, *Alcohol Use Among U.S. Ethnic Minorities*, Research Monograph No. 18. Washington, D.C.: Government Printing Office.

Caetano, R. (1987a). Acculturation and drinking patterns among U.S. Hispanics Forthcoming, *Br. J. Addict.* 82:789–99.

Caetano, R. (1986e). Acculturation and attitudes on appropriate drinking among U.S. Hispanics. Working paper F-199. Berkeley, Calif.: *Alcohol Research Group*.

Caetano, R. (1987b). Acculturation, drinking and social settings among U.S. Hispanics. *Drug Alcohol Depend.* 19:215–27.

Caetano, R. (1989). Drinking patterns and alcohol problems in a national sample of U.S. In Spiegler, D. L.; Tate, D. A.; Aitken, S. S.; and Christian, C. M. (eds.), *Alcohol Use among U.S. Ethnic Minorities*, NIAAA Research Monograph No. 18, DHHS Publication No. (ADM) 147–162. Washington, D.C.: U.S. Government Printing Office.

Caetano, R.; Campillo-Serrano, C.; and Medina Mora, M. E. Alcohol use and associated problems: A comparison between U.S. and Mexico communities. Prepared for presentation at the Meeting on Alcohol Use in Latin America: *Cultural Realities and Policy Implications*, Providence, R.I., October 11–12, 1985.

Caetano, R., and Medina Mora, M. E. (1986). *Immigration, acculturation and alcohol use: A comparison between people of Mexican descent in Mexico and the U.S.* Prepared under contract for the National Institute on Alcohol Abuse and Alcoholism. San Francisco: Alcohol Research Group, Medical Research Institute of San Francisco.

Cahalan, D. (1970). *Problem Drinkers*. San Francisco: Jossey-Bass.

Cahalan, D.; Cisin, I. H.; and Crossley, H. M. (1969). *American Drinking Practices: A National Study of Drinking Behavior and Attitudes*. New Brunswick, N.J.: Rutgers Center of Alcohol Studies.

Cahalan, D., and Room, R. (1974). Problem drinking among American men aged 21–59. *Am. J. Public Health* 62:1473–82.

Canino, G. J.; Bird, H. R.; Shrout, P. E.; Rubio-Stipec, M.; Bravo, M.; Martínez, R.; Sesman, M.; and Guevara, L. M. (1987). The prevalence of specific psychiatric disorders in Puerto Rico. *Arch. Gen. Psychiatry* 44:727 35.

Canino, G. J; Bird, H. R.; Shrout, P. E.; Rubio-Stipec, M.; Bravo, M.; Martínez, R.; Sesman, M.; Guzman, A.; Guevara, L. M.; and Costas, H. (1987). the Spanish Diagnostic Interview Schedule: Reliability and concordance with clinical diagnoses in Puerto Rico. *Arch. Gen. Psychiatry* 44:720–26.

Canino, G.; Bird, H.; Shrout, P.; Rubio-Stipec, M.; Geil, K.; and Bravo, M. (1987). The prevalence of alcohol abuse and/or dependence in Puerto Rico. In M. Gaviria and J. Arana (eds.), *Health and Behavior: Research Agenda for Hispanics*. Research Monograph Series, vol. 1. Chicago, Illinois: Publication Services of the University of Illinois at Chicago, pp. 127–144.

Clark, W., and Midanik, L. (1981). Alcohol use and alcohol problems among U.S. adults: Results of the 1979 National survey. In *Alcohol Consumption and Related Problems, Alcohol and Health Monograph I*. DHHS Publication No. ADM82-1190. Washington, D.C.: U.S. Government Printing Office.

De la Parra, A.; Terroba, G.; and Medina Mora, M. E. (1980). Prevalencia del consumo de alcohol en la ciudad de San Luis Potosi. *Enseñanza e Investigación en Psicología* 2(12):236–45.

Department of Health of Puerto Rico. *Annual Report of Vital Statistics*. Administracion de Facilidadesy Servicios de Salud, Oficina de Estadisticas de Salud. San Juan, Puerto Rico.

Eaton, W. W.; Holzer, C. E.; Von Korff, M.; Anthony, J. C.; Helzer, J. E.; George, L.; Burnam, M. A.; Boyd, J. H.; Kessler, L. G.; and Locke, B. Z. (1984). The design of the Epidemiologic Catchment Area surveys. *Arch. Gen. Psychiatry* 41:942–48.

Escobar, J. I.; Burnam, A.; Karno, M.; et al. (1986). Use of the minimental state examination (MMSE) in a community population of mixed ethnicity. *J. Nerv. Ment. Dis.* 174:607–14.

Folstein, M. F.; Robins, L. N.; and Helzer, J. E. (1983). The minimental state examination. *Arch. Gen. Psychiatry* 40:812.

García, C. S. (1976). *Magnitud del Problema de Alcoholismo en Puerto Rico*. Unidad de Investigación Cientifica. Recinto de Ciencias Médicas. Rio Piedras, Puerto Rico: Universidad de Puerto Rico.

Gilbert, J. (1986). Alcohol related practices, problems and norms among Mexican-Americans: An overview. Forthcoming in U.S. National Institute on Alcohol Abuse and

Alcoholism, *Alcohol Use Among U.S. Ethnic Minorities,* Research Monograph No. 18. Washington, D.C.: Government Printing Office.

Gilbert, M. J., and Cervantes, R. C. (1986). Patterns and practices of alcohol use among Mexican Americans: A comprehensive review. *Hispanic J. Behav. Sci.* 8:1–60.

Gomberg, E. S. L. (1982). Special populations. In Gomberg, E. L., White, H. R., Carpenter, J. A. (eds.), *Alcohol, Science and Society Revisited.* Ann Arbor: University of Michigan Press.

Gonzalez, E. (1983). *Magnitud y patrones de consumo de alcohol en Puerto Rico.* Departamento de Servicios Contra la Adicción, Secretaria Auxiliar del Instituto y Servicios Especiales.

Haberman, P. W., and Sheinberg, J. (1967). Implicative drinking reported in a household survey: A corroborative note on subgroup differences. *Q. J. Stud. Alcohol* 28:538–43.

Hayes-Bautista, D. E. (1980). Identifying "Hispanic" populations: The influence of research methodology upon public policy. *Am. J. Public Health* 70:353–56.

Hayes-Bautista, D. E. (1983). On comparing studies of different Raza populations. *Am. J. Public Health* 73:274–76.

Heath, D. (1982). Historical and cultural factors affecting alcohol availability and consumption on Latin America. In *Legislative Approaches to Prevention of Alcohol-related Problems: An Inter-American Workshop* pp. 128–88.

Helzer, J. E.; Canino, G. J.; Hwu-H. G.; Bland, R.; Newman, S.; and Yeh, E. K. (1989). Alcoholism: A cross-national comparison of population surveys with the DIS. In R. M. Rose and J. Barret (eds.), *Alcoholism: A Medical Disorder.* New York: Raven Press. 33–47.

Holck, S. E.; Warren, C. W.; Smith, J. C.; and Rochar, R. W. (1984). Alcohol consumption among Mexican-American and Anglo women: Results of a survey along the U.S.-Mexican Border. *J. Stud. Alcohol* 45:149–54.

Karno, M.; Hough, R.; Eaton, W. (1983). Development of the Spanish language—version of the National Institute of Mental Health Diagnostic Interview Schedule. *Arch. Gen. Psychiat.* 40:1183–1188.

Kish, L. (1965). *Survey Sampling.* New York: John Wiley & Sons.

Maril, R. L., and Zavaleta, A. N. (1979). Drinking patterns of low-income Mexican-American women. *Q. J. Stud. Alcohol* 40:480–84.

Marrero, O. (1980). Comment on "Identifying Hispanic Populations." *Am. J. Public Health* 70:1112.

Masur, J., and Jorge, M. R. (1985). Alcohol-related data in Brazil: A Review. Presented at a meeting on "Alcohol use in Latin America: Cultural Realities and Policy Implications." Providence, R.I.: Brown University, October 11–12.

Medina-Mora, M. E.; De la Parra, C. A.; and Terroba, G. G. (1980). *Extensión del consumo de alcohol en la población de la Paz,* B. C. (Encuesta de Hogares). Cuadernos Cientificos CEMESAM 12:193–204.

Merikangas, K.; Leckman, J. F.; Prusoff, B. A.; Pauls, D. L.; and Weissman, M. M. (1985). Familial transmission of depression. *Arch. Gen. Psychiatry* 42:367–72.

Miguez, H. A. (1980). *Consideraciones acerca de la ingestión del alcohol en Costa Rica.* San José, Costa Rica: Instituto Nacional Sobre Alcoholismo, Departmento de Investigaciones.

Natera, G., and Terroba, G. G. (1982). Prevalencia del consumo de alcohol y variables demográficas asociados en la ciudad de Monterrey, N.L. *Salud Mental* 1(5):82–86.

Regier, D. A.; Myers, J. K.; Kramer, M.; Robins, L. N.; Blazer, D. G.; Hough, R. L.; Eaton, W. W.; and Locke, B. Z. (1984). The NIMH Epidemiologic Catchment Area program. *Arch. Gen. Psychiatry* 41:934–41.

Roberts, R. E., and Lee, E. S. (1980). Comment on "Identifying Hispanic Populations." *Am. J. Public Health* 70:1111.

Robins, L. N.; Helzer, J. E.; Weissman, M. M.; Orvaschel, H.; Cruenberg, E.; Burke, J. D.; and Regier, D. A. (1984). Lifetime prevalence of specific psychiatric disorders in three sites. *Arch. Gen. Psychiatry* 41:949–58.

Roizen, R.; Campillo-Serrano, C.; Medina-Mora, M. E.; Howard, A.; Riston, E. B.; Room, R.; and Rottman, I. (1983). Community Response to alcohol related problems: Four-country analysis. World Health Organization Study Draft. Berkeley, Calif.: Alcohol Research Group.

Rosovsky, H. (1985). Public health aspects of the production, marketing, and control of alcoholic beverages in Mexico. *Contemp. Drug Problems* 12:659–78.

Rosovsky, H. (1981). Panorama del Impacto del Consumo de Alcohol en Mexico. Read at Reunion International "Las estrategias preventivas ante los problemas relacionados con el alcohol." Mexico, D.F., June 6–7.

Sartorious, W. (1979). *Cross Cultural Psychiatry*. Berlin, Heidelberg: Springer Verlag.

Schaefer, J. M. (1982). Ethnic and racial variations in alcohol use and abuse. In U.S. National Institute on Alcohol Abuse and Alcoholism, *Alcohol and Health Monograph 4: Special Population Issues*. Rockville, Md: Department of Health and Human Services.

Schuckit, M. (1983). Alcoholism and other psychiatric disorders. *Hosp. Community Psychiatry* 34.

Schuckit, M. A. (1981). Genetic and clinical implications of alcoholism and affective disorder. *Am. J. Psychiatry* 143:140–47.

Selby, M. L.; Lee, E. S.; Tuttle, D. M.; and Loe, H. D., Jr. (1984). Validity of the Spanish surname infant mortality rate as a health status indicator for the Mexican-American population. *Am. J. Public Health* 74:998–1002.

Taylor, W. B. (1979). *Drinking Homicide and Rebellion in Colonial Mexican Villages*. Stanford, Calif.: Stanford University Press.

Terroba, G. G.; Medina-Mora, M. E.; and Saltijeral, M. T. (1977). *Estudio epidemiológico sobre el consumo de drogas, medicamentos y alcohol en la ciudad de Mexico, B.C., a través de encuestas de hogares*. Reporte Interno IMP. Mexico: Mexican Institute of Psychiatry.

Treviño, F. M. (1982). Vital and health statistics for the U.S. Hispanic population. *Am. J. Public Health* 72:979–82.

U.S. Bureau of the Census. (1985). 1980 Census of Population and Housing, Advance Reports PHC-80-V-1. Bureau of the Census.

U.S. Bureau of the Census. Persons of Spanish Origin in the United States (Series P-20, No. 403). Washington, D.C.: U.S. Department of Commerce, Current Population Reports.

Vaillant, G. E., and Milofsky, E. S. (1982). Natural history of male alcoholism. *Arch. Gen. Psychiatry* 39:127–33.

White, H. R. (1982). Sociological theories of the etiology of alcoholism. In Gomberg, E. L.; White, H. R.; and Carpenter, J. A. (eds.), *Alcohol, Science, and Society Revisited*. Ann Arbor: University of Michigan Press, pp. 205–32.

[III] Europe

[10] Alcohol Use, Abuse, and Dependency in West Germany: Lifetime and Six-Month Prevalence in the Munich Follow-up Study

HANS-ULRICH WITTCHEN AND THOMAS BRONISCH

Despite many regional differences, central European countries including Austria, West Germany, East Germany, and some German-speaking parts of Switzerland have shared for almost 2 centuries quite similar patterns of alcohol consumption. This holds true not only for the amount of alcohol consumed and drinking habits, but also for attitudes towards alcoholism. Moderate drinking is encouraged, even demanded, and alcoholism is condemned as manifest "lack of will power." Consumption patterns were strongly influenced in the first half of the nineteenth century by the humanistic and puritanical ideals of a strong temperance movement. It was at this time that the first inpatient facilities for the treatment of alcoholics ("Trinkerheilstätte" or drinkers' sanatoria), were

The authors would like to thank Dipl. Inf. Hildegard Pfister for the statistical analyses and her advice on an earlier draft of this paper.

The data reported here are part of the Munich Follow-up Study (MFS), funded by the Robert Bosch Foundation. The MFS is a comprehensive 6–8 year follow-up investigation of former psychiatric inpatients and a general population sample. Principal investigators are Prof. Dr. H. U. Wittchen and Prof. Dr. D. von Zerssen. The following researchers and interviewers contributed significantly to this study: Sabine Dehmel, Rosmarie Debye-Eder, Toni Faltermaier, Heide Hecht, all Dipl.-Psych.; Christian Krieg, M.D.; Reinhold Laessle, Ph.D.; Wolfgang Maier-Diewald, Dipl.-Psych.; Hans-Ulrich Rupp, M.D.; Gert Semler, Dipl.-Psych.; Karin Werner-Eilert, Ph.D.; Monika Wueschner-Stockheim, Ph.D.; and Georg Wiedemann, M.D. The clinical reexaminations reported in this paper were done by Michael Zaudig, M.D., and Gerhard Vogl, M.D.

founded (Feuerlein & Küfner, 1986). Temperance organizations, mainly run by religious groups, such as the Blaues Kreuz (Blue Cross) and the Kreuzbund (Alliance of the Cross), were also formed at this time. Partly as a result of these influences, alcohol problems became also a subject of scientific concern, especially since the second half of the nineteenth century. In Switzerland, leading researchers were Eugen Bleuler and August Florel, and in Germany mainly Emil Kraepelin, who published at least seventeen papers on this subject between 1891 and 1921.

After World War I and particularly during the Nazi period, scientific interest in alcoholism came almost to a complete halt (Feuerlein & Küfner, 1986). Alcoholics Anonymous (AA), founded as early as 1935 in the United States by two former alcoholics, was not introduced into central Europe until after World War II (Feuerlein & Küfner, 1986). It was not until the 1960s that strong interest again developed in research and treatment of alcoholism, and this was due in particular to the decision of the German Supreme Court in 1968 to recognize alcoholism as a disease. Since then, all costs of treatment are covered under the statutory health insurance schemes. Thus, many specialized inpatient and outpatient institutions for the treatment of alcoholism and alcohol-related problems have been established during the last 20 years.

Alcohol Consumption and Drinking Habits

In Europe as a whole, alcoholic beverages have always been generally available to anyone over the age of 18, in restaurants and elsewhere. The average consumption rates of alcohol in most European countries are rather high and stable, with marked variations only in times of disaster.

Alcohol consumption rates in some German speaking, central European countries from 1900 to 1983 are shown in Figure 10–1 (Schweizerische Fachstelle für Alkoholprobleme, 1986). In all of these countries we find a rather high alcohol consumption. Only predominantly wine drinking countries like Portugal (13.5), France (13.1), Spain (12.8), and Hungary (11.7) display higher or equally high total alcohol consumption rates in Europe. With the exemption of Austria, where no such data on a year-by-year basis are available, stable consumption rates have prevailed since 1980.

Regional variations notwithstanding, beer can be regarded as a national drink of all four countries emphasized in this chapter (excluding the French- and Italian-speaking parts of Switzerland). Brewed according to regulations sometimes dating back many centuries, beer is produced by thousands of often small and localized breweries, each with its own long tradition. The breweries have helped shape many different local festivities that encourage specific drinking patterns, such as the annual springtime presentation of the new strong beer ("Starkbier" or

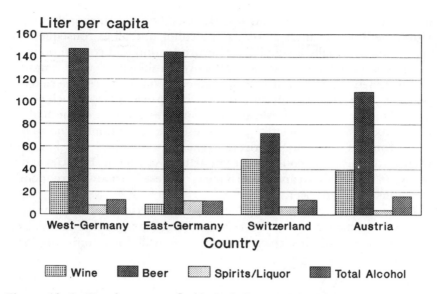

Figure 10–1a Development of Alcohol Consumption in Switzerland and Germany since 1900. Alcohol consumption in Switzerland is until 1975 averaged for a period of 5 years.

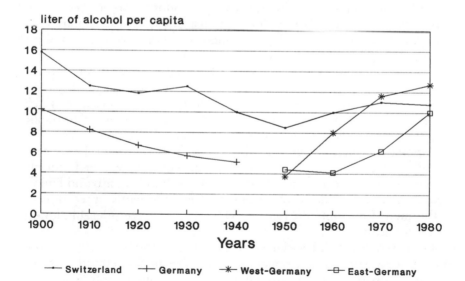

Figure 10–1b Alcohol Consumption in Central Europe (1983)—Alcohol/Year/Capita.

"Bockbier") and major festivals like the Octoberfest. During these festivities, the intake of huge amounts of alcohol, and all its consequences, is regarded as socially acceptable. The production and consumption of wine has an even longer tradition. However, unlike beer, wine is mostly not consumed daily, but more on special occasions or during periods of festivities. The trend is different in the wine growing areas, such as the Burgenland in Austria, the Mosel, and southwestern part of the Baden-Württemberg area in Germany, but these are exceptions. One major reason for this is its comparatively higher price. Spirits, whiskey, and other hard liquors are consumed regularly most often in East Germany, but also in the northern and eastern parts of West Germany—frequently in combination with beer.

These generalizations should be regarded as rough, and prevailing habits vary considerably within relatively small geographic areas. The remaining parts of this chapter, therefore, will focus only on West Germany.

Patterns of Alcohol Consumption in West Germany

Broadly, we can distinguish three types of areas with different patterns of alcohol consumption: (a) areas with a predominant use of beer (such as Bavaria), (b) areas with a predominant use of wine (western part, e.g., Mosel), and (c) areas with a high frequency of liquor consumers, most frequently together with beer (northern parts).

In an epidemiological survey of drinking habits in the adult population, Feuerlein & Küfner (1977) found that 51 percent of the adult population consumed alcohol daily or at least several times a week, 22 percent indicated that they almost never drink any kind of alcoholic beverages, and only 6 percent were completely abstinent.

Among the men, 60 percent drink primarily beer and 15 percent wine (Table 10–1). There is some overlap with 65 percent regularly drinking either beer or wine. Hard alcohol, such as Schnaps and liquor, is consumed "almost daily" by 21 percent, less frequently by 47 percent of the men. Consumption rates for females were considerably lower, except for wine.

Local festivities and social events, such as the Octoberfest in the Munich area, contribute dramatically to more or less episodic use of alcohol. Festivities and, in particular, the "Stammtisch" (56%), are the most frequent opportunities for the intake of larger amounts of alcohol. The "Stammtisch" is a primarily male institution, where a group of friends or small groups from social, sports, or professional organizations meet on the same evening each week in one special pub or bar always at the same specially designated table (thus the word Stammtisch or standing, regular table).

Alcohol consumption rates and drinking habits vary considerably

Table 10–1 Alcohol Consumption in the FRG (General Population survey 1974 (N = 1952) (from Feuerlein & Küfner, 1977)

	Males %	Females %	Total %
Frequency:			
Daily/almost daily	65	28	51
Almost never	10	32	22
Completely abstinent	—	—	6
Type of drink for those who drink at least several times a week:			
Beer	60	21	39
Wine	15	13	14
Beer and wine	65	28	47
Any hard drinks	29	15	21
Drinking Habits:			
Festivities	73	73	73
Regular "parties" (Stammtisch)	69	46	57
At work	14	3	17
TV	47	39	39
Lunch	15	10	12
Dinner	94	18	25
Alone	13	7	10

Not indicated.

Source: Feuerlein and Küfner (1977).

with age and sex. Wine and beer consumption is highest in the 30–39 year age group, with 72 percent of all men and 36 percent of women indicating almost daily consumption of at least one of these beverages. Hard drink consumption peaks at 40–49 years in men (35%) and at 50–59 in women (18%).

With regard to regional differences, the south German state of Bavaria would appear to have the highest number of regular wine and beer drinkers in Germany, with 82 percent of all Bavarian men and 38 percent of women indicating regular, daily consumption of either wine or beer. This compares to 56–64 percent of men and 22–29 percent of women in other geographical areas. Lower numbers for beer and wine consumption were also found for the northern states in Germany with an average of 58 percent for men and 23 percent for women. However, a higher number of subjects in the north regularly drink hard liquor, so there is no significant difference in the overall amount of alcohol consumed in the northern and southern German states.

Epidemiologic Studies

These data clearly indicate that alcohol is widespread, suggesting that alcohol-related problems might potentially constitute a major health issue. However, there are only few prevalence and incidence studies of alcohol dependence and abuse in the general population.

Feuerlein and Küfner's study (1986) consisted of a representative sample of the adult general population, which also constitutes Wave I of the Munich Follow-Up Study (MFS), described in detail below. The focus of this study was social and abusive drinking patterns, and relationships between drinking behavior, social variables, and physical and psychological complaints (see Table 10–4 for details of the assessment instruments). In addition to specific questions regarding consumption, alcohol-related problems and abuse were assessed by a self-rating scale, the "Kurzfragebogen für Alkoholgefährdete" (KFA) (Feuerlein et al., 1976; in English, 1980) and an "Index for Alcohol Abuse". The researchers found abuse rates of 7 percent for men and 1 percent for women (overall 3%), and described 22 percent as abstinent or nearly abstinent, 32–53 percent as modest consumers, 16–47 percent as heavy consumers, and 2–7 percent as pathological consumers.

Zintl-Wiegand et al. (1978) studied psychiatric morbidity in patients of general practitioners in the city of Mannheim. Using a semistructured interview approach, two research psychiatrists made diagnoses according to the ICD-8 and found a cross-sectional alcoholism rate of 5.9–6.6 percent.

Dilling et al. (1984) conducted a complex epidemiological survey between 1975 and 1979 in the upper Bavarian, predominantly rural county of Traunstein. Using a semistructured instrument, psychiatrists assigned diagnoses according to ICD-8. An overall illness prevalence of 24.1 percent was found, with 2.7 percent for alcoholism, and a further 2.4 percent with a high risk for having this diagnosis with a lower severity (p. 96).

In addition to these three studies, there exist some studies of the frequency of alcoholism in institutional settings. These show even more variation ranging from markedly lower to markedly higher rates. For example, in a separate analysis, Dilling et al. (1984, p. 106) reported markedly higher treated prevalence rates for alcoholism of 3.8 percent for psychiatric outpatient services, 10.8 percent for inpatient services, and 3.6 percent for general practitioners. In his review of general hospitals, Trojan (1980) reported rates varying between 0.4 and 1.2. However, Feuerlein and Küfner (1977), using a well validated instrument, the Munich Alcoholism Test (MALT), found rates as high as 10 percent of all inpatients. There are similar variations between other nonrepresentative studies, such as ones by Wieser (1973), Antons and Schulz (1976, 1977), and Wieser and Feuerlein (1976). Much of this variation can be explained by 1) the tremendous differences in the questions used to assess alcoholism, and 2) differences in the definitions for this disorder. Such variation argues for the use of a standardized diagnostic instrument, such as the DIS, and consistent definitions in order to make comparisons between studies more comparable.

Aims of this Chapter

The conclusions drawn in this chapter are based on results from the Munich Follow-Up Study adult general population sample, using the DIS to assess alcoholism and alcohol-related problems. The questions this chapter addresses are:

1. What is the prevalence of alcohol abuse and dependence according to the DIS/DSM-III criteria as assessed with the German version of the DIS (II)?
2. Which of the other mental disorders assessed by the DIS co-occur with alcoholism?
3. What type of alcohol is consumed?

Finally, some remarks on risk factors and stability of drinking patterns will be made.

Methods

The results reported are taken from a general population survey based on a random sample of the adult, West German population. This survey is part of a larger clinical and epidemiological follow-up study of former psychiatric patients and subjects from the general population, called the Munich-Follow-up Study (MFS).

Description of the MFS

The MFS is a comprehensive, 7-year follow-up of 1) 291 former psychiatric patients not dealt with here, and 2) a random sample of the adult general population of West Germany. The latter originally consisted of 2,524 subjects aged 16–65, who were selected for an initial examination in 1974. In this paper, we restrict the data presentation to those general population subjects who were followed-up over a 7-year period. (For more details compare Witchen et al., 1988.)

First Wave (1974): General Population Sample

At the index examination in 1974, 77.3 percent (1,952) of the subjects of the random population sample of 2,524 were successfully interviewed (Table 10–2). The interviews were done by a health research survey company using psychologists and other social professionals. The examination included questions about status, lifestyle, and attitudes; the assessment of psychopathology was made using self-administered rating scales and a brief IQ test.

The wave II examination, 7 years later, was planned as a more de-

Table 10–2 MFS-Wave I General Population Survey Response Rate, Attrition and the Selection (Exclusion Criteria) Process for Wave II

Wave I (1974)	Number	%
Number of subjects drawn in the original study:	2,524	100.0
Systematic drop-out (rejections, etc.):	533	21.1
Uncompleted interviews:	39	1.6
Completed interviews:	1,952	77.3
Selection for Wave II		
Application of exclusion criteria (IQ and Age)	487	—
Not eligible	99	—
Number of subjects for Wave II	1,366	—

tailed clinical follow-up; thus interviews were conducted exclusively by clinicians (psychiatrists and clinical psychologists). For economy, we excluded 487 subjects who were younger than 18, older than 57, or had an IQ below 85 (Figure 10–2). To ensure that we had both a representative random sample and a high number of "probable cases," a stratification method was used.

Wave II with the DIS (Version II)

Of the 657 subjects selected, 501 (76.3%) were interviewed, and this time the examination included the German translation of the DIS. Data analyses for the current paper were done on the 455 subjects with a full dataset, that is, no missing values in any of the "key" instruments (DIS, ICD checklist).

All selected subjects of the Wave I sample could be traced. At follow-up, 3.3 percent of the Wave I sample had died, 14.8 percent refused the reinterview completely, and 5.6 percent refused parts of it. Many refused the interview primarily because of an ongoing public discussion at the time about the possible misuse of personal data by state or federal supported research programs and a new privacy act, proposed by the federal government. For that reason, special attention was given both to the demographic characteristics of refusers, as well as their reasons for refusal. Based on Wave I data and a brief (usually telephone) interview with the refusers, it did not appear they differed significantly from nonrefusers in demographic distribution or psychopathology.

The sociodemographic characteristics of the 455 subjects reported in

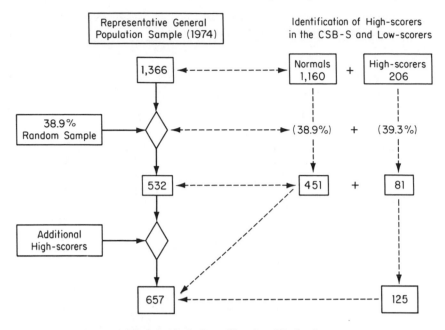

Figure 10–2 Stratification Method.

this chapter are shown in Table 10–3. Compared with the adult general population, there is a slight preponderance of women. Most of the subjects were married, living in inner city areas, and employed.

The German Version of the DIS

To summarize the design and to give a complete overview of the instruments used, Table 10–4 lists all assessment instruments. The German version of the DIS (Version II), its translation process, its reliability, and how its results compare to diagnoses according to the ICD have been extensively described elsewhere (Wittchen, 1984; Wittchen & von Zerssen, 1987). In order to meet our specific needs, some sections of the DIS were omitted or modified. Omitted were anorexia nervosa, pathological gambling, tobacco use disorder, ego-dystonic homosexuality, transsexualism, and cognitive impairment. The alcoholism section was modified to maintain a high degree of comparability with the instruments used in Wave I seven years earlier (before the DIS was available). Only one-quarter of the DIS questions in the alcohol section remained unmodified. Table 10–5 summarizes the modifications item by item. For most items, the self-report version of the MALT was used, and for some items DIS data were supplemented with health records. It can be seen that for some questions no clear equivalence is listed, as for the DIS item

Table 10–3 Sociodemographic Characteristics of Subjects (N = 455, Unweighted) in the MFS—1981—Wave II

			N	%
Sex:	Male		223	49.0
	Female		232	51.0
Age:		(Mean S.D.)	44.67 (9.53)	
Age groups:	25–45		256	56.3
	46–65		199	43.7
Marital status:	Single		35	7.7
	Married		370	81.3
	Other		50	11.0
Residence:	Innercity		256	56.3
	Suburb		108	23.7
	Rural		91	20.0
Professional status:	Working-full time		238	52.3
	Housewife		163	35.8
	Sickness status		5	1.1
	Unemployed		6	1.3
	Pension		31	6.8
	Other		11	2.4
	Missing value		1	0.2
Social class:	Lower		159	34.9
	Middle		278	61.1
	Upper		17	3.7
	Missing value		1	

154. Questions 152 and 153 were modified profoundly. These latter are of course only poor approximations of the item content of the original DIS. In spite of these modifications we applied the DIS diagnostic algorithm to our data in order to calculate the prevalence rates. These changes in the assessment procedure for alcoholism have to be taken into account when interpreting the diagnostic results and possible differences with other studies.

In addition to the DIS, social functioning of all subjects was assessed using the Social Interview Schedule (SIS) (Clare & Cairns, 1978; Hecht et al., 1987) and the Global Assessment Scale (GAS) (Spitzer et al., 1978). Utilization of in- and outpatient general and mental health services was assessed over the follow-up period.

Interviewers and Clinical Reexamination

Although the DIS is designed for use by either lay or clinician interviewers, only psychiatrists and clinical psychologists were used as interviewers in our study (Wittchen et al., in press). All subjects with a DIS diagnosis, plus other randomly selected subjects, were blindly reinterviewed by a psychiatrist from 2 days to 4 weeks after the DIS interview using the AMDP-DIASIKA Checklist (see Schmid-Bode et al., 1982; Guy and Ban, 1980) and all additional information the subject could make available to him. After the interview, the psychiatrist assigned a current (6-month) and a lifetime principal and secondary ICD-9 diagnosis, which will be compared here with the results obtained according to the DIS/DSM-III criteria. It has to be mentioned that the clinicians were not specifically told to screen for alcohol abuse and dependence, nor were items of this sort included in the AMDP/DIASIKA List.

Analysis

Diagnoses according to the DSM-III were generated by the DIS diagnostic computer program, which we modified to accommodate the changes we had made in the interview. The German DIS data were analyzed with the same program packages as used in the ECA to ensure an optimum of comparability. Prevalence rates for diagnoses were

Table 10–4 Design and Instruments Used in the MFS

	Index-Evaluation (wave I)		Course	Follow-up (wave II)	
	Patients (1973– 1975)	General Population Sample (1974)	(1974– 1981)	Patients (1981)	General Population Sample (1981)
Socialpsychological Assessment:					
Basic sociodemographic variables	*	*		*	*
Social data/Social Interview Schedule (SIS)	◄ *			*	*
Life Event Assessments (MEL)	◄ * ————————————		◄————— ◄	* ––––◄–*	
Psychological Assessment:					
Personality (PPI)	*			*	*
Paranoid-Depression-Scale (PD)	A* E *	*	* A * E *	*	*
Somatic Complaint List (BL)	A* E *	*	* A * E *	*	*
Global Assessment Scale (GAS)					*
IQ Test (MWT)	*				
Biographical data	◄ *				
Psychopathological Assessment:					
Basic records	◄A* E *		* A * E *◄	*	◄—*
Syndrome checklist (AMDP/DIASIKA)	*			*	
Diagnostic Interview Schedule (DIS)	◄————————————————		———◄	*	◄—*
Assessment of Illness Behavior:					
History of illness	◄ *————————————			◄–*––––◄–*	
Use of health services/type of treatment/course of treatment	◄ *—————————		•	*———◄–*––––◄–*	
Help-seeking behavior		*		*	*
Health behavior/health insurance		*		◄–*	◄–*

• in case of rehospitalization or utilization of medical/psychotherapeutic services
◄ retrospective assessment
A at admission
* assessment

Table 10–5 Comparison of the Original DIS (Version 2) Items with the Modified Items Used in MFS[a]

DIS No.	Text of Question in the DIS	Text in the Modification (MFS)
150	no modification except for self report	
151	no modification	
152	Have you ever drunk as much as a fifth of liquor a day, that would be about 20 drinks, or three bottles of wine or as much as 3 six-packs of beer in one day?	How often do you drink a lot of the following (beer, wine, spirits, liquor)? Rating options: almost daily (1), more than once a week (2), more than once a month (3), once or twice in the life, never (4). If coded 1–3—yes.
153	Has there ever been a period of two weeks when every day you were drinking 7 or more beers, 7 or more drinks or 7 or more glasses of wine?	as above: however, only codes of (1) and (2) were considered.
	How long has it been since?	No equivalence for this item.
154	not included	
155	Have you ever told a doctor about a problem you had with drinking?	Have you ever talked with your doctor about alcohol-related problems?
156	no modification, except for self report	
157	Have you ever wanted to stop drinking, but couldn't?	I have already tried unsuccessfully to stop drinking.
158	Some people promise themselves not to drink before 5 o'clock or never drink alone, in order to control their drinking. Have you ever done anything like that?	I have already tried a drinking system schedule (for example not to drink before certain hours).
159	Did you ever need a drink just after you had gotten up (that is before breakfast)?	I sometimes drink before breakfast.
160–163	no modification except for self report	
164	not included.	
165A	Not included, except: Did you neglect some of your usual responsibilities then (binges and benders)?	When I drink over longer time period I can't work or do my housework anymore.
166	Have you ever had blackouts while drinking, that is, where you drank enough, so that you couldn't remember the next day what you had said or done	It happened sometimes that I couldn't remember the next day, what happened after drinking alcohol.
167A–C	no modification	
168A	no modification	

(*continued*)

Table 10–5 (*Continued*)

DIS No.	Text of Question in the DIS	Text in the Modification (MFS)
168B	Alcohol-related health problems: vomiting blood or other stomach troubles?	Sometimes, especially in the morning, I have to vomit or have a lot of stomach problems.
168C	Trouble with tingling or numbness in your feet?	Sometimes I have a feeling of numbness in my feet or hands.
168	Memory trouble when you haven't been drinking?	During periods, when I have been drinking too much, I sometimes have memory problems.
168	Inflammation of your pancreas or pancreatitis?	Data taken from the medical records.
169	Have you ever continued to drink when you knew you had a serious physical illness, that might be made worse by drinking?	I have sometimes drunk alcohol, even when it was forbidden by the doctor.
170	no modification except for self report	
171	no modification	

ªOnly modifications are listed; for the remaining, see text.

weighted back to the total population from which the sample was obtained.

Results

Prevalence of Alcohol Abuse and Dependence

According to the DIS/DSM-III criteria, 13.0 percent of the adult general population (25–64) was found to fulfill the lifetime criteria for alcohol abuse, alcohol dependence, or both (Table 10–6). As expected, the rates for men (21.0%) were markedly higher than those for women (5.1%). The rates for alcohol abuse were considerably lower than those for dependence. This is quite surprising from the standpoint of European researchers, who usually find an inverse relationship when using the ICD, but presumably reflects the DSM-III definition. Alcohol dependence rates were highest for the 45–64 age group for both males and females.

Symptoms of Alcoholism

Among those meeting criteria for alcohol abuse or dependence, the most frequent symptoms are those that are considered classic signs for

Table 10–6 MFS: Lifetime Prevalence of Alcohol Abuse and Dependence in the Adult (Aged 25–64) Population Across Sex and Age Groups Based on the DIS (German Version)

		DIS/DSM-III Diagnoses			
		Alcohol Abuse	Alcohol Dependence	Alcohol Abuse and Dependence	Overall Prevalence
Males:	25–44	4.2	9.4	5.1	18.6
	45–64	1.7	17.3	4.9	23.9
	Total	3.0	13.0	5.0	21.0
Females:	25–44	0.8	0.8	1.4	2.9
	45–64	1.1	3.3	3.3	7.7
	Total	1.0	1.9	2.3	5.1
Total		2.0	7.4	3.7	13.0

alcoholism: not being able to do ordinary work without drinking, self-evaluation of being an excessive drinker, the wish to stop drinking, blackouts, and withdrawal symptoms (Table 10–7). The number of respondents who admitted alcohol-related job troubles (40%) and/or losing a job because of alcohol is particularly striking. It may be that such job troubles are confined to periods of extended alcohol-related festivities. During these festivities, many people miss work or are severely handicapped because of hangovers. Because no specific additional questions were asked with regard to this topic, however, no further data are available.

Similarly, the number of respondents with alcohol-related medical problems can be judged as extremely high. There might be several explanations for this finding. 1) The information on alcohol-related physical problems was partly assessed clinically in a separate part of the follow-up interview as well as by the health insurance records, and not by self report data in the DIS. Thus, we might assume that with the self-report there is a tendency to underestimate alcohol-related physical problems, whereas clinicians might be more sensitive or overinclusive, especially with regard to physical illnesses that might not have been caused but only "complicated" by alcohol. 2) This finding might also reflect the higher average age of our cohort, associated with a presumably higher risk for the development of physical disorders. This would be partly supported by the finding that the overall high number of alcohol-related lifetime symptoms can be mainly explained by men over 44.

Onset and Severity

The mean onset of the first alcohol symptom is well above 30 for the alcohol abuser group and just above 30 for the larger dependent group (Table 10–8). There are relatively few subjects indicating an onset before

Table 10–7 Symptom Frequencies (Unweighted Data) of Those with a Diagnosis of Abuse and/or Dependence (N = 67)

DIS (Version 2) Item Number[a]	Symptom	Proportion of Those with Alcohol Abuse and/or Dependence (N = 67) %
150	Family objected to respondent's drinking	36
151	Respondent thought himself an excessive drinker	61
152	Fifth of liquor in one day	b
153/54	Daily or weekly heavy drinking	b
155	Told physician about drinking problem	b
156	Friends or professionals said drinking too much	36
157	Wanted to stop drinking but couldn't	51
158	Efforts to control drinking	12
159	Morning drinking	55
160	Job troubles due to drinking	40
161	Lost job	40
162	Trouble driving	36
163	Arrested while drinking	36
164	Fights while drinking	b
165	Two or more binges	b
166	Blackouts while drinking	49
167	Any withdrawal symptom	49
168	Any medical complication	75
169	Continued to drink with serious illness	32
170	Couldn't do ordinary work without drinking	65

[a]See Appendix I for DIS Alcohol Section.

[b]Not assessed in the MFS or profoundly modified.

age of 25 (9%), but surprisingly more with a later onset in the 40s and 50s. This was unexpected, because the DIS determines onset of the disorder by asking, "What's the earliest age any of these things (the symptom questions asked) happened?" It does not ask at what age the respective symptoms clustered together for the first time. At first sight we thought that the relatively high average age of onset of the disorder could be explained by a cohort effect (because the youngest subjects in our study at the time of the interview were just about 25 years of age). However, this is unlikely because the age of onset for other disorders, such as phobias and other anxiety disorders, were well in the expected range. Other hypotheses, difficult to test, however, are memory prob-

Table 10–8 Onset, Severity and Duration of Alcohol-related Problems in the MFS

	Abusers (N = 10)		Dependents (N = 57)	
Mean age of onset	34.9	(7.6)	30.6	(12.1)
Mean number of symptoms	10.5	(2.1)	8.1	(4.2)
Mean duration	3.8	(4.5)	6.2	(5.9)

lems or the active attempt of the respondents to make a potential episode of alcoholism as short as possible ("denial effects"—see below).

The "severity," determined by a simple count of symptoms, revealed
a high mean symptom score for both groups. Abusers had even slightly
higher (NS) counts than dependers, due to a higher number of lifetime
psychosocial symptoms. In the dependency group, the high number of
subjects with symptoms of withdrawal is expected since the definition
requires this. Dependents also have a higher rate of alcohol-related
physical problems. The mean duration—that is, the time lapse between
the first occurrence and the last of any of the alcohol symptoms mentioned—was 3.8 years for abusers and 6.3 years for the dependency
group. The range varies from 1–13 years for abusers and 1–19 years for
dependents.

Six-Month Prevalence Rates and the Comparison with ICD Diagnoses

Whereas from the literature discussed in the Introduction and the
standpoint of European psychiatrists the DIS lifetime rates for alcoholism could be regarded as unusually high, there are considerable
changes when the 6-month prevalence rates are used. Only 1.3 percent
of all men and 0.9 percent of the women interviewed received a 6-month
DSM-III diagnosis of alcohol abuse or dependence Table 10–9. This
drop from lifetime to 6-month prevalence is dramatic and it may reflect
less willingness to admit current than past alcoholic symptoms. This
suggestion was partly supported by the clinical impression of the interviewers, who indicated a much higher percentage (overall 7.5%) of some
kind of current alcohol-related problem, including possibly alcohol-
related physical symptoms. However, consistent with the DIS, in most of
these cases the clinicians did not feel the reported symptoms were indic-
ative of clinical alcoholism. Furthermore, due to our modifications of the
DIS alcohol section, we included fewer symptoms in the inquiry about
recency, since twelve out the twenty-one DIS symptoms were covered in
other sections of our follow-up interview.

It is interesting to note that the 6-month rates of the DIS were very

*Table 10–9 MFS: Six-Month and Lifetime Prevalence of
DIS/DSM-III Alcohol Abuse and Dependence as Compared to the
ICD-Clinical Diagnosis (N = 455)*

	6-Month DSM-III	Lifetime DSM-III	Diagnosis ICD[a]
Male	1.3%	21.0%	0.98%
Female	0.9%	5.1%	0.46%
Total	1.2	13.0	0.8

[a]International Classification of Disease.

close to the results of the psychiatrists' reexamination. All but one current DIS/DSM-III case of alcohol abuse/dependence received a corresponding ICD-9 diagnosis, whereas for the lifetime comparison of ICD and DSM-III, extremely divergent results were found. This independent reexamination of all subjects revealed low ICD lifetime rates of about 1 percent for men and 0.5 percent for women, although the clinicians were encouraged to mention and code past as well as present diagnoses.

In order to learn more about these differences, we asked the psychiatrists to review all positive lifetime DIS/DSM-III alcoholism cases on the basis of DSM-III criteria (and not ICD) for alcoholism in order to see whether they might have overlooked the diagnosis, or whether they thought that the DIS criteria produced false positive diagnoses. Although there were a few cases where the clinician tended to change his judgment with regard to a past positive diagnosis, in most cases he claimed to have insufficient grounds for a positive diagnosis of either alcohol abuse or dependence. Although the clinicians agreed in 50 percent of the DSM-III alcoholism cases that there were some signs for alcohol abuse or possibly alcohol-related physical symptoms, these were not regarded as serious enough to justify a clinical ICD diagnosis.

This result does not throw into question the validity of the DIS approach to diagnose alcoholism; it merely points up the basic problem of reliable diagnosis, if clear criteria and diagnostic guidelines are missing, as is the case for the ICD-9. Based on the comments of the clinicians, we can furthermore assume that the clinical diagnostic decision process is primarily oriented towards the cross-sectional symptoms (possibly more often neglecting past symptoms) and is implicitly hierarchical. The latter includes the likelihood that alcoholic symptoms, especially if they are not clearly present at the time of the clinical examination, are usually not diagnosed if they occur together with other mental disorders (Wittchen & Von Zersson, 1987).

Comorbidity with Other Disorders

Respondents with either alcohol abuse or dependence have a slightly higher frequency of other DSM-III mental disorders (Table 10–10). Compared to the respective rates in the nonalcoholic group, the most frequent other disorders are panic disorder (8.7%), dysthymia (6.8), and medication abuse or dependence (5.9%). There was no indication of an association between alcoholism and major depression. In the majority of cases, other DSM-III disorders had an earlier onset than alcohol abuse or dependence. This applies especially to dysthymia and all phobic disorders, but it is difficult to draw any conclusions about causal connections between alcoholism and these other disorders.

Table 10–10 *Comorbidity of DIS/DSM-III Lifetime Diagnoses with Alcohol Abuse/Dependence*

	Weighted Percent with Positive DSM-III Diagnosis Among	
	Nonalcoholics %	Alcoholics %
Phobic disorders	11.8	14.7
Panic disorders	1.3	8.7
Dysthymia	3.3	6.8
Major depression	9.0	9.8
Drug disorders	1.5	5.9
Obsessive-compulsive disorder	2.2	2.0
Somatisation disorders	0.9	1.0
Any of the above DIS-Core diagnosis	22.5	29.2

Source: Feuerlein and Küfner (1977).

Drinking Patterns

When the current drinking habits of subjects with a lifetime diagnosis of alcohol abuse and/or dependence are analyzed, some significant, however not impressive, differences between the two groups can be seen. First, Table 10–11 indicates that there are more DIS alcoholics that drink daily beer, wine, and/or spirits. Second, the number of nonalcoholics who never drink beer is higher: 45.6 percent as compared to 22.8 percent in the alcoholic group. The clearest differentiation between groups, however, is found with regard to alcohol-associated problems as assessed in the MALT. The average number of alcohol-related psychosocial symptoms is significantly higher in the alcoholic group, with almost no overlap between groups.

The drinking pattern is generally quite stable over time. Of the few subjects who indicated in Wave I that they almost never drink alcohol, 51.8 percent gave the same answer at Wave II, seven years later. The respective numbers for moderate consumers were 63.1 percent, and for heavy consumers (see definition below), 56.4 percent. The risks for getting a lifetime DIS diagnosis of alcohol abuse/dependence was 8.1 percent for those who reported at Wave I that they almost never drank, 8.3

Table 10–11 *Use of Alcoholic Beverages and MALT-Mean Score in Alcoholics (Abuse and/or Dependence) and Nonalcoholics*

	Alcoholics %				Nonalcoholics %			
	Daily	Several times/ week	Several times/ month	Almost never	Daily	Several times/ week	Several times/ month	Almost never
Beer	44.6	15.8	16.8	22.8	15.6	20.3	18.5	45.6
Wine	16.8	7.9	27.7	47.5	3.7	11.2	39.6	45.6
Hard drinks	8.9	7.9	27.7	55.5	1.3	4.6	29.5	64.6
MALT-Score x̄ (s)		5.40	(4.0)			0.63	(1.21)	

Table 10–12 Some Selected Risk Factors and Correlates for Heavy Drinking and Alcoholism in the MFS Sample

	Proportion of All Drinkers Who Are Heavy Drinkers	Proportion of Heavy Drinkers Who Are Alcoholics
Total sample	32.7%	49.7%
Sex		
male	43.4%	52.7%
female	18.9%	40.7%
Marital Status		
single	36.5%	62.9%
married	32.7%	48.4%
separated/divorced/widowed	30.0%	50.0%
Years of education		
<8	33.2%	57.8%
8–12	30.7%	34.9%
>13	34.8%	35.6%
Social class (Moore and Kleimig)		
1,2 upper	39.1%	19.7%
3 middle	28.4%	48.4%
4 lower	35.2%	76.1%
Residence		
Urban	33.9%	41.8%
Rural	21.7%	78.7%
Mixed/suburban	39.5%	51.8%
Professional status		
not working	25.1%	70.2%
working	35.3%	44.8%
Drinking Habits at *Wave I* (seven years earlier)		
Heavy drinker	61.0%	50.1%
Drinks often at work	62.6%	63.5%
Drinks alone often	49.0%	52.7%
Drinks primary at dinner or meal	49.2%	39.8%
Any substance disorder		
no	32.2%	48.6%
yes	57.2%	75.3%
Any anxiety disorder		
no	32.3%	47.0%
yes	35.8%	65.8%

percent for Wave I moderate drinkers, and 28.3 percent for heavy drinkers.

Risk Factors

The analysis of correlates and the search for risk factors for alcoholism (see second column in Table 10–12) revealed the highest risk for unmarried, less skilled, lower class male subjects, especially if they have no jobs.

A slightly higher risk was found for rural than for suburban and inner city areas.

On the psychopathological level, having any other mental disorder and any other substance disorder or anxiety disorders in particular, increases the likelihood of getting a DIS/DSM-III diagnosis of alcohol abuse or dependence.

Of particular interest in our MFS was the question whether there are any specific patterns of alcohol consumption at Wave I that are related to the development of alcoholism as assessed in the DIS 7 years later. Of the four risk factors examined, only those subjects who drink often during work (63.5%) had a remarkably higher risk. "Heavy drinking" at Wave I as well as "often drinks alone" were only moderately associated with an alcoholism diagnosis in the DIS. With regard to risk factors for "heavy drinking at Wave II," no clear association was found, except for "heavy drinking" 7 years earlier at Wave I and "drinking during work."

Concluding Remarks

Before discussing these findings, the limitations of our study should be addressed. With regard to the diagnostic instrument, the DIS, it first has to be mentioned that a slightly modified way to assess the alcoholism criteria was used that seems to have affected at least some of the symptom counts. From these important differences we can learn how important it is to follow with great strictness the wording and the interview rules of the DIS. For some items, even a small deviation from the wording obviously affected the answers obtained.

Second, there are three factors that might have resulted in a diminished representativeness of our data: (1) As part of a follow-up study with two waves of interviews, we had attrition of subjects at both occasions. Although this does not seem to have damaged the representation of our sample, as discussed in the methods section, it might be that the rather low ICD rate for alcoholism could partially be explained by the loss of some "true" alcoholics, who have either died or refused the Wave I interview. (2) The sample size of the MFS is rather small; consequently, our error margins for the prevalence figures are rather large. (3) It has to be taken into account that our findings are based on an older age cohort. The youngest of the subjects was 25, the oldest 64, at the time of the examination with the DIS.

Aside from these methodological considerations stands the fact that the MFS, unlike other studies, offers two sets of data: the clinical findings as assessed by psychiatrists and psychologists, and the findings on the basis of the DIS.

With these aspects and methodological considerations in mind, it is surprising how similar our MFS lifetime results are to the data found in the ECA program. This applies not only to the overall rates, but also to the male–female ratio, some of the psychosocial risk factors, and the comorbidity aspects. The slightly lower overall prevalence might well be explained by the differences in the ethnic constitution of the samples as well as the higher mean age in our study. One important difference, however, is that unlike the ECA data, we do find the highest rates of abuse and/or dependence in the young or middle age groups. This result is in accordance with our finding that the most frequent DIS/DSM-III diagnostic criteria symptoms were those that were possibly alcohol-related. Because lifetime symptoms are cumulative, the increasing prevalence with age is not surprising.

It is important for further studies to examine specifically whether the higher frequency of physical alcohol-related symptoms in our cohort is just a simple product of our clinical assessment strategy (as opposed to the original self-report based DIS strategy) or whether this finding indicates a "true" difference. Since the overall alcohol consumption rates in Germany seemed to be higher than in the United States, it might be possible that the prevalence of alcohol-related physical problems is indeed higher in Germany.

In addition to the variation in the alcohol-related physical symptoms, we also found differences in the rank order of the most frequent symptoms. These may be related to cultural differences, such as greater permissiveness towards alcohol resulting in lower rates of subjects indicating that their environment objected to their drinking, and higher rates of subjects who drink daily or sometimes even in the morning and at work. These DSM-III symptoms may not have the same implications in Germany as elsewhere because they apply to a rather high number of non-alcoholic subjects during the times of the beer and wine festivals.

This may also help account for the differences between the DSM-III lifetime rates and the ICD rates found in our MFS. From the standpoint of European psychiatrists and their clinical understanding of alcohol abuse and dependence, our high DSM-III rates would probably be regarded with some caution. These reservations do not question primarily the validity of the DIS approach, but refer more to the DSM-III concept and its explicit criteria for alcohol abuse and dependence. Most DIS/DSM-III cases would not be regarded as "clinical cases" in Germany, even with a generous broad ICD concept of alcoholism.

This difference may be contributed to by the following factors:

1. A different understanding of alcohol abuse and maybe less pronounced also for dependence, that also relates to nosologic differences in the ICD-9 and DSM-III. As an example, it can be mentioned that in ICD the diagnosis of abuse is probably more a subthreshold diagnosis, whereas in DSM-III it constitutes a group of its own.

2. The way in which alcoholism criteria are specified in the DSM-III. Since the necessary symptom criteria for abuse and dependence do not have to cluster together but might occur consecutively in the subject's life, the higher rates might result from an accumulation of temporally unrelated symptoms or problems.
3. With the similar and lower DIS 6-month rates in mind, it is also plausible that many respondents with alcohol problems denied the presence of symptoms, but more easily admitted past symptoms and so were missed by the clinicians, since they did not systematically inquire about this.
4. Because of the clinician's traditional focus on a subject's present condition, there would also likely be less emphasis on a past diagnosis of alcoholism when some other current diagnosis is present. The good concordance between the clinician's ICD and the DIS/DSM-III 6-month diagnosis for alcohol abuse/dependence also seems consistent with this.

With these differences in mind, we can state that using the DSM-III criteria and adopting the DIS lifetime approach results in findings similar to the US-ECA program: Alcohol abuse and dependence are the most frequent disorders in men. Despite the fact that German society is obviously more permissive towards alcohol than many others, the rates are not higher than in the ECA. This permissiveness may, however, influence the symptom structure, which does seem to be different from that found in the ECA. This may be an important explanation, for example, of the higher rate of physical symptoms that can be related to alcohol.

References

American Psychiatric Association Committee on Nomenclature and Statistics (1980). *Diagnostic and Statistical Manual of Mental Disorders*, third ed. Washington, D.C.: American Psychiatric Association.
Antons, K., Schulz, W. (1976 and 1977). Normales Trinken und Suchtentwicklung. Theorie und empirische Ergebnisse interdisziplinärer Forschung zum sozialintegrierten Alkoholkonsum und süchtigem Alkoholismus. Bd. I und II, Hogrefe, Göttingen.
Bronisch, T.; Wittchen, H.-U.; Krieg, C.; Rupp, H.-U.; and von Zerssen, D. (1985). Depressive neurosis—A long-term prospective and retrospective follow-up study. *Acta Psychiatr. Scand.* 71:237–48.
Clare, A. W., and Cairns, V. E. (1978). Design, development and use of a standardized interview to assess social maladjustment and dysfunction in community studies. *Psychol. Med.* 8:589–604.
Degkwitz, R.; Helmchen, H.; Kockott, G.; and Mombour, W. (1975). Diagnosenschlüssel und Glossar psychiatrischer Krankheiten: ICD-8. New York: Springer.
Dilling, H.; Weyerer, S.; and Castell, R. (1984). Psychische Erkrankungen in der Bevölkerung. Stuttgart: Enke.
Feuerlein, W.; Küfner, H.; Ringer, C.; and Antons, K. (1976). Kurzfragebogen für Al-

koholgefährdete (KFA). Eine empirische Analyse. *Archiv. Psychiatr. Nervenkr.* 222:139–52.

Feuerlein, W., and Küfner, H. (1977). Akloholkonsum, Alkoholmissbrauch und subjektives Befinden: Ergebnis einer Repräsentativerhebung in der Bundesrepublik Deutschland. *Arch. Psychiatr. Nervenkr.* 224:89–106.

Feuerlein, W.; Ringer, C.; Küfner, H.; and Antons, K. (1980). Diagnosis of Alcoholism: The Munich Alcoholism Test (MALT). In M. Galanter (ed), *Currents in Alcoholism,* Volume VII. London: Grune and Stratton, Inc.

Feuerlein, W., and Küfner, H. (1986). Alcohol and alcohol problems research. II. Federal Republic of Germany. *Br. J. Addict.* 81:613–19.

Guy, W., and Ban, T. A. (1980). The AMDP-System Manual for the Assessment and Documentation of Psychopathology. New York: Springer.

Hecht, H.; Faltermaier, T.; and Wittchen, H.-U. (1987). Social Interview Schedule (SIS). Ein Verfahren zur Beschreibung sozialer und sozialpsychologischer Faktoren der Lebenssituation. (Deutsche überarbeitete Version, 3. Fassung). . . . : Roederer Verlag.

Schmid-Bode, W.; Bronisch, T.; and von Zerssen, D. (1982). A comparative study of PSE/Catego and DiaSika: Two psychiatric computer diagnostic systems. *Br. J. Psychiatry* 141:292–95.

Schweizerische Fachstelle für Alkoholprobleme (1986). *Zahlen und Fakten zu Alkohol—und Drogenproblemen 1985/1986.* Verlag Schweizerische Fachstelle für Alkoholprobleme, Bern.

Semler, G., and Wittchen, H.-U. (1983). Das Diagnostic Interview Schedule—Erste Ergebnisse zur Reliabilität und differentiellen Validität der deutschen Fassung. In D. Kommer, and B. Röhrle (eds.), *Gemeindepsychologische Perspektiven* (3), Köln, 109–17.

Spitzer, R. L.; Endicott, J.; and Robins, E. (1978). Research Diagnostic Criteria. Rationale and reliability. *Arch. Gen. Psychiatry* 35:773–82.

Trojan, A. (1980). Epidemiologie des Alkoholkonsums und der Alkoholkrankheit in der Bundesrepublik Deutschland. *Suchtgefahren* 26:1–17.

Wieser, A. (1973). *Das Trinkverhalten der Deutschen.* Nicolai, Herford.

Wieser, S., and Feuerlein, W. (1976). Über die Prävalenz des Alkoholismus (Alkoholmissbrauch und Alkoholabhängigkeit) im Bundesland Bremen. *Fortschr. Neurol. Psychiatr.* 44:447–61.

Wittchen, H.-U. (1984). *The German Version of the Diagnostic Interview Schedule* (DIS Version 2)–Reliability and Results from a General Population Survey, Report to the Division of Biometry and Epidemiology, NIMH.

Wittchen, H.-U. (1988). Natural cause and spontaneous remissions of untreated anxiety disorders—results of the Munich Follow-up Study (MFS). In I. Hunt and H.-U. Wittchen (eds.), *Panic and Phobias 2*: Treatments and variables affecting cause and outcome. Springer: Berlin, Heidelberg, New York, Tokyo.

Wittchen, H.-U.; Hecht, H.; Zaudig, M.; Vogl, G.; Semler, G.; and Pfister, H. (1988). Häufigkeit und Schwere psychischer Störungen in der Bevölkerung.—Eine epidemiologische Feldstudie—. In H.-U. Wittchen, and D. von Zerssen, (Eds.), *Verläufe behandelter und unbehandelter Depressionen und Angststörungen.* Springer, Berlin, Heidelberg, New York, Tokyo (in press).

Wittchen, H.-U., and von Zerssen, D. (1987). *Verläufe behandelter und unbehandelter Depressionen und Angststörungen.* Springer: Berlin, Heidelberg, New York, Tokyo.

Zerssen, D. v., unter Mitarbeit von Koeller, D. M. (1976). *Klinische Selbstbeurteilungsskalen (Ksb-S) aus dem Münchner Psychiatrischen Informationssystem* (PSYCHIS München). Manuale. a) allgemeiner Teil. b) Paranoid-Depressivitätsskala. c) Befindlichkeitsskala. d) Beschwerdenliste. Beltz, Weinheim.

Zintl-Wiegand, A.; Schmidt-Manshart, C.; Leisner, R.; and Cooper, B. (1978). Psychische Erkrankungen in Mannheimer Allgemeinpraxen. Eine klinische und epidemiologische Untersuchung. In Häfner, H. (Ed.), *Psychiatrische Epidemiologie.* Springer: Berlin, Heidelberg, New York, Tokyo.

[11] Alcoholism, Culture, and Psychopathology: A Comparative Study of French, French Canadian, and American Alcoholics

THOMAS F. BABOR, AMY WOLFSON, DENYSE BOIVIN,
SIMONE RADOUCO-THOMAS,
AND WILLIAM CLARK

This chapter departs considerably from others in this book in that it approaches the subject of alcohol and culture from the viewpoint of clinical samples of diagnosed alcoholics. Although emphasis is given to the prevalence and patterning of alcohol problems in France and other French-speaking countries, this will be approached from a comparative perspective in an effort to highlight some important but highly speculative notions about the patterning of alcoholism and how it is affected by cultural and psychological variables. These notions will first be summarized to set the stage for subsequent comparisons of French, American, and French Canadian alcoholics. These groups are particularly appropriate for such a comparative analysis because they represent different points on a continuum of cultural permissiveness toward alcohol that has often been cited in sociocultural theories of alcoholism.

The French have long been notorious for their affinity to alcohol and their affliction with alcohol-related problems. Their daily pattern of consumption and preference for wine has undoubtedly contributed to a

This work was supported in part by a grant from the National Institute on Alcohol Abuse and Alcoholism (P50-AA03510). The authors would like to thank Michie Hesselbrock, Roger Meyer, Jean Yves Benard, and Meredith Weidenman for their assistance in the collection and analysis of the data.

more quiescent form of alcoholism, characterized by later onset and physical, rather than psychosocial, consequences of drinking. Other chapters in this volume have described the history of drinking and alcohol problems in the United States. Cultural diversity, geographic mobility, the frontier style of drinking to intoxication, and the long history of alcohol control efforts in the United States have all been implicated in the development of a national drinking pattern that is more erratic and socially disruptive than that observed in wine-producing countries like France. Although Quebec was settled by French Protestants in the seventeenth century and remains close to France in language and culture, it also shares many features in common with the English-speaking provinces of Canada. In particular, the beverage preferences and drinking patterns are more similar to the English than the French.

Alcoholism, Psychopathology, and Culture

In this chapter we will use data collected from clinical samples of diagnosed alcoholics in three countries as a means of testing hypotheses derived from two related sociocultural theories of alcoholism proposed by E. M. Jellinek (1960, 1962) and Benjamin Kissin (1977). These rather loosely constructed theoretical notions describe a set of relationships among cultural variables, psychological disorder, and patterns or types of alcoholism. Jellinek's formulation was based on his observations of the prototypical types of excessive drinkers found in France and the United States. The "inveterate drinker" typical of France is characterized by daily heavy drinking in the absence of overt intoxication. Sociocultural and economic factors, rather than psychological vulnerability, are thought to predominate in the development of this type of heavy drinking pattern. In contrast, the symptomatic drinker, thought to be typical of the United States and the "Anglo-Saxon" countries, is characterized by impaired control of alcohol consumption, frequent intoxication, and drinking to escape from psychological problems. When these patterns of excessive drinking occur in the presence of physical dependence symptoms (i.e., tolerance and withdrawal), they are termed by Jellinek the delta and gamma varieties of alcoholism, respectively. According to Jellinek (1960, pp. 28–29):

In societies which have a low degree of acceptance of large daily amounts of alcohol, mainly those will be exposed to the risk of addiction who on account of high psychological vulnerability have an inducement to go against the social standards. But in societies which have an extremely high degree of acceptance of large daily alcohol consumption, the presence of any small vulnerability, whether psychological or physical, will suffice for exposure to the risk of addiction.

Jellinek's sociocultural theory of alcoholism has been reformulated by Kissin (1977) in terms of the "psychosocial principle." This hypothesis

states that the degree of psychopathology associated with the development of alcohol dependence is inversely related to the level of acceptance of alcohol abuse in that individual's subculture. A corollary of this
hypothesis (Kissin, 1983) is that "the degree of psychopathology necessary to develop alcoholism is inversely proportional to the strength of
the biological and social influences tending in that direction" (p. 104). In
this conceptualization, the etiological origins of alcoholism in a given
individual may be biological, psychological, social, or a combination of
each. The summation of these factors represents an index of predisposition. The more that one factor is operative, the less others need to be
present to precipitate the development of alcoholism. On the aggregate
level, the rate and type of alcoholism will reflect the relative contributions of biological, psychological, and social influences. In France, where
social encouragement is given to heavy drinking, psychopathology can
be expected to play less of a role in the clinical profile of alcoholism than
it does in countries such as the United States, where drinking is viewed
more as an escape from unpleasant feelings or circumstances.

Given the intermediate position of Quebec between French and
Anglo-American culture, one would expect that French Canadian alcoholics would represent an amalgam of both patterns of alcoholism.

While our own analyses will by no means provide a definitive test of
hypotheses derived from these sociocultural theories, they will help to
illustrate an approach that could serve as a model for future research.
The data sets were obtained from alcoholic patients at representative
treatment facilities in Hartford, Connecticut; Quebec City, Canada; and
Tours, France. These patients, particularly the French and American
alcoholics, belong to national cultures that differ markedly in the general
acceptance of heavy drinking by men. According to the psychosocial
principle, one would predict a lower prevalence of psychopathology
among French male alcoholics, and higher rates among American and
French Canadian men. A second hypothesis concerns the relative differences between men and women in the prevalence of psychopathology. Regardless of national culture, the prevalence of psychopathology should be higher among women than men, given the
subcultural norms that discourage heavy drinking by women in almost
all societies. A third prediction concerns the relationship between psychopathology and the patterning of alcoholism in different cultural
groups. One explanation for the more intensive, rapid, and socially disruptive type of alcoholism observed among men in countries like the
United States is that psychopathology plays a more significant role in the
etiology of gamma alcoholism than of delta alcoholism. If this is the case,
then regardless of culture, the degree of psychopathology should be
associated with earlier onset, more rapid course, more severe symptoms,
and worse prognosis. These relationships, if demonstrated, might ex-

plain why French alcoholism is considered to be qualitatively different from American alcoholism.

Methods and Procedures

Sample Selection and Patient Characteristics

Male and female alcoholic patients were recruited randomly from representative alcoholism treatment facilities in three comparable urban areas located in the United States, Canada, and France. The facilities were chosen to recruit patients from a broad range of socioeconomic backgrounds. The American patients ($N=321$) were recruited from three facilities in the area of Hartford, Connecticut. Approximately 55 percent of the sample came from a university-affiliated health center, 21 percent from a Veterans Administration Medical Center, and 24 percent from a state-funded freestanding treatment facility for alcohol and/or substance abuse patients. The sample of French alcoholics (65 males, 82 females) was drawn from Centre Louis Sevestre, one of the largest alcoholism treatment facilities in France, located near the city of Tours in the Loire Valley. These patients were part of a larger sample ($N=306$), of which 147 were interviewed with the Diagnostic Interview Schedule for the purpose of the present study. Patients were referred from a large variety of medical facilities and social service agencies. The majority were identified in work settings. Although the region around Tours accounted for the largest proportion of patients, approximately one-half were referred from other parts of France.

The French Canadian alcoholics (58 males, 28 females) were recruited from the inpatient and outpatient services of the Department of Alcohology, Hopital Saint-François d'Assise, Quebec, Canada. Approximately 1,500 patients are admitted each year for treatment of alcohol- and drug-related disorders, making this facility the largest public alcoholism treatment hospital in eastern Quebec.

Table 11–1 summarizes the personal and demographic characteristics of the three samples. The male patients in each sample were comparable in mean age (39 years), but the French females (40.5 years) were slightly older than the Americans (37.2 years). Despite the overall similarity in age among men and women in the three samples, reported onset of DSM-III alcoholism symptoms was approximately 5 years earlier in each of the male samples. While the American and French Canadian patients indicated similar onset ages, the French men and women reported first alcoholism symptoms approximately 6 years later than their North American counterparts. The samples also differed with respect to marital status. The American alcoholics had a higher proportion

Table 11–1 Personal and Demographic Characteristics of American, French Canadian, and French Alcoholics

	Males			Females		
	Hartford (N = 231)	Quebec (N = 58)	Tours (N = 65)	Hartford (N = 90)	Quebec (N = 28)	Tours (N = 82)
Current age	39.5	39.7	38.5	37.2	39.9	40.5
Age onset DSM-III alcoholism	24.9	25.9	31.4	30.8	30.3	36.1
% Married	26.8%	36.8%	49.2%	34.4%	38.5%	50.7%
% Post-secondary education	31.6%	16.3%	10.0%	22.5%	22.5%	21.4%

of patients who were single, divorced, and separated, while the French had the greatest proportion of married persons. There were no significant cross-national differences in educational achievement. The Americans had a slightly greater proportion with post-secondary education and the French had greater representation in the technical/secondary category. It is impossible to determine whether these samples are representative of the population of alcoholics within the three countries. This question is of less concern to the present investigation because, as described below, the samples were chosen primarily to test for cross-national similarities in the relationship between psychopathology and drinking, rather than to identify cross-cultural differences in behavior and symptoms.

Procedure

An extensive battery of assessments was administered to each patient as part of a multidisciplinary, cross-national, longitudinal study of alcoholic subtypes. The assessments of primary interest to the present study are the NIMH Diagnostic Interview Schedule (DIS) (Robins et al., 1981; Helzer et al., 1981) and the Last Six Months of Drinking Questionnaire (Hesselbrock et al., 1983). The first version of the DIS was used to interview the French sample, while the second revision was used in the American and French Canadian samples. Both the French and French Canadian translations were accomplished by bilingual speakers using back translation as a method of checking accuracy. The DIS was scored using DSM-III criteria to obtain information about the prevalence and ages of onset of major psychiatric disorders. This information was used to classify patients according to "primary" or "secondary" alcoholism. In primary alcoholism, either there is no psychiatric disorder, or alcoholism antedates the onset of other disorders. Primary alcoholics were therefore defined by the presence of DSM-III alcoholism symptoms prior to, or in the absence of, the onset of other DSM-III disorders. In secondary alcoholism, the onset of psychiatric disorders (that are not related to alcohol abuse) precedes the onset of alcohol problems.

The Last Six Months of Drinking Questionnaire was used to assess reasons for drinking, recent dependence symptoms, quantity and frequency of drinking, and the consequences of heavy alcohol consumption. The reliability and validity of responses measured by representative parts of this questionnaire have been established in separate validation studies of the U.S. sample (Hesselbrock et al., 1983) and the French sample (Babor et al., 1981). The questionnaire was designed to obtain information about behaviors, signs, and symptoms that are: a) amenable to verbal description, b) within the patient's realm of awareness or knowledge, and c) capable of being rated on frequency or intensity scales. Self-report items measuring recent drinking experiences and problems were selected from the criteria proposed by the National Council on Alcoholism (Criteria Committee, 1972) or were derived from sources where previous research (Edwards & Gross, 1976; Perrin, 1964; Mulford & Miller, 1960) had demonstrated their usefulness as measures of relevant constructs (e.g., alcohol dependence, alcohol-related problems). Most items are phrased in the first person to facilitate comprehension and personal identification by the patient, and are rated on a 5-point scale of frequency ranging from never (in the last 6 months) to very frequently (i.e., every day).

Additive scales were created from the results of parallel factor analyses that identified common sets of items conforming to the following content areas (see Hesselbrock et al., 1983, and Babor et al., 1987, for discussion of scale development):

1. *Alcohol dependence.* This scale includes fourteen items measuring tolerance, withdrawal symptoms, impaired control, morning drinking, and preoccupation with alcohol. These symptoms conform closely to the alcohol dependence syndrome concept as proposed by Edwards and Gross (1976).
2. *Social problems.* Six items dealing with various alcohol-related social consequences comprise this scale. These items ask about the frequency of family complaints, job problems, threats from spouse, legal difficulties, violent behavior, and accidents or injuries.
3. *Physical consequences.* Five items were combined to measure physical and neurological changes associated with chronic drinking: black and blue spots on skin, flushed face, impotence, difficulty in concentrating, and problems with abstract thinking.
4. *Social reasons for drinking.* This scale includes four items measuring social reasons for drinking: to celebrate special occasions, to be with other people, to conform with other people's expectations, and as a mealtime beverage.
5. *Psychological reasons for drinking.* Nine items were added to operationalize the concept of "escape" drinking for psychological motives: helps to relax, helps to forget worries, improves bad

mood, relieves tension, to feel better, to mix better with people, to get the effect of alcohol, to relieve tiredness, to get to sleep.

The questionnaire also included a set of items measuring the quantity and frequency of alcohol consumption. These were derived from interview items used in national surveys (e.g., Cahalan, Cisin, & Crossley, 1969) to estimate how often the respondent drinks, and the usual amount consumed on a typical day of drinking. The response categories were modified so that the upper limits of consumption would be more sensitive to alcoholic drinking patterns. The Americans and Canadians were asked to report on three beverages (beer, wine, liquor). The French responded to questions about these beverages as well as cider and aperitifs. After multiplying the quantity and frequency responses for each beverage, an estimate is obtained of the daily amount of absolute alcohol consumed each day during the 6 months prior to hospitalization.

As in all cross-national research, the problem of translating the instrument to achieve semantic equivalence was crucial. Initially developed in English, all items were first translated into French by a bilingual native French translator. The modified translation was then studied by three monolingual treatment personnel at the Centre Louis Sevestre. Appropriate modifications were again made to assure that the items were comprehensible to patients in French-speaking Canada.

Follow-up evaluations were conducted using an extensive interview schedule. Eighty-four percent ($N=266$) of the American patients known to be alive were located and interviewed at one year, while 74 percent were reinterviewed at 3 years. In the French sample, twenty-two patients in the DIS interview sample were located 4 years after discharge. These patients were chosen because of their proximity to Tours. Although the sample is small, it represents more than 90 percent of the interviews attempted and is therefore considered representative of the larger DIS sample. The French Canadian sample was reinterviewed at 1 year post-discharge. Fifty-four percent ($N=31$) of the male patients were located. As with the French follow-up sample, this group is considered too small to provide anything more than a tentative replication of the findings from the larger American sample.

Results

Table 11–2 summarizes information pertaining to the prevalence of major DSM-III diagnoses in the three samples. Among women alcoholics, depression was the most prevalent psychiatric disorder, while antisocial personality (ASP) and/or drug dependence were most often diagnosed in men. Although phobias and other anxiety disorders were also prevalent, the psychoses were infrequent, possibly because these

Table 11–2 Prevalence[a] of Major DSM-III Psychiatric Disorders in Samples of French, French Canadian, and American Alcoholics

	Hartford		Quebec		Tours	
	Males	Females	Males	Females	Males	Females
Alcoholism only	25%	20%	21%	10%	50%	37%
Depression	32%	52%	42%	41%	20%	60%
Antisocial personality disorder	49%	20%	16%	14%	30%	6%
Drug abuse/dependence	45%	38%	27%	38%	2%	2%
Phobia	20%	44%	34%	38%		
Average number of DSM-III psychiatric diagnoses	2.46	2.46	2.83	2.64	2.68	1.63

[a]Percentages can total more than 100% within a sample of males or females because of multiple diagnoses in some individuals.

patients are typically treated in psychiatric settings. Although greater proportions of the males than females were diagnosed as having "alcoholism only" (i.e., no psychiatric co-morbidity), there were no significant differences in the average number of psychiatric diagnoses between the sexes within each sample.

Table 11–3 describes the results of statistical comparisons between primary and secondary alcoholics within each sample. Among males, ASP was the most frequent psychiatric diagnosis that occurred before the onset of alcoholism. This group was therefore chosen as the most representative type of male secondary alcoholic in order to test the hypothesis that antecedent psychiatric disorder in alcoholics predisposes individuals to a more virulent and severe form of alcoholism. Similarly, the occurrence of antecedent depression in women was used to classify a group of secondary alcoholics in each of the female samples. It should be noted that the samples of primary and secondary alcoholics are very small in the Quebec sample. Caution is therefore recommended in the interpretation of these data.

Another reason that antisocial personality disorder and depression were chosen to define the primary/secondary distinction is because these disorders have most often been implicated in etiological theories of male and female alcoholism, respectively (Kissin, 1977). By choosing males with primary ASP and females with primary depression, it becomes possible to evaluate the contribution of the same types of antecedent psychopathology across the three national samples. To the extent that the relationships are consistent across national groups, this would be evidence for the cross-national generalizability of the psychopathology-drinking relationship.

The groups were compared within categories of sex and nationality by means of the Student's *t* test. The results, shown in Table 11–3, indicate that primary male alcoholics differ consistently across all three samples from patients having antecedent ASP with respect to age of

Table 11–3 Comparison of Primary and Secondary Alcoholism in Samples of American, French Canadian, and French Alcoholics

		Males		Females	
		Primary Alcoholics	ASP Alcoholics	Primary Alcoholics	ASP Alcoholics
Number of patients	Hartford	79	102	24	17
	Quebec	20	7	8	7
	Tours	29	15	34	34
Age of onset	Hartford	31.31	21.65[a]	31.63	32.91
	Quebec	29.55	19.71[b]	27.25	34.43
	Tours	31.69	28.47[c]	37.88	36.38
Alcohol dependence	Hartford	2.88	3.34[a]	2.81	3.01
	Quebec	2.72	3.37[b]	2.40	2.45
	Tours	3.22	3.49	2.26	2.54
Physical consequences	Hartford	1.72	1.85	1.69	1.80
	Quebec	1.33	1.37	1.51	1.56
	Tours	2.02	2.20	1.89	2.09
Social problems	Hartford	1.83	2.09[c]	2.06	1.47[a]
	Quebec	1.32	1.56[a]	1.41	1.36
	Tours	1.52	2.46[a]	1.50	1.88[c]
Daily oz. alcohol consumption	Hartford	6.47	8.70[a]	6.53	6.37
	Quebec	8.10	7.04	3.68	6.49
	Tours	4.93	10.18[a]	3.11	3.87
Psychological reasons for drinking	Hartford	2.14	2.25	2.40	2.37
	Quebec	1.77	1.66	1.65	1.52
	Tours	1.93	2.41[a]	2.06	2.09
Social reasons for drinking	Hartford	1.42	1.45	1.57	1.47
	Quebec	2.44	2.54	2.53	2.68
	Tours	1.53	1.64	1.24	1.41

[a]p, $< .01$, one-tailed t-test

[b]$p < .05$, one-tailed t-test

[c]$p < .10$, one-tailed t-test

onset of alcohol problems and degree of alcohol-related social problems. In two of the three samples, primary alcoholics differ significantly from ASP alcoholics in terms of severity of alcohol dependence and amount of daily alcohol consumption. In all samples, ASP alcoholics experienced alcohol problems earlier than primary alcoholics, and manifested more severe dependence and social problems. There was no such discrimination among the females classified according to primary alcoholism and antecedent depression. Although there were significant differences in social problems within the Hartford and Tours samples, the direction of the differences was not consistent. In one sample, primary alcoholics manifested more problems, while in the other they manifested fewer problems. The results indicate that only antecedent ASP is associated with a more serious form of alcoholism, regardless of nationality.

Table 11–4 presents the results of a correlational analysis that evalu-

Table 11–4 Correlations Between Lifetime Psychological Severity and Various Drinking Variables

	Males			Females		
	Hartford (N = 187)	Quebec (N = 58)	Tours (N = 65)	Hartford (N = 69)	Quebec (N = 28)	Tours (N = 82)
Alcohol dependence	.36[a]	.35[a]	.43[a]	.25[b]	.41[b]	.19[b]
Physical consequences	.22[a]	.23[a]	.17	.52[a]	−.10	.09
Social problems	.36[a]	.27[a]	.55[a]	.31[a]	−.02	.24[b]
Daily alcohol consumption	.11	.01	.41[a]	−.04	.53[a]	.17
Psychological reasons	.33[a]	.32[a]	.45[a]	.29[a]	.17	−.04
Social reasons	.03	.04	.08	.00	.02	.20
Outcome[c]						
(One year)	.19[a]			−.06		
(3–4 years)	.18[a]		−.24[d]	−.19		.37[d]

[a]p < .01

[b]p < .05

[c]Outcome status was quantified according to the following ordinal scale: 1 = Abstinent; 2 = Drinking without problems; 3 = Drinking with problems; 4 = One or two inpatient treatment episodes; 5 = Three or more inpatient treatment episodes; 6 = Death from alcohol-related causes.

[d]Because the follow-up evaluation in the French sample was restricted to patients living in the area near Tours, not all patients who were located had been interviewed previously with the DIS. These correlations are therefore based on smaller numbers of men (N = 12) and women (N = 10) than were used in the other analyses.

ates the association between psychiatric severity and various alcohol-related problems, behaviors, and reasons for drinking. Psychiatric severity is defined by a simple count of the number of DSM-III categorical diagnoses recorded for each patient in addition to alcoholism by means of the DIS. This measure reflects the cumulative severity of lifetime psychiatric symptomatology, regardless of whether it was developed independent of, in conjunction with, or as a consequence of drinking. The results show that psychiatric severity correlates significantly with alcohol dependence, social problems, and psychological reasons for drinking in all three samples of male alcoholics. In general, the greater the lifetime psychiatric severity, the higher the degree of alcohol dependence, the more social consequences associated with alcohol use, and the more the patient reported drinking for psychological reasons. With regard to outcome status following treatment, only the American patients indicated a significant correlation between psychiatric severity and poor outcome. Although the correlation coefficients of the French patients were larger than those for American patients, the lack of statistical significance is attributable to the small size of the French sample.

Discussion

The results of the present research provide some support for the theory that psychopathology accounts for a pattern of male alcoholism characterized by early onset, more rapid course, and more serious symptomatology. But contrary to prediction, antecedent depression and degree of psychopathology were not associated with the patterning of alcoholism in women. These results are consistent with previously reported findings obtained from earlier analyses of the same French and American patient samples (Babor & Dolinsky, 1988; Rounsaville et al., 1987; Babor et al., 1987; Hesselbrock et al., 1984).

The general consistency of these relationships across all three national samples of male and female alcoholics gives evidence of the robustness of these findings. It also provides support for Jellinek's hypothesis that psychological vulnerability may account for the different patterns of alcoholism observed in France and America, and for Kissin's theory that psychological factors are relatively less prominent in the etiology of alcoholism in countries where heavy drinking is encouraged by social custom.

The role of personality disorder, particularly antisocial personality, has long been implicated in the etiology of alcoholism in men (Kissin, 1983). The present study indicates that ASP may also contribute to a more socially disruptive manifestation of alcoholism that is reflected in the severity of alcohol dependence as well as the frequency of alcohol-related social problems. Additional support for this interpretation is provided by the positive correlation between degree of psychiatric severity, which was heavily influenced by the contribution of ASP in males, and psychological reasons for drinking. Although psychiatric severity proved to be a significant predictor of treatment outcome only in the American sample, it should be noted that the number of French alcoholics actually located at follow-up who had participated in the earlier DIS interview was quite small. In reviewing the outcome data from the larger sample ($N=91$), it is interesting to point out that the abstinence rate among the French male alcoholics at 4 years post-treatment (36.2%) was far higher than that observed among the American male patients at 3 years (18%). Although the presence or absence of psychopathology cannot be inferred as the sole explanation for these differences, it should certainly be considered as a hypothesis for future research on the relative efficacy of alcoholism treatment in different countries.

In contrast to the findings on male alcoholics, the data obtained from the female samples did not support the hypothesized role of antecedent depression and psychiatric severity in the etiology and patterning of alcoholism in women. These results suggest that both drinking and psychopathology are more complex phenomena in women, and indicate that cross-cultural theories developed primarily on the basis of experience with male alcoholics do not easily generalize to women. In a more intensive analysis of the outcome data presented in this report (Rounsaville et al., 1987), it was found that depression in women was associated with *better* outcome when more specific indicators of outcome status are employed.

Despite findings that provide at least partial confirmation of a little investigated but often repeated theory of alcoholism, the present study illustrates some of the problems and pitfalls of conducting cross-national research on alcoholism. Among the problems encountered in the course of this research were difficulties in translating instruments, finding suitable numbers of patients with different types of psychopathology, and locating patients at follow-up. Coordinating and funding cross-national research is a difficult enterprise, one that often relies on the voluntary contributions of numerous dedicated researchers. It is not always possible to translate concepts like drunkenness into precise equivalents in different languages, where the connotations of the terms may have different degrees of social acceptability. The recruitment of patient volunteers for a time-consuming series of interviews and questionnaires often results in missing data when a patient terminates participation after providing only some of the data. The low prevalence of some disorders makes it difficult to find sufficient numbers of patients for planned comparisons. Finally, locating patients for follow-up is a tedious and risky undertaking that sometimes produces only ambiguous findings.

In spite of these problems, the present study provided useful data to test our hypotheses. Nevertheless, caution should be exercised in the interpretation of the findings. The prevalence data, for example, could be the result of sampling bias rather than cross-national differences. Similarly, the lack of significant differences and correlations in the female samples could be the result of small sample size.

In many respects the French are an ideal national group to test cross-cultural theories because their drinking patterns are relatively distinct, and hypotheses have been proposed to explain them. Recent international trends in the choice and consumption of alcoholic beverages may make such research more difficult in the future because of a general homogenization of drinking customs in the Western industrialized countries. As Osterberg (1986) and others have noted, wine drinking is declining in France as beer and distilled beverages take on popularity with younger drinkers. In the future, the classic wine drinking *buveur d'habitude* may no longer account for the typical pattern of alcoholism in the wine-producing countries, even as the liquor-drinking relief drinker may no longer represent the typical symptomatic alcoholic in the "Anglo-Saxon" countries of northern Europe and North America. Under these conditions, it may become necessary to search for new drinking cultures to test theories of alcoholism.

One implication of the present study for the future planning of cross-national research on alcohol concerns the relative merits of investigating similarities rather than differences. Another way of describing these different research styles is in terms of the distinction between pancultural generality versus cultural relativity. The concept of cultural relativity implies that the differences among countries in social organization and child rearing practices are related to differences in drinking behavior. This leads to the expectation of wide variations in attitudes toward alcohol, drinking practices, alcohol-related problems, and patterns of alcoholism. The pancultural-generalist view emphasizes similarities in the effects and functions of drinking across societies. Biologically, all humans are members of the same species, susceptible in the same way to intoxication, dependence and liver damage. Socially, almost all humans find alcohol reinforcing. Psychologically, drinking is a means of coping with environmental stress. This would lead one to expect certain common features in drinking behavior, especially at the biological and psychological levels of analysis. The beauty of the comparative method is that it allows researchers to explore both similarities and differences related to culture. The present research suggests that the comparative method may be useful in the identification of "pancultural" influences on the patterning of alcoholism (e.g., the relationship between psychopathology and drinking behavior in male alcoholics), and that these psychological "universals" may help to explain cross-national differences in the predominant types of alcoholism observed in different countries.

References

Babor, T. F., and Dolinsky, Z. S. (1988). Alcoholic typologies: Historical evaluation and empirical evaluation of some common classification schemes. In R. Rose and J. Barrett (eds.), *Alcoholism: Origins and Etiology.* New York: Raven Press, pp. 245–65.

Babor, T. F.; Martinay, C.; Benard, J. Y.; Ferrant, J. P.; and Wolfson, A. (1987). Homme alcoolique, femme alcoolique: Etude comparative sur l'alcoolisme feminin. (Male alcoholic, female alcoholic: A comparative study on female alcoholism.) *Bulletin de la Societe Française d'Alcoologie* 9(1), 20–30.

Babor, T. F.; Weill, J.; and Ferrant, J. P. (1981). Enquete sur la credibilite et la coherence des responses donnes par les alcooliques aux questions portant sur la consommation d'alcool. (A study of the validity and reliability of responses given by alcoholics to questions about their alcohol consumption.) *La Revue de l'Alcoolisme* 27(2), 87–96.

Cahalan, D.; Cisin, I. H.; and Crossley, H. M. (1969). *American Drinking Practices.* New Brunswick, N.J.: Rutgers Center for Alcohol Studies.

Criteria Committee, National Council on Alcoholism (1972). Criteria for the diagnosis of alcoholism. *Am. J. Psychiatry* 129:127–35.

Edwards, G., and Gross, M. M. (1976). Alcohol dependence: Provisional description of a clinical syndrome. *Br. Med. J.* 1:1058–61.

Helzer, J. E.; Robins, L. N.; Croughan, J. L.; and Welner, A. (1981). Renard diagnostic interview. *Arch. Gen. Psychiatry* 38:393–98.

Hesselbrock, M.; Babor, T. F.; Hesselbrock, V.; Meyer, R. E.; and Workman, K. (1983). "Never believe an alcoholic?" On the validity of self-report measures of alcohol dependence. *Int. J. Addict.* 18:593–609.

Hesselbrock, M.; Hesselbrock, V.; Babor, T. F.; Stabenau, J.; Meyer, R. E.; and Weidenman, M. (1984). Antisocial behavior, psychopathology, and problem drinking in the natural history of alcoholism. In D. Goodwin, K. Van Dusen, and S. Mednick (eds.), *Longitudinal Studies of Alcoholism.* Nijhoff Publishing Co., Boston, pp. 197–214.

Jellinek, E. M. (1962). Cultural differences in the meaning of alcoholism. In: D. J. Pittman and C. R. Snyder (eds.), *Society, Culture and Drinking Patterns*. Carbondale, Ill.: Southern Illinois University Press, pp. 382–88.

Jellinek, E. M. (1960). *The Disease Concept of Alcoholism*. New Haven, Conn.: College and University Press.

Kissin, B. (1983). The disease concept of alcoholism. In R. G. Smart, F. B. Glaser, Y. Israel, H. Kalant, R. E. Popham, and W. Schmidt, (eds.), *Research Advances in Alcohol and Drug Problems*, vol. 7. New York: Plenum Press, pp. 93–126.

Kissin, B. (1977). Theory and practice in the treatment of alcoholism. In B. Kissin and H. Begleiter (eds.), *Treatment and Rehabilitation of the Chronic Alcoholic*. New York: Plenum Press, pp. 1–51.

Mulford, H. A., and Miller, D. E. (1960). Drinking in Iowa: IV. Preoccupation with alcohol and definitions of alcohol, heavy drinking and trouble due to drinking. *Q. J. Stud. Alcohol* 21:279–91.

Osterberg, E. (1986). Alcohol-related problems in cross-national perspective: Results of the ISACE study. In T. F. Babor (ed.), *Alcohol and Culture: Comparative Perspectives from Europe and America*, vol. 472. New York: New York Academy of Sciences, pp. 10–20.

Perrin, P. (1964). De la perte de liberte envers l'alcool. *La Revue de l'Alcoolisme* 10:1–8.

Robins, L. N.; Helzer, J. E.; Croughan, J. L.; Williams, J. B. W.; and Spitzer, R. L. (1981). NIMH Diagnostic Interview Schedule (DIS), Version III. St. Louis, Missouri: Department of Psychiatry, Washington University School of Medicine.

Rounsaville, B.; Dolinsky, Z. S.; Babor, T. F.; and Meyer, R. E. (1987). Psychopathology as a predictor of treatment outcome in alcoholics. *Arch. Gen. Psychiatry* 44:505–13.

[IV] Asia and the Pacific

[12] Alcohol Abuse and Dependence in New Zealand

J. Elisabeth Wells, John A. Bushnell,
Peter R. Joyce, Andrew R. Hornblow,
and Mark A. Oakley-Browne

New Zealand lies east of Australia and from 33 to 53 degrees south in the Pacific Ocean. It consists of two main islands and a number of smaller ones, with a combined land area of 268,000 square kilometers, about the size of the British Isles or Japan. Much of the country, particularly the South Island, is mountainous; however, the temperate climate has enabled great agricultural productivity on the 54 percent of the land that is arable. New Zealand's traditional export products have been frozen lamb carcasses, butter, and cheese, but there has been considerable diversification in the last 20 years.

New Zealand was first discovered by Polynesians, probably before 1000 A.D., with major migration taking place about 300 years later. These New Zealand Polynesians came to be known as Maori. The first European sighting of New Zealand was by Abel Tasman in 1642, but there is no record of any other European stop here until the first of Cook's visits in 1769. From 1792 onward, whaling stations were established and there was trade with Australia in whale oil, seal skins, flax, and timber. Missionary activity also began. A British Resident was appointed in 1833 and in 1840 British Sovereignty was proclaimed. From 1853 until 1875 there were elected provincial councils of limited power, as well as a national parliament, but since the provincial system was abolished there has been only one legislature for New Zealand.

At the 1986 census, the population of New Zealand was just under 3.3 million and predominantly European in ethnic origin (86%) with 9 percent Maori, 3 percent Pacific Island Polynesian, and 1 percent other. Two-thirds of the population live in the seventeen main urban areas, and only 4 percent are classified as rural dwellers. There has been a tradition of full employment in New Zealand, and in the 1950s and 60s the unemployment rate was only about 1 percent. It has climbed steeply since the oil shocks of the early 1970s to reach 6 percent in the 1980s, which is still moderately low in comparison with other Western countries (N.Z. Official Year Book 1986–1987).

The city of Christchurch lies on the east coast of the South Island in the province of Canterbury. Its population in 1986 was nearly 300,000. Being in the south it has fewer Maoris and Pacific Islanders (3% versus 12% for the country as a whole). Very little information is available about regional differences in alcohol consumption in New Zealand, and there is no folklore suggesting that Christchurch is different from other parts of the country. Regional beer figures for the late 1970s and early 1980s (Williams, 1982) show the Canterbury region to have an average consumption, with the West Coast of the South Island being the only region markedly higher than the rest. A general mortality atlas for 1974–1978 (Borman & Leiataua, 1984) showed Christchurch to have a lower than average rate of cirrhosis of the liver, but it is not known if this has been true in other time periods, or to what extent it is influenced by lower rates of Hepatitis B. In summary, what limited evidence there is indicates that alcohol consumption in Christchurch is fairly typical of that for most parts of New Zealand, perhaps a little lower than for some other areas.

Alcohol Legislation and Drinking Practices

It is possible to divide the history of liquor legislation of New Zealand into five phases—a laissez-faire approach from 1846 to 1873, early efforts at regulation from 1873 to 1893, the rising tide of prohibition and restriction from 1893 to 1918, a long stalemate between 1918 and 1948, and a gradual trend toward liberalization since 1948, extremely cautious at first but more marked since 1960 (Royal Commission of Inquiry, 1974, quoted in Park, 1985).

The hard-drinking of the earliest settlers, whalers, traders, and ex-convicts continued throughout the gold rushes of the 1860s, but as more stable settlement developed, there were increasing attempts to curb the worst excesses of alcohol consumption. The move for temperance and prohibition was linked with that for women's suffrage, which was granted in 1893 in spite of opposition from the liquor trade (Sutch, 1969:134–35). From 1894 on, a number of local areas were voted "dry." A triennial national prohibition poll was introduced in 1881 and prohibition gained more than half of the votes at all elections from 1902 to 1914 but was never enacted because of the requirement for a two-thirds majority. A special poll in 1919 required only a 50 percent majority but lost 49 to 51 percent by the 4:1 vote against prohibition among servicemen overseas who had not yet returned from the First World War.

The vote for prohibition has declined ever since (Park, 1985; Bollinger, 1959). The 6 o-clock closing of bars, which was introduced as part of the war effort in 1917, continued until 1967, a victory for both the temperance movement and for the liquor trade who could sell more liquor during the shorter opening hours. Many other aspects of the complex morass of alcohol legislation were also the result of attempts to restrict alcohol and reduce consumption, but nevertheless enabled the liquor trade to increase its profits (Bollinger, 1959).

The moves to liberalization since the Second World War have often been hailed as moves toward civilization, France being regarded as an example to be emulated. However, since the early 1970s there has been an enormous growth in inpatient and outpatient treatment facilities for alcoholics. With the formation of the Alcoholic Liquor Advisory Council in 1976, there has been much greater awareness of the costs of higher alcohol consumption, even though the barbaric 5 to 6 o'clock "swill" no longer exists.

The social meaning of alcohol in New Zealand has not been extensively explored (Park, 1985), although there have been some studies of particular work or ethnic groups. Hodges (1987) attempted to investigate the meaning of drunkenness for young men and their obsession with chundering (vomiting) and other bodily functions.

Alcohol Consumption

Figure 12–1 shows the adult per capita consumption of alcohol in New Zealand from 1888 to 1985. The liberalization of drinking laws since the Second World War has been matched by a marked increase in consumption; the 1981 level was one-and-one-half times that for 1955. The price of alcohol relative to disposable income decreased over this period (Ashton & Casswell, 1987), and this undoubtedly also played a major role in the consumption increase. Since 1980, however, there has been some increase in the real price of alcohol and a drop in consumption (Ashton & Casswell, 1987).

In 1978 there was a national study of current alcohol consumption and attitudes with a sample of 10,000. The majority (65%) reported drinking moderately (<20 ml. absolute alcohol/day), with a minority (9%) of heavy drinkers who reported drinking more than 60 ml. per day and who accounted for almost two-thirds of the total alcohol consumed (Casswell, 1980). Males drank more than females, and for both sexes consumption was highest in the late teens and early twenties (Casswell, 1980; Gregson et al., 1981). Although heavy drinkers were found in almost all social groups, there were some social class differences with a lower class pattern for less frequent drinking but larger quantity per

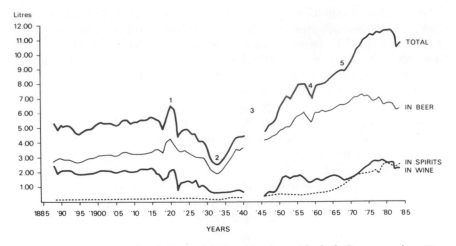

Figure 12–1 New Zealand Since 1888—Absolute Alcohol Consumption Per Capita Aged 15+. Key: 1—World War I, 1914–1918, 2—Depression, 3—World War II, 1939–1945, 4—Nordmeyer's "Black" Budget increased taxes on alcohol, 5—Six o'clock closing ended. [*Source:* Alcohol Research Unit, Auckland and the Alcoholic Liquor Advisory Council, Wellington, New Zealand.]

occasion contrasting with a higher class pattern of more regular consumption of smaller amounts (Casswell & Gordon, 1984).

In 1981 New Zealand was ranked fifteenth in per capita consumption of alcohol in those aged 15 and over (Brown et al., 1982), just ahead of Canada and the United States and below most European countries and Australia.

Methods

The results presented in this chapter come from 1,498 interviews carried out from April to December 1986 in the Christchurch Urban Area. The sampling area included the central city, neighboring suburban boroughs and extended to the semirural margin of the city. In March 1986 the census count of persons usually resident in this area was 181,000 for adults aged 18–64 years out of a total population of 295,000 (New Zealand Census, 1986). People in long term institutional care were not included in this survey. However, employee quarters and other forms of group living were included in the sampling frame, along with private residences.

A three stage sampling design was used. First, 250 primary sampling units were systematically selected with probability proportional to size from census tract areas called mesh blocks. After enumeration, dwellings were systematically selected so that the overall probability of selection of all dwellings was equal (Kish, 1965). One member from each selected household was also chosen by Kish selection (Kish, 1965). For two out of three dwellings any usually resident occupant between 18 and 64 years of age was eligible; for every third dwelling only a young woman (18–44 years) was eligible. This oversampling was carried out to collect more cases of eating disorders and depression, disorders of particular interest to some of the research team. No interviews by proxy or using an interpreter were allowed. Version III of the DIS was used with the addition of generalized anxiety and bulimia from Version IIIA and an adaptation of the Health Services Questionnaire used in the U.S. ECA survey.

Interviewers attended a 75-hour training course and reported weekly to their supervisors. Supervisors inspected completed interviews, discussed difficulties, and reported back any problems found by editors or by the extensive computer "cleaning" programs that checked for acceptable/out-of-range codes, illogical skips, and consistency. A sample of questionnaires underwent further verification, which showed that very few errors got through the entry and checking process. The SAS diagnostic program provided by NIMH for Version IIIA of the DIS was used with minor modification to make diagnoses. Analyses were carried out using the BMDP statistical package (Dixon, 1985).

Results

Table 12–1 shows the demographic composition of the Christchurch sample after weighting for age and sex to the 1986 census results. The response rate was calculated without weighting. Unoccupied dwellings were excluded from calculations. There was a 94 percent response rate for household listings and 74 percent of designated respondents agreed to interview which, by the method of Von Korff et al. (1985), gives an overall response rate of 70 percent. Loss of designated respondents was nearly always due to respondent refusal (93%).

In comparison to the 1986 census, our survey results showed males and those under 25 to be relatively underrepresented. Post-stratification adjustments to correct for response loss ranged from 2.07 for males 18 to 24 years, to 1.39 for females aged 45 to 64 years. After weighting, the age and sex distributions are the same as those for the Christchurch Urban Area in the 1986 census, the oversampling of young women having been dealt with through design-weights.

Christchurch has a predominantly white population with only about 3 percent Maori and Pacific Island people (N.Z. Official Year Book, 1986–1987). The survey results reflect the racial mix in Christchurch even though there was no post-stratification for race.

Table 12–1 *Sample Size and Demographic Composition,*
Christchurch (Weighted Except Where Indicated)

Category	Number or %
Number of subjects interviewed	1,498
Overall response rate	70%[a]
Age	
18–24	22%
25–44	47%
45–64	32%
Sex (% female)	51%
Race	
Maori	2%
Pacific Islander	<1%
White	96%
Other	2%
Years at school: proportions with	
<10 years	30%
11 years	26%
12 years	31%
13+ years	14%
Number of marriages	
0	27%
1	65%
2 or more	8%
Residence at time of interview	
Urban	100%
Rural	0%
Socioeconomic status for recent or current full time work	
SES 1 or 2	29%
SES 3 or 4	51%
SES 5 or 6	19%

[a]This percentage is unweighted; all others are weighted (see text).

In New Zealand children start school at 5 years old and are required to remain in school until they turn 15, so that the standard minimum of schooling is 10 years. Although the survey recorded qualifications gained after leaving school, it was not possible to convert these to equivalent full-time years of education, so Table 12–1 reports only years of schooling from age 5.

The majority of Christchurch adults are married and living with their spouse; those never married are predominantly young. The entire sample is urban as defined by the New Zealand Department of Statistics, even though a few are living on small holdings on the outskirts of the city.

Occupation was coded separately for males and females according to a standardized system for New Zealand (Johnston, 1985). For Table 12–1, only current or recent (the last 3 years), full-time (30+ hrs./week) work is reported. Only 69 percent of the sample was classifiable in this way (weighted estimate). Compared with national figures based on the 1976 census (Johnston, 1985), this sample has an excess at the top in classes 1 and 2 (29% versus 21%) whereas classes 5 and 6 are underrepresented (19% versus 23%). These differences may be due to differing definitions of full-time work, secular trends, urban/rural differences, or differences between Christchurch and other urban areas. However, it may be that there was some social class effect on the response rate.

The Symptoms of Alcoholism

Apart from a few modifications in the alcohol consumption questions so as to use quantity designations known to New Zealand drinkers, the wording of the DIS alcohol section for our survey was as it appears in Appendix 2. Excessive consumption symptoms were those reported most frequently. Twenty-four percent of the whole sample reported that at some time in their life they had drunk heavily, either daily (Question 153) or weekly (Question 154), and 20 percent reported that they had drunk the equivalent of a fifth of liquor in one day at least once. Blackouts and the respondent considering himself to be an excessive drinker were the next most common symptoms (13%), closely followed by family objections to the respondent's excessive drinking (11%).

The least commonly reported symptoms were losing a job (1%), continuing to drink in the face of an illness which might be made worse by drinking (1%), or being unable to do ordinary work without drinking (1%).

Table 12–2 shows the proportion of those with alcohol abuse or dependence reporting each symptom. The rank order correlation for symptom frequency between alcoholics and nonalcoholics is 0.85, indicating a similar ordering in the two groups although very different absolute rates. The correlation in rank frequency for male and female alcoholics is also moderately high—0.80—but there is a pattern for women alcoholics to be more likely to consider their drinking excessive and to tell others about their problems, whereas males are more likely to have experienced legal or violent consequences of drinking, and to have binged or consumed high amounts on a single occasion. Regular heavy consumption, blackouts, withdrawal symptoms, medical consequences and morning drinking occurred equally often for male and female alcoholics.

Table 12–2 Individual Symptom Frequencies Among Those with Alcohol Disorders Christchurch (Weighted Percentages)

DIS Item Number	Symptom	Proportion of Those with Alcohol Abuse and/or Dependence Who Endorsed This Item %	Rank
150	Family objected to respondent's drinking	45	5
151	Respondent thought himself an excessive drinker	47	4
152	Fifth of liquor in one day	74	1
153/154	Daily or weekly heavy drinking	70	2
155	Told physician about drinking problem	10	16
156	Friends or professionals said drinking too much	29	8
157	Wanted to stop drinking but couldn't	9	17
158	Efforts to control drinking	15	13
159	Morning drinking	11	14.5
160	Job troubles due to drinking	11	14.5
161	Lost job	3	20
162	Trouble driving	23	9
163	Arrested while drinking	18	12
164	Physical fights while drinking	38	6
165	Two or more binges	22	10
166	Blackouts while drinking	53	3
167	Any withdrawal symptom	31	7
168	Any medical complication	20	11
169	Continued to drink with serious illness	7	18
170	Couldn't do ordinary work without drinking	6	19

Drinking Patterns

Everyone in the sample has been classified into one of the six lifetime drinking patterns as shown in Table 12–3, and the current (6-month) prevalence rate for alcohol abuse and/or dependence is also given.

Although a temperance movement still exits in New Zealand, we found that lifetime total abstention is not common in Christchurch; only 2 percent fell into this category. More than half the respondents are social drinkers who have not drunk heavily or had problems. Heavy drinkers without problems are not common either (4%). Table 12–3 shows that the mean age at interview for nonproblem heavy drinkers is similar to that for drinkers with problems, that is, those without problems are not just a young group. Nonetheless, it is likely that many of them will go on to develop problems. Heavy drinking, as defined in questions 153 and 154, is not a necessary prerequisite for problems. Although 90 percent of those with alcohol dependence were heavy drinkers, only 47 percent of those with alcohol abuse and 36 percent of nonalcoholic problem drinkers were heavy drinkers.

Problem drinkers are those who reported at least one symptom but

Table 12–3 Lifetime Rates of Various Drinking Categories,
Christchurch (Weighted Estimates)

Drinking Category	Christchurch	
	%	Mean age
Total abstention	2	42
Nonheavy/nonproblem	57	40
Heavy/nonproblem drinkers	4	36
Problem drinkers	17	34
Alcohol abuse only	9	35
Dependence with or without abuse	10	38
Six-month prevalence of alcoholism (Abuse and/or dependence)	8	—

did not meet DSM-III criteria for abuse or dependence. Their mean age is close to that for abusers and only 4 years younger than that for alcohol dependence, so they are a less severe group rather than a much younger group.

Alcohol abuse without dependence is a little less prevalent than alcohol dependence (9% and 10% respectively), and the combined lifetime prevalence is 18.9 percent. This is considerably higher than for any of the other core disorders as shown in Table 12–7, and was exceeded only by generalized anxiety (31%) and sexual dysfunction (33%). The 6-month prevalence of alcoholism is also high relative to other disorders.

The Course of Alcoholism

Some information about the course of alcoholism can be obtained from the reports of respondents in this cross-sectional survey. Two percent are lifelong abstainers, 19 percent have drunk alcohol but report never becoming intoxicated, and most (79%) report having become intoxicated at some time in their lives.

Table 12–4 shows that on average men become intoxicated earlier than women, and alcoholics earlier than nonalcoholics, the differences being only two years with all means falling in the late teenage years. For alcoholics, the mean age at which the first symptom occurred is around 20, four to five years after the first intoxication. There is a trend for women alcoholics to have a longer incubation period and fewer symptoms.

For Table 12–4, alcoholics in remission are defined as those with no symptoms in the last year. Fifty-one percent of those with a lifetime diagnosis were in remission. The mean age of remission is in the late 20s. The mean number of symptoms ever is similar for those in remission (4.4) and for those who are still alcoholic (4.1). The average number of symptoms for current alcoholics is almost identical whether or not they

Table 12–4 Onset, Severity, and Course of Alcoholism, Christchurch (Weighted Estimates)

	Men	Women	Total
Mean Age First Intoxicated (If Ever)			
Total sample	17	19	18
Alcoholics only	16	17	16
Nonalcoholics	18	19	18
Mean Value Among Alcoholics			
Age of onset of alcoholism	20	22	20
Number of years from first intoxication to first alcohol symptom	4.2	5.6	4.4
Mean number of lifetime symptoms	4.3	3.8	4.3
Mean Value Among Alcoholics in Remission[a]			
Age last symptom	28	29	28
Duration of alcoholism in years	8.7	6.6	8.3
Lifetime symptoms	4.5	3.6	4.4

[a]Remitted alcoholic = no alcohol symptoms for at least one year prior to interview (proportion = 51% of those with a lifetime diagnosis of alcohol abuse and/or dependence).

N.B. 0.5 aded to all mean ages before rounding to allow for years being truncated, i.e., age x is on average age x + ½.

have been alcoholic for more than 10 years—4.1 versus 4.2 symptoms, respectively. Among those who have remitted, those with a duration of more than 10 years had 5.3 symptoms on average, whereas those with shorter duration had a mean of 4.1 symptoms.

The mean duration of alcoholism among those in remission is 8.3 years, but the distribution is very skewed so that 50 percent had a duration of 5 years or less (unweighted estimate). Thus, for many remitted alcoholics, the time from their first to their last symptom is just a few years, but about one-quarter experienced symptoms for more than a decade.

Risk Factors and Correlates of Alcoholism

We have defined risk factors as those that are clearly antecedent to alcoholism and affect its prevalence, examples being sex or childhood conduct disorders. Correlates are associated factors that are not necessarily antecedent—other psychiatric disorders, for example.

Lifetime prevalence rates by age and sex are shown in Table 12–5. Overall, men have an alcoholism rate 5 times that for women, but this ratio is highest for the oldest age group (8:1) and declines to 3:1 in the 18–24 age group. For males, lifetime prevalence does not vary much with age, although the 25–44 age group has the highest rate. For women, lifetime prevalence decreases with age.

Life table analysis of age of onset of first symptom shows very clear cohort effects. From age 15 on, more recent cohorts show a higher prevalence at each age of onset. For men, the lifetime prevalence rate is

Table 12–5 Lifetime Prevalence of Alcohol Abuse
and/or Dependence (Design-Weighted and Post-stratified)

Sex	Age (Years)			
	18–24	25–44	45–64	Total
Male	29.7	34.8	29.3	32.0
Female	9.1	6.3	3.9	6.1
Total	19.6	20.4	16.3	18.9

almost flat across the current age groups because the cohort effect appears to be almost completely balanced by the greater number of years at risk for alcoholism. For women, the cohort effect dominates, resulting in a decline in rates in the older age groups.

Table 12–6 shows the effects of some other possible risk factors and correlates of alcoholism. The first column presents these factors as predictors of heavy drinking among drinkers, lifetime abstainers being excluded. The second column presents the same factors as predictors of alcoholism among heavy drinkers. Overall, 24 percent of drinkers are or have been heavy drinkers and 56 percent of those heavy drinkers have met DSM-III criteria for alcohol dependence or abuse. Multiplying the probability of these outcomes together and allowing for abstainers (2%) underestimates the prevalence of alcoholism (13% versus 19%) because many abusers (53%) were not heavy drinkers. Nonetheless, the two-stage pattern of prediction yields some useful insights about pathways into alcoholism.

We have already seen that sex is an important risk factor and that alcoholism is over 5 times more common in men than women (Table 12–5). The male/female ratio for heavy drinking is not quite as large, although still substantial at 3.5 (Table 12–6). However, the ratio falls to 1.4 when we look at the proportion of heavy drinkers who are alcoholic. Thus, New Zealand women who drink heavily are more like their male counterparts in terms of their risk of developing alcoholism. The number of marriages and the number of years at school show little association with heavy drinking or alcoholism. However, for full-time workers, socioeconomic status shows a consistent effect with lower rates of heavy drinking and alcoholism in groups with higher status. The last three variables in Table 12–6 are strong predictors of heavy drinking and of alcoholism in heavy drinkers. Early intoxication could be thought of as a marker of early alcohol problems rather than a risk factor. The number of childhood conduct disorder groups is a more conventional risk factor, although it does include early intoxication. Drug disorder is a correlate; it may have developed earlier or later than alcoholism or heavy drinking or in tandem with them.

The relation between alcoholism and other psychiatric disorders is shown in Table 12–7. Of the disorders listed, alcoholism is the most

Table 12–6 Risk Factors and Correlates for Heavy Drinking and Alcoholism, Christchurch (Weighted Percentages)

	Proportion of All Drinkers Who Are Heavy Drinkers %	Proportion of Heavy Drinkers Who Are Alcoholic %
Nonabstaining sample (N = 1462)	24	56
Risk factor or correlate		
Sex		
Men	38	60
Women	11	42
Number of marriages		
0	26	52
1	23	57
2+	29	60
Years at school		
≤10 years	30	57
11 years	24	61
12 years	19	46
13+ years	24	60
Socioeconomic status for current or recent full-time work		
SES 1 and 2	24	48
SES 3 and 4	32	57
SES 5 and 6	35	65
Childhood conduct groups positive		
None	15	38
1 or 2	30	55
3 or more	49	78
Intoxicated before age 15		
No	26	48
Yes	48	81
Any drug disorder		
No	22	51
Yes	58	84

prevalent. Because of the personal, family, social, and health problems resulting from alcohol abuse and dependence, it is clear that it presents a major public health problem. The rank order of the lifetime prevalence of disorders is similar in the Christchurch sample and the combined ECA samples with two major exceptions: cognitive impairment is much less common in Christchurch because no one over 64 years of age was interviewed, and depression and dysthymia are much more frequent in Christchurch than in the ECA samples.

The second column of Table 12–7 shows the lifetime prevalence of disorders among alcoholics, namely those who met DSM-III for alcohol abuse or dependence during their lifetime. The third column shows one measure of the extent to which alcoholics are at greater or lesser risk for

Table 12–7 Lifetime Prevalence Rates of Core Diagnoses and Risk Ratios Among Alcoholics, Christchurch (Weighted Percentages)

Diagnosis in Order of Lifetime Prevalence in the Combined ECA Sample	Lifetime Prevalence in Total Sample %	Lifetime Prevalence in Alcoholics %	Risk Ratio Prevalence in Alcoholics/Prevalence in Nonalcoholics %
Alcoholism	18.9	—	—
Phobic disorder (any)[a]	10.7	14.1	1.4
Drug abuse and/or dependence (any)	5.7	18.7	7.2
Cognitive impairment (mild or severe)	1.1	0.8	0.6
Major depression	12.5	17.3	1.5
Dysthymic disorder	6.4	8.9	1.5
Anti-social personality disorder	3.1	12.1	12.7
Obsessive compulsive disorder	2.2	2.9	1.4
Panic disorder	2.2	2.3	1.1
Schizophrenia	0.3	0.5	1.5
Mania	0.7	0.9	1.4
Somatization disorder	0.0	0.0	0.0
Schizophreniform	0.0	0.2	—[b]
Anorexia nervosa	0.1	0.1	0.9
Any core DIS diagnosis apart from alcoholism	27.6	44.1	1.9

[a]Including social phobia.

[b]Ratio undetermined because of zero denominator.

each disorder than nonalcoholics—the ratio of the prevalence in the two groups. By far the highest ratio (12.7) is for antisocial personality disorder. While this partly reflects the antisocial consequences of alcoholism, there is also a strong antecedent component as shown in Table 12–6 by the predictive power of the number of childhood conduct disorder symptoms.

Drug abuse or dependence is the disorder with the second highest risk ratio (7.2). All other risk ratios are less than two. The three other common disorders—depression, dysthymia, and phobia—all show some association with alcoholism with risk ratios close to 1.5. The remaining disorders show no strong associations with alcoholism, but it must be remembered that the total sample size is 1,498 with only 232 alcoholics, so that there is considerable imprecision in estimating the prevalences and hence their ratios. For example, for a disorder like mania with 1 percent prevalence among alcoholics, the standard error of this estimate is about 0.7 percent. Overall, alcoholics were 1.9 times more likely than nonalcoholics to have at least one of the other diagnoses listed in Table 12–7.

The prevalence of alcoholism and antisocial personality disorder is higher for males than for females, whereas the reverse is true for phobia, depression, and dysthymia. However, calculating risk ratios separately for males and females does not reduce the association between antisocial personality and alcoholism (overall ratio = 12.7, male ratio = 12.3, female ratio = 17.1). For the predominantly female disorders, calculating risk ratios separately for each sex has the expected effect of increasing the risk ratios. For depression, there is an overall ratio of 1.5, a male ratio of 2.9, and a female ratio of 1.6. For dysthymia, the three ratios are 1.5 overall, 3.6 and 1.9 for men and women, respectively, and for phobia the overall ratio is 1.4, with 5.0 for males and 2.3 for females.

Discussion

The moderately high level of alcohol consumption in New Zealand would be expected to lead to a moderately high prevalence rate for alcoholism. Certainly this is true for Christchurch, with 32 percent of men and 6 percent of women meeting lifetime criteria for alcohol abuse or dependence. Furthermore, the 50 percent increase in consumption from the 1950s to the 1980s would suggest a strong cohort effect, with more recent cohorts experiencing higher rates. The survey results show clear evidence of such a cohort effect, particularly for women. It may be that this apparent cohort effect is partly the result of forgetting by older respondents or greater mortality among those with alcohol problems so that few of them survive into the older age groups. However, it seems unlikely that these factors could be the entire explanation for our findings. The implication of a real cohort effect is that not only is there a current major health problem with alcohol, but that it can be expected to get worse.

The most common symptoms reported by both alcoholics and non-alcoholics are those of excessive consumption, either at one time (Question 152) or regularly (Questions 153 and 154). Not surprisingly, blackouts are a relatively common outcome of such high consumption. Job loss is extremely rare, which is to be expected from the low unemployment rate. Labeling drinking as excessive, whether in oneself or others, is related to the drinking norms of the group one identifies with. Therefore, if alcoholism rates are high, as in Christchurch males, then less labeling may occur for the same behavior than would happen for a group with a lower alcoholism rate such as women. The symptom frequencies for male and female alcoholics in Christchurch demonstrate this pattern, with less self-labeling or objections by others being reported by males. Also, seeking help from others and attempts to control drinking are unlikely to occur while drinking and its problems are seen as normal; low frequencies of these behaviors are reported in Christchurch.

The onset of alcoholism occurs mainly in the late teens and early 20s, with only 4 to 6 years between first intoxication and the first symptom. This means that primary prevention efforts need to be focused on or before this period.

It is encouraging to note that there are quite high rates of remission—of those ever meeting criteria for alcoholism, 51 percent have had no symptom in the last year and 42 percent have had no symptom in the last 3 years. However, even if half can be expected to remit under the status quo, whether by self-help or sometimes with professional help, that still would leave about 9 percent who become alcoholic and never recover. Of the core diagnoses in Table 12–7, only depression and phobia have lifetime prevalence rates that are higher than this estimated rate for alcoholics who continue to have problems. Therefore, while remission rates are encouraging, alcoholism still remains what is perhaps our most serious psychiatric disorder in New Zealand. Even those who remit experience symptoms for several years. There is a need for extensive secondary prevention work with those who have developed alcohol problems, whether or not they have met criteria for alcoholism, to diminish problems and improve remission rates.

Apart from age and sex, the major predictors of heavy drinking and alcoholism are early intoxication, childhood conduct disorders, and any drug disorder. Similarly, the main psychiatric disorders that tend to occur with alcoholism are antisocial personality disorder and drug abuse or dependence. There appears to be a weak association with most of the other core diagnoses.

In closing, it is important to reiterate that ours is not a national sample from New Zealand, but rather from one city only. Results for Christchurch do not necessarily apply to the rest of New Zealand. However, there is no reason to suspect that Christchurch is greatly different, and our findings are probably a reasonable estimate of psychiatric disorder for demographically similar groups throughout the remainder of these islands.

References

Ashton, T., and Casswell, S. (1987). Alcohol taxation as a public health policy: the New Zealand experience. *Community Health Stud.* 108–19.

Bollinger, C. (1959). *Grog's Own Country: History of Liquor Licensing in New Zealand.* Wellington, New Zealand: Price Milburn.

Borman, B., and Leiataua, S. (1984). *A General Mortality Atlas of New Zealand.* Wellington, New Zealand: National Health Statistics Center, Department of Health.

Brown, M. M. ; Dewar, M. F.; and Wallace, P. (1982). *Alcoholic Beverage Taxation and Control Policies: International Survey.* Ottawa, Canada: Brewers Association of Canada.

Casswell, S. (1980). *Drinking by New Zealanders.* Wellington and Auckland, New Zealand: Alcoholic Liquor Advisory Council and the Alcohol Research Unit.

Casswell, S., and Gordon, A. (1984). Drinking and occupational status in New Zealand men. *J. Stud. Alcohol* 45:144–48.

Dixon, W. J. (1985) BMDP Statistical Software. Berkeley, Calif. University of California.

Gregson, R. A. M.; Elvy, G. A.; and Stacey, B. A. (1981). Attitudes, age and sex as correlates and predictors of self-reported alcohol consumption. *Aust. J. Psychol.* 33: 345–53.

Hodges, I. D. (1987). "Off our faces": Drinking and the dissolution of the public man. A paper read at the workshop, Research Today Health Tomorrow, held in Wellington, New Zealand, August 1987.

Johnston, J. (1985). A revision of socio-economic indices for New Zealand. Wellington, New Zealand: New Zealand Council for Educational Research.

Kish, L. (1965). *Survey Sampling.* New York: Wiley.

New Zealand Census of Population and Dwellings (1986) Regional Summary Series, Report 24. Wellington, New Zealand: Department of Statistics.

New Zealand Official Yearbook (1986–1987). Wellington, New Zealand Department of Statistics.

Park, J. (1985). Towards an ethnography of alcohol in New Zealand. Auckland, New Zealand: Department of Anthropology, University of Auckland, Working Paper No. 66, rev. ed.

Sutch, W. B. (1960). *Poverty and Progress in New Zealand.* Wellington, New Zealand: Reed.

Von Korff, M.; Cottler, L.; George, L. K.; Eaton, W. W.; Leaf, P. J.; and Burnam, A. (1985). Nonresponse and nonresponse bias in the ECA surveys. In W. W. Eaton and L. G. Kessler (eds.), *Epidemiologic Methods in Psychiatry: The NIMH Epidemiologic Catchment Area Program.* New York: Academic Press.

Williams, J. (1982). New Zealand beer consumption by region, 1978, 1980–81. Wellington, New Zealand: Lion Breweries [unpublished].

[13] Alcoholism in Taiwan Chinese Communities

ENG-KUNG YEH AND HAI-GWO HWU

Alcoholism among the Chinese has been reported to be rare and there have been few prevalence studies in community populations. An epidemiological study conducted from 1946 to 1948 has so far been the only available survey of the Taiwan Chinese population in the literature. Only two cases of alcoholism (0.01%) were identified in that study (Lin, 1953).

This finding has been supported by the infrequency of alcoholic cases seen in psychiatric clinical settings. The rarity of alcoholism among the Chinese has been explained from a biological point of view: that the Chinese are highly sensitive to alcohol and have low tolerance (Ewing, 1974; Wolff, 1972); and from a sociocultural point of view: that the Chinese generally drink only with meals and on ceremonial occasions, that alcohol-induced behavior is rejected by the Chinese, and that the absence of popular drinking places (such as taverns or bars) discourages the regular and excessive consumption of alcoholic beverages (Hsu, 1955; Singer, 1972). Similar suggestions were made in a survey of Chinatown in San Francisco (Chu, 1972). More recently in a report of the mainland Chinese, also a low-risk population for alcoholism, Lin and Lin have proposed a "substitution hypothesis:" that gambling and narcotic addiction might play important roles as substitutes for other psychosocial pathology among the Chinese (Lin & Lin, 1982).

Taiwan has undergone rapid industrialization and social changes during the past three decades. The increased production of alcohol beverages together with economic prosperity of the country have made the intake of alcoholic beverages more popular in daily life with rapidly increasing opportunities for excessive drinking in social settings. This has been supported by the sharp and consistent increase of annual total national consumption and, to a lesser extent, the per capita consumption

215

of alcoholic beverages during the past 3 decades in Taiwan as shown in Figures 13–1 and 13–2, respectively.

Though the rate of alcohol-induced mental disorders in clinical settings is generally still lower than would be expected, there has been a trend toward an increase in the proportion of outpatients with alcoholic psychoses at the Taipei City Psychiatric Center, from 0.7 percent of the total outpatients during 1970–1974 to 1.9 percent in 1980–1985. A higher rate of alcoholism among inpatients has been reported from a medium-size teaching general hospital in central Taiwan (Wu and Shen, 1985). However, out of the 130 patients with diagnosis of alcoholism during 1982–1984, 68 cases (58%) were primarily admitted to medical wards for physical disorders. In a recent survey of the total inpatients in the medical, surgical, and gynecological wards of a private general hospital in Taipei city, 12 cases (7.1%) and 11 cases (6.5%) were diagnosed as alcohol abuse and dependence, respectively, according to DSM-III (Chen et al., 1986). The low rate of alcoholism in psychiatric outpatient settings may be due to the attitudes of the patients and their families toward psychiatric disorders in general, and alcoholism in particular, that is, that they would not seek psychiatric treatment unless their symptoms become severe. A comparative study of outpatients by means of a structured diagnostic interview schedule between Taipei and Los Angeles has shown that there were only 6 male alcoholic cases identified at

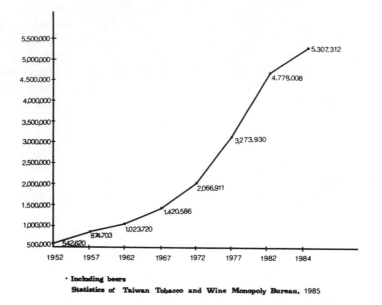

* Including beers
Statistics of Taiwan Tobacco and Wine Monopoly Bureau, 1985

Figure 13–1 Annual Total Consumption of Alcoholic Beverages in Taiwan (including beer) (1952–1984). [*Source:* Statistics of Taiwan Tobacco and Wine Monopoly Bureau, 1985.]

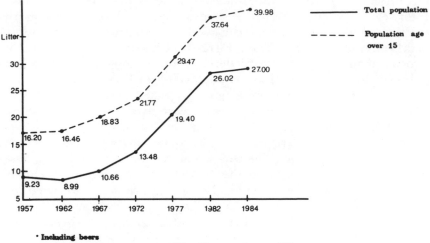

* Including beers
Statistics of Taiwan Tobacco and Wine Monopoly Bureau, 1985

Figure 13–2 Annual per capita consumption of alcoholic beverages in Taiwan (including beer) (1957–1984). [*Source:* Statistics of Taiwan Tobacco and Wine Monopoly Bureau, 1985.]

the Taipei City Psychiatric Center out of 100 randomly selected outpatients during a 3-month period in 1980. Though this number was considerably smaller than that in Los Angeles (sixteen males and nine females) during the same period of time, the Chinese alcoholics showed significantly higher scores in impairment of social functions than their American counterparts (Yeh et al., 1980).

The above findings suggest that alcoholism among the Chinese is not as rare as has been reported, and that its prevalence in the community might have increased under the impacts of rapid industrialization and social changes that have taken place during the past 3 decades in Taiwan.

In order to obtain up-to-date findings on the incidence and prevalence of mental disorders and the related data in community population, the Department of Health of the Executive Yuan (Cabinet) in 1981 initiated a nationwide epidemiological study project known as the Taiwan Psychiatric Epidemiologic Project (TEPE). This paper reports some of the major findings on alcoholism in three different sites of a Taiwan Chinese community as obtained from the TEPE.

Method of Study

The Taiwan Psychiatric Epidemiologic study (TEPE) was designed to study the community population age 18 years and over covering three different areas, namely, an urban area, townships, and rural villages. The special value and uniqueness of this study project is in its case-identification method by the Chinese version of the NIMH Diagnostic Interview Schedule (NIMH-DIS), an example of a third generation psychiatric epidemiologic study as classified by Dohrenwend (Dohrenwend and Dohrenwend, 1982). The NIMH-DIS consists of a series of highly structured questions with clearly defined criteria designed to reach diagnoses of specific mental disorders according to DSM-III clinical diagnosis through computer processing of the interview data. The schedule has been reliably used by nonprofessionals in psychiatric case-identification after a short course of training, and is thus useful for epidemiological study on large size samples in the community (Robins et al., 1981; Robins et al., 1982). The DIS was originally developed as the case-finding interview schedule in the NIMH Epidemiological Catchment Area (ECA) project (Regier et al., 1984), and has been translated into several major languages in European, Asian, and Latin American countries for application in psychiatric epidemiological studies (Helzer, 1985).

Case Identification Method

Version II of the DIS was first translated into Chinese by one of the authors of this chapter (Hwu) with modifications to form the Chinese modification of DIS-CM-I (Hwu et al., 1983). The DIS-CM-II was later developed to correspond to Version III of the DIS and further modification of the items from the DIS-CM-I with poor inter-rater reliability. A series of studies of the agreement between psychiatrist's clinical diagnosis and those derived from the DIS-CM on 100 inpatients and outpatients, and on ninety-five cases with DIS-CM-II positive diagnosis and ninety-two cases with DIS-CM-II negative diagnoses, have revealed that the kappa values for each diagnostic category are satisfactory, except for phobic disorders. The McNemar test has shown significant false negative bias for manic episode in the clinical cases and for tobacco dependence in the community sample as shown in Table 13–1 (Hwu et al., 1984; Hwu et al., 1986).

The development of DIS-CM, its inter-rater reliability, and validity of case-identification are reported in more detail in other chapters of this book and elsewhere. The DIS-CM-II was used in the above mentioned study of Taipei City in 1982, the DIS-CM-III in the study of the townships in 1984, and a DIS-CM-IV in the study of villages in 1985, with further questions of physical sensitivity to alcohol intake and help-seeking behavior.

Training of the Interviewers

Forty-eight to fifty senior students of medicine, psychology, and health education in the first study, and of medicine in the second and third studies, selected from seventy to eighty applicants served as interviewers

Table 13–1 Agreement Between DIS-CM Diagnosis and Clinical Diagnosis

	DIS-CM(+) Clinical(+)	DIS-CM(+) Clinical(−) (False Positive)	DIS-CM(−) Clinical(+) (False Negative)	DIS-CM(−) Clinical(−)	K-value
Clinical cases					
Schizophrenia	42	6	17	35	0.54
Manic episode	18	0	9	73	0.82
Depressive episode	4	1	1	94	0.96
Community samples					
Manic episode	3	4[a]	0	180	0.59
Depressive episode	10	7	3	167	0.67
Anxiety state	26	20	17	125	0.44
Phobic disorder	6	27[a]	5	149	0.18
Obsessive-compulsive disorder	1	18[a]	0	168	—
Psychosexual dysfunction	6	4	2	175	0.70
Tobacco dependence	11	4	17[a]	155	0.45
Alcohol abuse/ dependence	7	10[a]	1	169	0.53
Schizophrenic disorder	0	1	0	186	—
Cognitive impairment	1	1	0	185	—
Any diagnosis covered	64	30	25	68	0.42

[a]McNemar test for bias in over diagnosis between two diagnostic systems $p < .05$.

Quoted from Hwu, Yeh, and Chang (1986). Chinese diagnostic interview schedule. I. Agreement with psychiatrist's diagnosis. *Acta Psychitr. Scand.* 73:225–33, Table 1, p. 227.

in all three parts of the TEPE after a carefully and comprehensively designed 2-week full-time training course. The training program consisted of general orientation to the TEPE, didactic lectures on the applications of the DIS-CM, observation of videotaped interviews with the DIS-CM, practice in interview with clinical and community samples, exercise in scoring with mutual analysis, and assigned homework. The interrater reliability with the DIS-CM-II in the first study and with the DIS-CM-III in the second study after the training were highly satisfactory as shown in Table 13–2.

Sampling Method

The sample size of 5,000 for a metropolis and 3,000 for the townships and rural villages was based on consideration of 1) reported prevalences of mental disorders in literature, 2) the nature of the case-finding method and the expected duration of each interview, and 3) the problems and difficulties anticipated in the field work.

A multi-staged stratified sampling method was employed to draw the study samples, which represented all general population members of the study sites age 18 and over (Chang et al., 1984).

Table 13–2 Agreement Between Interviewers on Scoring of DIS-CM After Training

Degree of Agreement	Mean % of Number of Questions with Agreement	
	First study site: metropolis	Second study site: townships
100	32.2	62.3
90–99	45.9	34.2
85–89.9	10.8	1.8
80–84.9	4.7	1.5
75–79.9	2.5	0.1
70–74.9	3.8	0.1
Below 70	0	0
Beyond 90%	78.2	96.5
Beyond 85%	89.0	98.3
Beyond 80%	93.8	99.8

In the study of Taipei city, eight "Chi" (administrative districts) were drawn out of a total of sixteen according to the distribution of inhabitants and the level of urbanicity. Within these, we randomly sampled 40 "Li" (census tracts) and 200 "Lin" (blocks). Rosters from records of sociodemographic data and addresses of all inhabitants over age 18 in the 200 sample "Lin" were then constructed. One respondent per household was then sampled and contacted by mail or in person to assess their willingness to participate. Those who failed to respond or refused were replaced by repeated sampling from the rosters to obtain the subjects with similar demographic background until the target number was achieved. In order to facilitate the proceeding of field work, the so-called "Direct Approach Method" (Mitchell, 1980) or "Foot-In-The-Door-Method" (Graves & Magilavey, 1981) were employed in addition to the so-called "Research Team Control Method" (Moser & Kalton, 1971), as described above, to allow the interviewers to draw other subjects when the prospective subject could not be interviewed.

For the second segment of the TEPE, two townships were selected to represent the two typical types in present-day Taiwan. One (Su-Lin) is geographically near to Taipei city and has experienced a rapid population increase associated with industrialization during the past 6 years. The other (Tsau-tung) is geographically isolated from Taipei and has experienced a more gradual population increase.

For the third segment of the TEPE, six counties (two each from northern, central, and the southern parts of Taiwan) with a total of ninety villages (Tsung) were drawn to represent three types of rural villages in present-day Taiwan, namely a mixture of farming and/or fishing villages.

The sampling procedure in the two townships and in six counties were the same as in Taipei city, but with more flexibility. As shown in

Table 13–3 Response and Incompletion Rate for Interview

	Total Sample Drawn		Interview Completed		Nonrespondent			
					Refusal		Other Reasons	
	N	%	N	%	N	%	N	%
Taipei city	8,156	100	5,005	61.4	543	6.7	2,608	32.0
Su-lin	1,989	100	1,505	75.6	26	1.3	458	23.0
Tsau-tung	1,759	100	1,499	85.2	8	0.5	252	14.3
Villages	3,831	100	2,995	78.2	30	0.8	806	21.0

Table 13–3, the refusal rate at the time of interview was quite low, lowest in Tsau-tung, next lowest in villages and Su-Lin, and higher in Taipei. The great majority of nonrespondents for interview were absent from the household due to change of job, schooling, and military enlistment but who had not yet reported the changes to the population Registration Office. For the very small number of expired or hospitalized nonrespondents, mental disorders as causes of death or hospitalization were carefully ruled out.

The sample sizes in the completed study are 5,005 for Taipei, 3,004 for townships, and 2,995 for rural villages. As shown in Table 13–4, there are minor differences in the distribution by sex and age between the study samples and the general population age over 18 in each study site.

Results

Sociodemographic Findings

The sociodemographic distributions of the study samples into four age groups, and by educational levels, marital status, domicile of origin, and occupations are significantly different between each of three study sties (Table 13–5). This indicates the different sociodemographic composition of the inhabitants in the metropolis, townships, and rural villages in present day Taiwan, and illustrates the necessity of selecting populations in each of the three areas in order to have a study sample that is representative of the full range of the Taiwanese population.

Lifetime Prevalence

The unweighted lifetime prevalence of alcohol abuse and of total alcohol dependence are 3.4 and 1.5 percent respectively in the metropolis, 8.0 and 1.8 percent in the townships, and 6.3 and 1.2 percent in the villages (Table 13–6). When alcohol dependence is subclassified into that without or with abuse, dependence without abuse is much lower in both

Table 13–4a Demographic Characteristics of Study Samples in Three Sites

	Taipei (%)		Townships (%)		Villages (%)	
Sex	Sample	General population age over 18[a]	Sample	General population age over 18[a]	Sample	General population age over 18[a]
Male	49.3	51.4	52.6	51.6	54.9	55.2
Female	50.7	48.6	47.4	48.4	45.1	44.8

Table 13–4b Sample and General Population (%)

	Taipei				Townships				Villages			
	Male		Female		Male		Female		Male		Female	
Age	Sample	G.P.[a]	Sample	G.P.[a]	Sample	G.P.[a]	Sample	G.P.[a]	Sample	G.P.[a]	Sample	G.P.[a]
18–24	17.6	20.6	21.2	22.4	22.0	23.1	24.3	24.7	27.2	28.2	29.8	28.0
25–44	41.9	44.6	49.4	50.6	49.4	47.3	46.7	46.6	39.8	39.5	38.1	38.2
45–64	31.5	27.9	22.8	20.8	22.6	23.8	21.0	21.0	25.7	25.6	24.5	25.1
65+	8.9	6.9	6.7	6.3	6.0	5.8	8.0	7.7	7.3	6.8	7.7	8.7

[a]Population registered in Household Registration Office in 1982 for Taipei; 1984 for townships, and 1985 for rural.

Table 13–5 *Sociodemographic Distribution of Study Samples in Three Sites*

	Metropolis			Townships			Villages		
Sociodemographic Data	Male $N = 2466$ %	Female $N = 2539$ %	Total $N = 5005$ %	Male $N = 1579$ %	Female $N = 1425$ %	Total $N = 3004$ %	Male $N = 1643$ %	Female $N = 1352$ %	Total $N = 2995$ %
Age-group[abc]									
18–24 years	17.6	21.2	19.4	22.0	24.4	23.1	27.1	29.8	28.3
25–44 years	41.9	49.6	45.7	49.5	46.6	48.1	39.8	38.0	39.0
45–64 years	31.5	22.8	27.1	22.5	20.9	21.8	25.7	24.5	25.2
65+ years	8.9	6.6	7.8	6.0	8.1	7.0	7.3	7.7	7.5
Education[abc]									
9th grade and lower	40.4	50.7	45.6	63.5	73.5	68.1	72.7	82.6	77.2
10th grade and higher	59.6	49.3	54.2	36.5	26.5	31.9	27.3	17.4	22.8
Marital status[b]									
Married	68.4	69.9	69.1	70.4	72.1	71.2	65.8	69.7	67.5
Never married	26.6	21.8	24.2	26.2	18.3	22.4	30.1	20.8	25.9
Others	5.0	8.3	6.7	3.4	9.6	6.4	4.1	9.5	6.5
Domicile of origin[abc]									
Native Taiwanese	62.3	73.9	68.2	92.2	94.3	93.2	96.4	97.9	97.1
Others	37.7	26.1	31.8	7.8	5.7	6.8	3.6	2.1	2.9
Occupation[abc]									
Upper four[d]	52.1	33.1	42.5	29.3	18.1	24.0	16.2	10.7	13.7
Lower three[e]	32.8	19.3	25.9	64.3	42.7	51.4	77.8	45.7	63.3
Housewife, student, and unemployed	15.1	47.6	31.6	6.4	39.2	21.9	6.0	43.6	23.0

[a]Metropolis vs Townships $p < .05$

[b]Townships vs Villages $p < .05$

[c]Villages vs Metropolis $p < .05$

[d]Professionals: Executive of large or medium-sized enterprise, Administrator, Onwer of store; clerical, sales or service worker

[e]Skilled worker, Semiskilled worker, Non-killed worker

223

Table 13–6 Lifetime Prevalence of Alcohol Abuse and Alcohol Dependence With or Without Abuse

	Metropolis						Townships						Villages					
	Male N = 2,466		Female N = 2,539		Total N = 5,005		Male N = 1,579		Female N = 1,425		Total N = 3,004		Male N = 1,643		Female N 1,352		Total N = 2,995	
	N	%	N	%	N	%	N	%	N	%	N	%	N	%	N	%	N	%
Alcohol abuse	158	6.4	11	0.4	169	3.4 (3.5)[a]	232	14.7	8	0.6	240	8.0 (7.8)	185	11.3	3	0.2	188	6.3 (6.3)
Alcohol dependence without abuse	15	0.6	1	0.04	16	0.3 (0.3)	5	0.3	1	0.07	6	0.2 (0.2)	6	0.4	—	—	6	0.2 (0.2)
Alcohol dependence with abuse	55	2.2	2	0.1	57	1.2 (1.2)	45	2.9	3	0.2	48	1.6 (1.6)	29	1.8	—	—	29	1.0 (1.0)

[a]Numbers in parentheses are weighted %.

sexes and in all three sites. The weighted prevalences are shown in the same table and differ little. The prevalences of alcohol abuse and/or dependence are clearly exceeded only by those for tobacco dependence in the three sites, and are about equal to the rates of general anxiety disorders in townships and villages (Table 13–7). The lifetime prevalences of alcohol abuse and dependence with or without abuse by sex in 5-year age intervals are shown in Table 13–8, and into the four age groups used elsewhere in this volume in Table 13–9. In the latter table it can be seen that the rate of abuse for males is generally higher in younger groups (44 and under) than in the older two groups, and is highest in the 25–44-year age group in all three sites. Alcoholism is so rare in females that age differences are not really detectible. The alcohol disorders are definitely and consistently male predominant in all three sites.

Table 13–9 also shows total rates for abuse and dependence. Only for abuse do the rates differ very much by site, being highest in the townships, next highest in villages, and lowest in the metropolis. These differences are more significant in males than in females. The rate of dependence is considerably lower and is much the same through all three sites.

Six-Month Prevalence

The unweighted 6-month prevalences for alcohol abuse and dependence are 1.1 and 0.5 percent in the metropolis, 3.9 and 1.0 percent in townships, and 2.8 and 0.5 percent in the villages, and again the weighted prevalences are essentially identical (Table 13–10). Differences by age group, site, and sex are much the same as those described above. There is a somewhat greater differential for dependence between the townships and the other two sites, but the differences are still not significant.

Educational Level

Generally, the lifetime prevalences of alcohol abuse and dependence are higher in lower educational level groups in all three sites. The differences are, however, significant only in metropolitan males and not significant for either sex in the townships and villages (Table 13–11).

Lifetime Prevalence and Marital Status

The relationship between the prevalence rates of alcohol abuse/ dependence and marital status is different in each of the study sites (Table 13–12). In the metropolis, the rate of alcohol dependence is highest in males listed as "other" marital status, next highest in the never-married, and lowest in the married group. The rate of alcohol abuse, however, shows no significant difference by marital status. In the townships, the signifi-

Table 13–7 Lifetime Prevalence of Specific Mental Disorders in Three Sites

	Metropolis			Townships			Villages		
	Male $N = 2,466$ %	Female $N = 2,539$ %	Total $N = 5,005$ % [a]	Male $N = 1,579$ %	Female $N = 1,425$ %	Total $N = 3,004$ % [a]	Male $N = 1,643$ %	Female $N = 1,352$ %	Total $N = 2,995$ % [a]
Psychotic disorders									
Schizophrenia	0.3	0.3	0.3 (0.3)	0.2	0.3	0.2 (0.2)	0.4	0.1	0.2 (0.2)
Manic episode	0.2	0.2	0.2 (0.2)	0.1	—	0.1 (0.1)	0.1	0.1	0.1 (0.1)
Bipolar disorder	0.1	0.2	0.2 (0.2)	—	0.4	0.2 (0.2)	—	0.1	0.03 (0.03)
Paranoid disorder	0.4	0.6	0.5 (0.5)	0.6	0.8	0.7 (0.7)	0.4	0.3	0.1 (0.3)
Depressions									
Major depressive episode	0.7	1.0	0.9 (0.9)	0.9	1.6	1.7 (1.7)	0.6	1.4	1.0 (1.0)
Dysthymic disorder	0.7	1.1	0.9 (0.9)	1.4	1.6	1.5 (1.5)	0.6	1.4	0.9 (0.9)
Anxiety/somatoform disorder									
General anxiety disorder	2.4	5.0	3.7 (3.7)	8.8	12.4	10.5 (10.5)	6.1	9.0	7.4 (7.5)
Phobic disorder	2.7	5.7	4.2 (4.2)	2.7	8.8	5.6 (5.7)	2.2	5.0	3.4 (3.4)
Obsessive-compulsive dis.	0.8	1.1	0.9 (0.9)	0.4	0.7	0.5 (0.5)	0.4	0.2	0.3 (0.3)
Panic disorder	0.1	0.3	0.2 (0.2)	0.3	0.4	0.3 (0.3)	0.1	0.2	0.1 (0.1)
Somatization disorder	—	—	0.04 (0.04)	0.1	0.1	0.1 (0.1)	0.1	0.2	0.1 (0.1)
Substance use disorder									
Alcohol abuse	6.4	0.4	3.4 (3.5)	14.7	0.6	8.0 (7.8)	11.3	0.2	6.3 (6.3)
Alcohol dependence	2.8	0.1	1.5 (1.5)	3.2	0.3	1.8 (1.8)	2.1	—	1.2 (1.2)
Tobacco dependence	14.3	1.3	7.7 (8.0)	22.6	0.7	12.2 (12.0)	24.1	0.7	13.6 (13.2)
Drug dependence	—	—	0.1 (0.1)	0.4	—	0.2 (0.2)	—	—	—
Personality disorder									
Antisocial personality	0.2	0.04	0.1 (0.2)	0.1	—	0.1 (0.1)	0.1	—	0.03 (0.03)
Pathological gambling	0.9	0.08	0.5 (0.5)	1.0	0.1	0.6 (0.6)	0.8	—	0.4 (0.4)
Psychosexual disorder									
Transsexualism	—	0.08	0.1 (0.1)	—	0.4	0.2 (0.2)	—	0.1	0.03 (0.03)
Psychosexual dysfunction	1.0	1.7	1.4 (1.3)	0.8	2.8	1.8 (1.8)	2.7	2.2	2.5 (2.5)
Cognitive impairment	0.1	0.7	0.4 (0.4)	1.3	2.2	1.7 (1.7)	1.2	1.7	1.4 (1.4)

[a]Numbers in parentheses are weighted %.

Table 13–8 Lifetime Prevalence of Alcohol Abuse, and Alcohol Dependence With or Without Abuse in Each Sex and 5-year Age Groups

Age group	Metropolis Male I	II %	III[a]	Female I	II %	III[a]	Total I	II %	III[a]	Townships Male I	II %	III[a]	Female I	II %	III[a]	Total I	II %	III[a]	Villages Male I	II %	III[a]	Female I	II %	III[a]	Total I	II %	III[a]
18–24	4.8	0.7	2.8	—	—	—	2.2	0.3	1.2	11.0	—	3.2	0.6	—	0.3	5.8	—	1.7	12.6	0.2	1.3	0.2	—	—	6.7	0.1	0.7
25–29	8.1	0.0	2.6	0.3	—	—	3.9	—	1.2	17.6	0.4	1.9	0.4	—	0.4	9.3	0.2	1.2	16.0	—	1.8	1.0	—	—	8.7	—	1.0
30–34	5.5	0.3	2.6	0.8	—	0.3	2.9	0.1	1.3	19.4	0.4	4.3	0.5	—	—	11.2	0.2	2.4	10.5	1.2	2.3	—	—	—	6.9	0.7	1.4
35–39	12.4	—	1.7	0.7	0.4	—	6.1	0.2	0.8	15.0	—	2.3	—	—	—	8.4	—	1.3	10.9	0.8	1.6	—	—	—	5.9	0.4	0.8
40–44	7.0	0.5	2.2	0.9	—	0.4	3.6	0.2	1.2	14.7	0.8	1.6	0.8	0.8	—	8.1	0.8	0.8	11.9	0.7	—	—	—	—	6.3	0.4	—
45–49	7.9	1.8	1.2	—	—	—	3.8	0.9	0.6	17.1	—	4.5	1.0	—	—	9.6	—	2.4	11.9	—	3.5	—	—	—	6.9	—	2.0
50–54	5.0	0.9	2.7	1.1	—	—	3.3	0.5	1.5	13.4	—	4.5	1.2	—	1.2	8.2	—	3.1	6.7	—	2.5	—	—	—	4.0	—	1.5
55–59	4.5	0.5	1.8	0.8	—	—	3.2	0.3	1.2	7.5	1.3	—	—	—	—	4.0	0.7	—	12.8	—	2.1	—	—	—	7.1	—	1.2
60–64	4.7	1.2	2.4	—	—	—	2.9	0.7	1.5	20.8	1.9	1.9	—	—	—	10.9	1.0	1.0	6.1	—	3.0	—	—	—	2.9	—	1.4
65–69	6.2	—	0.9	—	—	—	3.7	—	0.5	11.9	—	2.4	2.5	—	—	7.3	—	1.2	2.9	1.5	1.5	2.4	—	—	2.7	0.9	0.9
70–74	4.7	1.6	1.6	—	—	—	2.9	1.0	1.0	—	—	—	—	—	—	—	—	—	8.7	—	—	—	—	—	3.4	—	—
75+	2.3	2.3	2.3	—	—	—	1.0	1.0	1.0	10.3	—	3.4	—	—	—	4.1	—	1.4	3.4	—	—	—	—	—	1.8	—	—
Total	6.4	0.6	2.2	0.4	0.04	0.1	3.4	0.3	1.2	14.7	0.3	2.9	0.6	0.07	0.2	3.4	0.2	1.6	11.3	0.4	1.8	0.2	—	—	6.3	0.2	1.0

[a]I: Alcohol abuse

II: Alcohol dependence without abuse

III: Alcohol dependence with abuse

227

Table 13–9 Age-and-Sex-Specific Lifetime Prevalence of Alcohol Abuse/Dependence

		Metropolis			Townships			Villages			Comparison Between Study Site by t-test					
											I		II		III	
		Male N = 2,466 %	Female N = 2,539 %	Total N = 5,005 %	Male N = 1,579 %	Female N = 1,425 %	Total N = 3,004 %	Male N = 1,643 %	Female N = 1,352 %	Total N = 2,995 %	M	F	M	F	M	F
18–24	AA	4.8	—	2.2	11.0	0.6	5.8	12.6	0.3	6.7	<.001	<.001	n.s.	n.s.	<.001	<.01
	AD	3.5	—	1.5	3.2	0.3	1.7	1.6	—	0.8	n.s.	<.01	<.01	<.05	<.001	—
25–44	AA	8.1	0.6	4.0	17.3	0.5	9.5	12.7	0.2	7.2	<.001	n.s.	<.001	n.s.	<.001	<.1
	AD	2.5	0.2	1.3	3.1	0.3	1.8	2.1	—	1.2	n.s.	n.s.	<.1	<.01	n.s.	<.1
45–64	AA	5.4	0.5	3.3	14.3	0.7	8.1	9.7	—	5.4	<.001	n.s.	<.001	<.01	<.001	<.01
	AD	3.1	—	1.8	3.7	0.3	2.1	2.8	—	1.6	n.s.	<.01	n.s.	<.05	n.s.	—
65+	AA	5.0	—	2.8	8.4	0.9	4.3	4.2	1.0	2.7	<.001	<.001	<.001	n.s.	n.s.	<.001
	AD	2.3	—	1.3	2.1	—	1.0	1.7	—	0.9	n.s.	—	n.s.	—	n.s.	—
Total	AA	6.4	0.4	3.4 (3.5)a	14.7	0.6	8.0 (7.8)	11.3	0.2	6.3 (6.3)	<.001	n.a.	<.01	<.01	<.001	<.01
	AD	2.8	0.1	1.5 (1.5)	3.2	0.3	1.8 (1.8)	2.1	—	1.2 (1.2)	n.s.	n.s.	<.1	<.05	n.s.	n.s.
Comparison between age group	AA X² P	8.84 <.05	n.s.	n.s.	11.08 <.05	n.s.	13.36 <.005	9.17 <.05	n.s.	7.77 <.1	—	—	—	—	—	—
	AD X² P	n.s.	n.s.	n.s.	n.s.	n.s.	n.s.	n.s.	—	n.s.	—	—	—	—	—	—

I: Metropolis vs Townships

II: Townships vs Villages

III: Villages vs Metropolis

a Numbers in parentheses are weighted %.

Table 13–10 Age-and-Sex-Specific 5-Month Prevalence of Alcohol Abuse/Dependence

| | | Metropolis | | | Townships | | | Villages | | | Comparison Between Study Site by t-test | | | | | |
		Male N = 2,466	Female N = 2,539	Total N = 5,005	Male N = 1,579	Female N = 1,425	Total N = 3,004	Male N = 1,643	Female N = 1,352	Total N = 2,995	I M	I F	II M	II F	III M	III F
		%	%	%	%	%	%	%	%	%						
18–24	AA	1.6	—	0.7	5.5	0.3	2.9	7.0	—	3.7	<.001	<.01	<.1	<.05	<.001	—
	AD	0.9	—	0.4	2.3	0.3	1.3	0.7	—	0.4	<.001	<.01	<.001	<.05	n.s.	—
25–44	AA	3.2	0.4	1.7	9.3	—	5.0	5.8	0.2	3.4	<.001	<.01	<.001	<.1	<.001	n.s.
	AD	0.8	0.2	0.5	1.8	0.3	1.1	0.6	—	0.3	<0.1	n.s.	<.01	<.05	n.s.	n.s.
45–64	AA	1.2	—	0.7	6.2	0.7	3.7	3.1	—	1.7	<.001	<0.1	<.001	<.01	<.001	—
	AD	1.2	—	0.7	1.4	—	0.8	1.9	—	1.1	n.s.	—	n.s.	—	<.1	—
65+	AA	0.5	—	0.3	1.1	—	0.5	—	—	—	<.05	—	<.001	—	<.01	—
	AD	—	—	—	—	—	—	—	—	—	—	—	—	—	—	—
Total	AA	2.0	0.2	1.1 (1.2)[a]	7.3	0.2	3.9 (3.8)	5.1	0.1	2.8 (2.9)	<.001	n.s.	<.01	n.s.	<.001	n.s.
	AD	0.9	0.1	0.5 (0.5)	1.7	0.2	1.0 (1.0)	1.0	—	0.5 (0.5)	<.01	n.s.	<.1	n.s.	n.s.	n.s.
Comparison between age group	AA	<.005	n.s.	<.01	<.01	n.s.	<.005	<.005	n.s.	<.005						
	AD	n.s.	n.s.	n.s.	n.s.	n.s.	n.s.	<.1	—	<.1						

I: Metropolis vs Townships

II: Townships vs Villages

III: Villages vs Metropolis

[a]Numbers in parentheses are weighted %.

Table 13–11a Lifetime Prevalence of Alcohol Abuse/Dependence and Educational Level

| | Metropolis | | | | | | | | | Townships | | | | | | | | | Villages | | | | | | | | |
| | ≤9 yrs. | | | 10–15 yrs. | | | ≥16 yrs. | | | ≤9 yrs. | | | 10–15 yrs. | | | ≥16 yrs. | | | ≤9 yrs. | | | 10–15 yrs. | | | ≥16 yrs. | | |
	M	F	T	M	F	T	M	F	T	M	F	T	M	F	T	M	F	T	M	F	T	M	F	T	M	F	T
Alcohol abuse	6.1	0.7	3.1	8.1	0.1	4.2	3.9	0.5	2.9	15.6	0.7	7.8	13.6	0.3	8.0	7.1	—	5.0	11.2	0.3	5.9	11.9	—	7.8	6.4	—	5.9
Alcohol dependence	3.7	0.2	1.8	2.9	—	1.5	1.0	0.5	0.9	3.8	0.3	2.0	2.3	0.3	1.5	—	—	—	2.6	—	1.4	0.9	—	0.6	—	—	—

Table 13–11b Comparison between Educational Levels

| | Metropolis | | | Townships | | | Villages | | |
	Male	Female	Total	Male	Female	Total	Male	Female	Total
Alcohol abuse	$P < .01$	$P < .1$	n.s.	n.s.	n.s.	n.s.	n.s.	n.s.	n.s.
Alcohol dependence	$P < .05$	n.s.	n.s.	n.s.	n.s.	n.s.	$< .1$	—	n.s.

Table 13–12a Lifetime Prevalence of Alcohol Abuse/Dependence and Marital Status

	Metropolis									Townships									Villages								
	Never married			Married			Others[a]			Never married			Married			Others[a]			Never married			Married			Others[a]		
	M	F	T	M	F	T	M	F	T	M	F	T	M	F	T	M	F	T	M	F	T	M	F	T	M	F	T
Alcohol abuse	6.5	0.4	3.7	6.3	0.5	3.4	6.5	—	2.4	9.4	0.4	5.9	16.5	0.7	8.9	18.5	—	5.3	11.1	0.2	6.0	12.5	0.4	8.1	4.5	—	1.5
Alcohol dependence	3.2	—	1.7	2.4	0.2	1.2	7.3	—	2.7	3.4	0.4	7.2	3.1	0.3	1.7	3.7	—	1.1	2.1	—	1.1	2.0	—	1.3	3.0	—	1.0

Table 13–12b Comparison between Marital Status Group

	Metropolis			Townships			Villages		
	Male	Female	Total	Male	Female	Total	Male	Female	Total
Alcohol abuse	n.s.	n.s.	n.s.	$X^2 = 12.5$ $P < .005$	n.s.	n.s.	n.s.	n.s.	$X^2 = 12.2$ $P < .005$
Alcohol dependence	$X^2 = 10.56$ $P < .01$	n.s.	$< .1$	n.s.	n.s.	n.s.	n.s.	n.s.	n.s.

[a]Indicate separated, divorced, widows, or widowers.

cant difference is observed in male alcohol abusers, and neither in female abusers nor in either sex among those who are alcohol dependent. Again, the highest rate is seen in "other" marital status group, but next highest in the married group, and lowest in the never-marrieds.

Lifetime Prevalence and Occupation

Higher rates of both alcohol abuse and dependence are seen among workers' groups than in the other two occupational groups in the metropolis, while in townships and villages the rates in the workers and upper occupational groups are much the same (Table 13–13). In all three sites, the rates of alcohol abuse and dependence are lowest in occupational group III, which includes housewives, students, enlisted soldiers, and the unemployed. This low rate is found for males as well as for females.

Lifetime Prevalence and Domicile of Origin

The inhabitants in Taiwan can be classified into three major ethnic or subcultural groups. Native Taiwanese Chinese refer to the descendants of Chinese who migrated to the island primarily from Fukien and, to a lesser extent, from Kwangton province of China during the seventeenth and eighteenth centuries. This group, which constitutes approximately 70 percent of the current population, has lived on the island for generations, and has been influenced to some extent by Japanese culture during the 50 years of Japanese administration. The second group are Mainland Chinese and their descendents, who migrated to Taiwan after World War II. This group constitutes approximately 28 percent of the total population. The members of the first generation of this group had migrated from all parts of China and had gone through similar refugee experiences but maintained subcultures different from that of the Taiwanese Chinese. The third group, the aborigines, are ethnically Malayo-Polynesian, constitute about 2 percent of the total population, and are divided into nine tribes with varying degrees of acculturation to Chinese culture. Because they are such a small proportion in this study, the aborigines are grouped for convenience with the mainland Chinese as "others" in Table 14–1, but are disaggregated in the next table.

As a whole, the rate for alcohol dependence is higher in the "others" group than in the Taiwanese group in all three sites of study, but the difference is significant only for females in townships as shown in Table 13–14. The rate for alcohol abuse shows no differences across the sites. The rate of alcohol dependence in aborigines is 6.9 percent (2 out of 29 total subjects), which is significantly higher than that of the Chinese (1.5%—Table 13–15). Interestingly, the rate of alcohol abuse in aborigines as a whole (two cases, 6.9%) is fairly comparable with that of the

Table 13–13a Lifetime Prevalence of Alcohol Abuse/Dependence and Occupation

	Metropolis									Townships									Villages								
	I			II			III			I			II			III			I			II			III		
	M	F	T	M	F	T	M	F	T	M	F	T	M	F	T	M	F	T	M	F	T	M	F	T	M	F	T
Alcohol abuse	6.5	0.5	4.1	8.3	0.8	6.2	3.9	0.3	1.3	17.1	1.2	11.4	15.4	0.7	10.1	4.9	0.2	1.2	12.4	0.0	8.0	11.9	0.2	8.1	4.9	0.3	1.3
Alcohol dependence	2.9	0.4	1.9	3.2	0.0	2.3	2.3	0.0	0.6	2.6	0.8	1.9	3.6	0.0	2.3	2.2	0.3	0.7	2.3	0.0	1.5	2.4	0.0	1.6	0.0	0.0	0.0

Table 13–13b Comparison between Occupations

	Metropolis			Townships			Villages		
	Male	Female	Total	Male	Female	Total	Male	Female	Total
Alcohol abuse	$X^2 = 9.5$ $P < .01$	— n.s.	$X^2 = 51.0$ $P < .01$	16.47 $P < .01$	— n.s.	70.30 $P < .01$	7.25 $P < .1$	— n.s.	45.37 $P < .01$
Alcohol dependence	— n.s.	$X^2 = 6.08$ $P < .05$	$X^2 = 16.27$ $P < .01$	— n.s.	— n.s.	7.42 $P < .1$	— n.s.	—	12.66 $P < .01$

I Professionals: Executive of large or medium-sized enterprise, Administrator, Owner of store; clerical, sales or service worker

II Skilled worker, Semiskilled worker, Non-skilled worker

III Housewife, student, soldiers and unemployed

Table 13–14a *Lifetime Prevalence of Alcohol Abuse/Dependence in Each Domicile Group of Origin*

	Metropolis						Townships						Villages					
	Native Taiwanese			Others[a]			Native Taiwanese			Others[a]			Native Taiwanese			Others[a]		
	Male	Female %	Total	Male	Female %	Total	Male	Female %	Total	Male	Female %	Total	Male	Female %	Total	Male	Female %	Total
Alcohol abuse	6.4	0.5	3.1	6.5	0.3	3.9	14.8	0.6	8.0	13.8	0.0	8.3	11.1	0.2	6.2	15.3	0.0	10.2
Alcohol dependence	2.9	0.2	1.4	2.7	0.0	1.6	3.2	0.1	1.7	3.3	2.5	2.9	2.0	0.0	1.1	5.1	0.0	3.4

Table 13–14b *Comparison between Domicile Group*

	Metropolis			Townships			Villages		
	Male	Female	Total	Male	Female	Total	Male	Female	Total
Alcohol abuse	n.s.	n.s.	n.s.	n.s.	n.s.	n.s.	n.s.	n.s.	n.s.
Alcohol dependence	n.s.	n.s.	n.s.	n.s.	$X^2 = 14.7$ $P < .005$	n.s.	n.s.	n.s.	n.s.

[a]Indicates mainland Chinese and aborigines.

Table 13–15 Lifetime Prevalence of Alcohol Abuse/Dependence in Chinese and Aborigines

| | Metropolis | | | | Townships | | | | Villages | | | |
| | Chinese N = 4,995 | | Aborigines N = 10 | | Chinese N = 2,988 | | Aborigines N = 16 | | Chinese N = 2,992 | | Aborigines N = 3 | |
	N	%	N	%	N	%	N	%	N	%	N	%
Alcohol abuse	168	3.4	1	10.0	239	8.0	1	6.3	188	6.3	0	0.0
Alcohol dependence	73	1.5	0	0.0	52	1.7	2	12.5	35	1.2	0	0.0

Chinese (5.4%). Table 13–15 shows these two groups by domicile of origin, but the numbers of aborigines are quite small.

Symptom Profile

Both the alcohol abuse and dependence groups show significantly higher symptom rates in mode of and attitude toward drinking, alcohol-related social problems, and psychological or physical sequelae than do nonalcoholic cases (Tables 13–16 & 13–17). This well supports the diagnostic validity of the DIS-CM in differentiating the cases of alcohol abuse and dependence from nonalcoholic respondents. There are some differences in the mode of drinking, and alcohol-related physical diseases between the abuse and dependence cases. Those in the dependence group drink more heavily and for longer periods of time, and have more physical complications such as tremor and epileptic seizures, and hepatic, gastric, and pancreatic diseases than abuse cases. Interestingly, there are no significant differences in attitude to drinking and in social problems between these two alcoholic groups, except for a higher rate of losing a job or being fired in the dependence group in the metropolitan sample, and a higher rate of physical fights in the dependence group at all three sites. Differences in other categories of symptoms and consequences between study sites are sporadic and inconsistent. The age of onset of first intoxication and of any alcohol-related symptom is younger in the alcohol groups than in nonalcohol groups. Comparing alcohol abusers and those with dependence, the latter have a greater mean number of positive lifetime symptoms, more significant in townships and villages (Table 13–18), and have a younger age of onset (Table 13–19). As a whole, the mean number of alcoholic symptoms is higher in the dependence group than abuse group, and more significant in townships and villages as shown in Table 13–16. The difference in mean number of alcohol symptoms by sex is not consistent, except in the abuse group in the metropolis and the dependence group in townships, where males seem to have more symptoms than females.

Help-Seeking Behavior

In both abuse and dependence groups, the rate of prior medical consultation and of treatment seeking is surprisingly low. In the abuse group, visiting Western physicians and self-medication with Western drugs (particularly in townships) seem to be the most frequent behavior among the few help-seeking experiences. Surprisingly, in the dependence group, not a single case reported "visiting western physicians" in the metropolis compared to 20.4 and 8.6 percent in the townships and villages, respectively. Self-medication with Western drugs for alcohol dependence is higher in the townships than in the metropolis and villages.

Table 13–16 Symptom Profiles of Nonalcoholics, Alcohol-abusers and Alcohol Dependants

	Nonalcoholics			Alcohol Abuse			Alcohol Dependence		
	I	II %	III	I	II %	III	I	II %	III
Mode of drinking									
1. Ever drunk 1 bottle of strong liquor or 3 bottles of ordinary liquor or 18 bottles of beer in a day.	1.1	0.8	0.6	62.1	46.7	42.6	75.3	63.0	74.3
2. Ever drunk at least more than 7 big glasses of strong or ordinary liquor or 7 bottles of beer every day for 2 weeks.	0.1	0.1	0.0	0.0	0.0	0.0	84.9	66.7	85.7
3. Ever had one night of excessive drinking every week for 1–2 month period.	0.4	0.3	0.2	18.9	13.8	11.7	57.5	55.6	57.1
4. Need to drink on wakening in morning.	0.0	0.0	0.0	0.0	0.0	0.0	13.7	18.5	25.7
5. Ever had continuous and excessive drinking for 2 days or longer.	0.1	0.0	0.0	14.8	9.6	9.6	38.4	35.2	40.0
6. Continue drinking in spite of physical diseases.	0.0	0.0	0.0	7.7	11.7	10.6	12.3	31.5	17.1
7. Ever had a period of time in need of excessive drinking in order to work.	0.0	0.0	0.0	1.8	1.3	0.5	1.4	7.4	11.4
Attitude to drinking									
1. Family ever opposed drinking.	4.2	7.8	7.2	62.7	68.3	71.8	53.4	68.5	54.3
2. Ever considered yourself as excessive drinker.	1.3	2.3	2.1	39.6	48.3	39.4	50.7	61.1	57.1
3. Ever been persuaded to stop drinking.	4.1	7.6	6.5	89.4	91.7	92.3	78.1	83.3	91.4
4. Ever tried to stop drinking but failed.	0.2	0.2	0.3	26.0	37.5	40.4	24.7	42.6	40.0
5. Tried not to drink before 5:00 p.m. or not to drink alone.	0.2	0.3	0.4	18.9	42.9	33.5	11.0	44.4	14.3
Social problems due to drinking									
1. Ever had difficulties in working.	0.1	0.2	0.1	15.1	11.7	9.6	11.8	26.0	17.1
2. Ever been fired or lost job.	0.0	0.0	0.0	0.0	0.0	1.1	4.1	0.0	0.0
3. Ever had car accident.	0.1	0.4	0.3	12.4	13.3	13.8	13.7	9.3	22.9
4. Ever had trouble with police or been arrested.	0.0	0.0	0.0	4.1	1.7	2.7	4.1	7.4	11.4
5. Ever had fight.	0.1	0.3	0.3	12.4	10.8	12.8	21.9	25.9	22.9

More cases of help seeking from indigenous healers for alcohol dependence is reported from villages than from the other two sites, though the rate is quite low. With exception of alcohol abusers in the metropolis, there is no utilization of crisis intervention agencies for drinking problems at any of the sites.

Table 13–17 Symptom Profiles of Nonalcoholics, Alcohol-abusers and Alcohol Dependants

	Nonalcoholics			Alcohol Abuse			Alcohol Dependence		
	I	II %	III	I	II %	III	I	II %	III
Physical or psychic symptoms									
1. Loss of memory during drinking.	0.0	0.0	0.0	35.5	28.8	24.5	32.9	40.7	34.3
When stop drinking ever had									
2. Tremor	0.0	0.0	0.0	0.0	0.0	0.0	11.0	27.8	11.4
3. Epileptic seizure	0.0	0.0	0.0	0.0	0.0	0.0	1.4	1.9	0.0
4. Delirium tremens	0.0	0.0	0.0	0.0	0.4	1.1	1.4	13.0	0.0
5. Hallucinations	0.0	0.0	0.0	0.6	0.0	0.5	0.0	3.7	0.0
Had had the following diseases									
6. Liver	0.1	0.1	0.3	4.1	7.5	4.8	6.9	13.0	11.4
7. Vomiting of blood or stomach trouble	0.1	0.5	0.4	11.2	22.5	15.4	16.4	33.3	25.7
8. Peripheral neuropathy	0.0	0.0	0.0	2.4	2.1	1.6	2.7	7.4	0.0
9. Long standing memory impairment	0.0	0.0	0.1	3.6	11.3	9.0	9.6	11.1	14.3
10. Pancreatitis									

Age of onset

1. First experience of getting drunk.	23.0 ± 7.3	22.6 ± 7.8	21.8 ± 7.7	21.7 ± 8.7	21.2 ± 6.6	20.5 ± 6.2	20.9 ± 11.1	20.2 ± 8.1	19.8 ± 8.8
2. First experience of any AA or AD symptoms.	25.4 ± 8.3	24.6 ± 7.0	24.2 ± 7.4	26.4 ± 9.0	25.4 ± 8.7	24.7 ± 8.1	23.9 ± 8.6	24.0 ± 9.4	23.8 ± 9.4

Help-seeking behavior

1. Ever told you doctor about your drinking.	0.5	0.6	0.8	11.2	10.4	9.0	13.7	24.1	17.1
Ever consulted for drinking problems									
2. Western physicians	0.4	0.5	0.4	7.1	10.0	6.9	0.0	20.4	8.6
3. Traditional Chinese doctors	0.1	0.0	0.1	1.2	1.3	1.1	1.4	3.7	0.0
4. Self-medicated (Western drugs)	0.3	0.9	0.6	3.6	19.2	4.8	2.7	16.7	2.9
5. Self-medicated (Herb drugs)	0.1	0.1	0.0	0.6	2.9	1.6	1.4	1.9	2.9
6. Indiginous healers	0.0	0.0	0.0	0.0	0.8	0.0	1.4	0.0	2.9
7. Crisis intervention agencies	0.3	0.0	0.0	3.0	0.4	0.0	0.0	0.0	0.0

I: Taipei City

II: Townships

III: Villages

Risk of Other Mental Disorders in Alcoholic Cases

Alcohol abuse and dependence are associated with high risk for other lifetime mental disorders. The relative risk for specific mental disorders is shown in Table 13–20. There seem to be more mental disorders with a high relative risk ($RR > 2$) among alcoholics in the metropolis and townships than in the villages. Tobacco dependence (in all three sites), drug dependence (in the metropolis and townships), and antisocial personality (in the metropolis) are the disorders with considerably high comorbidity with alcoholism. A markedly high risk for manic episode is seen in the townships, while there is no such case found in the other two sites. Interestingly, the risk for major depression and schizophrenia is not consistent across the three sites, while the risk for dysthymic disorder is more consistent except for alcohol abuse in the metropolis. As for the anxiety disorders, comorbidities are higher for obsessive-compulsive disorder, but inconsistent for generalized anxiety disorder, phobias, and panic disorders.

Discussion

Compared with the prevalence of alcoholism reported in a 1946–1948 study, rates in this study show an increase of as high as 120–180 times. This surprising figure cannot be explained only by differences in diagnostic criteria, case-identification tools, and sampling methods. In the process of rapid industrialization, along with social change from a traditional, conservative society to a modern, democratic, pluralistic society with economic prosperity, alcohol intake has become increasingly popular in social intercourse, and excessive drinking has become socially sanctioned or even encouraged. From 1952 until 1984, the annual total consumption of alcohol beverages increased almost tenfold, and the annual per capita consumption almost threefold, as shown in Figures 13–1 and 13–2. These rates of increase are even higher than tobacco consumption for the same time period. It is important to recognize that although the annual per capita consumption by volume of alcohol beverages has increased as much as 3 times during the past 3 decades, the increase in per capita consumption in absolute alcohol in both total and age-over-15 population has been less significant, as shown in Figure 13–3. This is because the increase has largely been in the intake of light alcoholic beverages such as beer rather than strong liquors. However, even in terms of absolute alcohol, the annual per capita consumption in the total population has more than doubled since 1952. Though there are still no reliable data available, the sharp increase in accidental deaths in Taiwan during the past decade may be related to the increase in alcohol intake.

Table 13–18 Mean Number of Positive Lifetime Alcohol Symptoms

| | Alcohol Abuse | | | | | | | | | Alcohol Dependence | | | | | | | | |
| | Male | | | Female | | | Total | | | Male | | | Female | | | Total | | |
	N	Mean	SD	N	Mean	SD	N	Mean	SD	N	Mean	SD	N	Mean	SD	N	Mean	SD
Metropolis	158	3.7	± 1.7	11	2.7	± 0.8	169	3.6	± 1.7	70	4.9	± 2.3	3	5.3	± 2.5	73	4.9	± 2.2
Townships	232	3.7	± 1.5	8	4.0	± 1.5	240	3.8	± 1.6	50	6.1	± 2.5	4	4.3	± 3.2	54	6.0	± 2.6
Villages	185	3.6	± 1.4	3	4.3	± 1.5	188	3.6	± 1.0	35	5.7	± 2.4	0	—	—	35	5.7	± 2.5

Table 13–19 Mean Age of First Alcohol Symptoms

| | Alcohol Abuse | | | | | | | | | Alcohol Dependence | | | | | | | | |
| | Male | | | Female | | | Total | | | Male | | | Female | | | Total | | |
	N	Mean	SD	N	Mean	SD	N	Mean	SD	N	Mean	SD	N	Mean	SD	N	Mean	SD
Metropolis	105	26.3	± 9.1	5	28.0	± 7.4	110	26.4	± 9.0	56	23.8	± 8.7	3	25.7	± 9.0	59	23.9	± 8.6
Townships	195	25.3	± 8.5	7	29.9	± 13.0	202	25.4	± 8.7	46	24.0	± 7.5	3	23.7	± 7.0	49	24.0	± 7.4
Villages	162	24.7	± 8.2	3	26.0	± 6.6	165	24.7	± 8.1	29	23.8	± 9.4	0	—	—	29	23.8	± 9.4

Table 13–20 Relative Risk of Specific Mental Disorders in Alcoholic Cases[a]

	Metropolis			Townships			Villages		
	AA	AD	AD-AA	AA	AD	AD-AA	AA	AD	AD-AA
Manic episode	—	—	—	—	58.7	11.0	—	—	—
Major depression	1.5	4.8	2.5	—	—	—	1.7	—	1.5
Dysthymic disorder	—	4.8	2.0	2.7	4.3	3.0	1.3	3.4	1.6
Schizophrenia	4.1	—	2.9	—	8.4	1.6	—	—	—
Paranoid disorder	2.4	—	1.7	1.4	6.2	2.3	—	—	—
Obsessive-compulsive disorder	5.1	1.8	4.1	2.9	4.4	3.2	1.7	—	1.4
General anxiety disorder	1.0	—	—	1.1	2.0	1.3	1.4	—	1.3
Phobias	1.4	1.8	1.5	—	—	—	—	1.3	—
Panic disorder	—	—	—	—	—	—	4.7	—	4.0
Drug dependence	13.8	40.0	21.8	7.6	19.4	9.6	—	—	—
Tobacco dependence	4.5	5.7	5.1	4.1	4.6	4.2	3.3	2.7	3.2
Antisocial personality	9.7	240.5	140.5	—	—	—	—	—	—
Psychosexual dysfunction	2.3	—	1.6	—	1.0	—	2.6	2.6	2.6
Total number of disorder with RR > 2	8	6	7	5	9	6	3	3	3

[a]Relative Risk = $\dfrac{\text{Prevalence rate of a specific disorder in alcoholics}}{\text{Prevalence rate of the same disorder in nonalcoholic}}$

AA: Alcohol abuse only

AD: Alcohol dependence without abuse

AD-AA: Alcohol dependence with abuse

The lifetime prevalences of alcohol abuse and dependence in our three sites in Taiwan are, however, significantly lower than those reported from the NIMH ECA study sites for Caucasian, Black, and Hispanic ethnic groups in the United States (Robins et al., 1983; Escobar et al., 1985). They are also considerably lower than rates reported from Seoul and rural areas of Korea (Lee, 1987). The annual per capita consumption of alcoholic beverages in absolute alcohol in Taiwan is also significantly lower than that of Korea, where it was 5.4 liters in 1981 (Lee, 1987). The lifetime prevalence rates reported from Korea for alcoholism are even higher than those of the NIMH ECA study sites and Puerto Rico as shown in Table 13–21 (Canino et al., 1986).

Though the data are still preliminary, alcohol prevalence reported from Hong Kong is lower than that of rural villages and townships in Taiwan, but is fairly comparable with that in Taipei (Chen et al., 1986). Should it prove true that the prevalence of alcohol abuse/dependence in Hong Kong Chinese is lower than that of Taiwanese Chinese, this might provide an opportunity to test the "substitution hypothesis" to see whether the rates of pathological gambling and drug dependence might be higher in Hong Kong, and that they might serve as a substitution for alcoholism in the Hong Kong Chinese. However, the difference could also be a rural/urban one, with Taipei and Hong Kong both being densely populated metropolitan areas.

Regarding this latter difference, it is interesting to find in this study

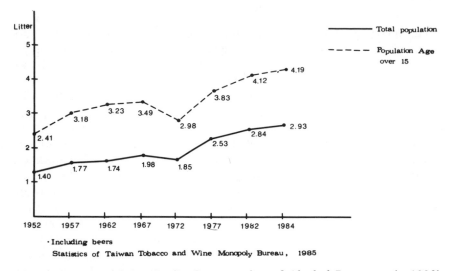

· Including beers

Statistics of Taiwan Tobacco and Wine Monopoly Bureau, 1985

Figure 13–3 Annual Per Capita Consumption of Alcohol Beverages in 100% Ethanol in Taiwan (including beer). [*Source:* Statistics of Taiwan Tobacco and Wine Monopoly Bureau, 1985.]

that while the prevalence of alcohol *abuse* in two townships is higher than rural villages, and that both townships and rural villages are higher than the metropolis, the rates for alcohol *dependence* across the three sites are nearly the same. It can, thus, be hypothesized from the above findings that etiologically alcohol dependence is more genetically determined,

Table 13–21 Lifetime Prevalence of Alcohol Abuse/Dependence in Different Study Sites (Weighted %)

Study Site	%
U.S.A.	
New Haven	11.5
Baltimore	13.7
St. Louis	15.7
Los Angeles	
Anglo	18.6
Hispanic	14.8
Puerto Rico	12.6
Korea	
Seoul	21.7
Rural	22.4
Hong Kong	3.3
Taiwan	
Taipei	5.0
Townships	9.6
Rural	7.5

while alcohol abuse is affected more by social and environmental factors than biological. That the prevalence of alcohol abuse in townships and rural villages are both higher than that of Taipei city as reported in this study seems to be in accord with the findings reported from rural area of the NIMH ECA study sites (Blazer, et al, 1985).

The lower rate of alcoholism among the Chinese compared to other ethnic groups and especially Caucasians has been explained by a higher rate of ALDH Isozyme deficiency among the Chinese, a factor that is genetically determined. This relationship has been discussed in a recent study by Omori et al. that included Taiwan (Omori et al., 1986), and our results reported here are consistent. The higher rate of alcohol dependence in aborigines compared to Chinese inhabitants in Taiwan is also consistent with previous work (Rin & Lin, 1962). This difference may also conceivably be due to a difference in ALDH Isozyme levels, and thus a genetically determined relative tolerance to alcohol among the aborigines compared to the Chinese. It is interesting to find that the rate of alcohol abuse in aborigines is higher than that of their Chinese counterparts in the metropolis. Whether or not this finding indicates severer psychosocial stress among aboriginal inhabitants in the metropolis compared to those in townships and villages in present-day Taiwan deserves further study. Such a comparative study between the aborigines and the Chinese inhabitants of Taiwan is currently underway (Chen et al., 1986). We obviously have too few aborigines in the current study reported here to do more than provide some speculation.

Looking at the symptom profiles, over one-third of alcohol abusers and more than half of dependents consider themselves to be "excessive drinkers." The families of both alcohol groups oppose, to the same extent, their drinking. Both alcohol groups had, in the same proportion, tried to stop drinking but failed. Generally speaking, social, legal, or job problems do not seem to be the serious problems among the Taiwan Chinese alcoholics. Tremor is the most frequently reported symptom among the group of withdrawal symptoms in the dependent group. By definition, there are no withdrawal symptoms reported in the abuse group, but physical diseases are reported in both dependent and abuse groups. The rather high rate of diseases of stomach, liver, and pancreas are noteworthy. The rates for physical diseases in both alcohol groups and withdrawal symptoms in the dependent group are both higher in townships than in Taipei city and villages.

The mean number of alcohol symptoms in this study is greatest in dependence cases in the townships. It will be of considerable interest to compare the symptom profile of Taiwan Chinese and aborigine alcoholics with those of the Koreans and of other ethnic groups.

The Taiwan Chinese alcoholics seldom seek help for their drinking problems. When they do, they go to Western physicians more often than to any other kind, but the infrequency of help-seeking may help to account for the high rate of alcohol-related physical diseases commented on above.

References

Blazer, D; George, L. K.; Landerman, R.; Pennybacker, M.; Melville, M. L.; Woodbury, M.; Manton, K. G., Jordan, K.; and Locke, B. (1985). Psychiatric disorders: A rural/urban comparison. *Arch. Gen. Psychiatry* 42:651–56.

Canino, G. J.; Bird, H. R.; Shrout, P.; Rubio, M.; Bravo, M.; Matinez, R.; Sesman, M.; and Guerara, L. M. (1986). The Prevalence of Specific Psychiatric Disorders in Puerto Rico. Unpublished paper.

Chang, L. Y.; Yeh, E. K.; and Hwu, H. G. (1984). Taipei Psychiatric Epidemiological Study: A Methodological Note. Paper presented at Symposium on Cross-Cultural Psychiatric Epidemiology, Hong Kong, May 11–12.

Chen, C. C.; Yeh, E. K.; and Hwu, H. G. (1986). Unpublished data from "A Study of Aldehyde Dehydrogenase Isozymes among Alcoholics and Non-Alcoholics in Taiwanese and Aborigines" Research Project NSC 76-0412-B109-01. Republic of China: National Science Council.

Chen, C. N.; Wong, J.; Lee, N.; and Lai, P. (1986). An On-Going Study of Alcoholism in Hong Kong. Paper presented at Symposium 109 on Alcoholism with the DIS: America, Europe, and Asia. Washington, D.C.: 139 Annual Meeting of the American Psychiatric Association, May 10–16.

Chu, G. (1972). Drinking pattern and attitudes of rooming-house Chinese in San Francisco. *Q. J. Study Alcoholics* (Suppl. 6): 58–68.

Dohrenwend, B. P., and Dohrenwend, B. S. (1982). Perspectives on the Past and Future of Psychiatric Epidemiology (The 1981 Rema Lapouse Lecture). *Am. J. Public Health* 72:1271–79.

Escobar, J. I.; Karno, M.; Burnam, A.; Hough, R. L.; Timbers, D. M.; and Santana, F. (1985). Psychiatric Epidemiology Across Ethnic Groups: The Los Angeles ECA Study. Paper presented at International Symposium on Psychiatric Epidemiology, Taipei, April 26–28.

Ewing, J. A.; Rouse, B., and Pellizziri, E. D. (1974). Alcohol sensitivity and ethnic background. *Am. J Psychiatry* 131:206–7.

Goethe, H. W.; Agarwal, D. P.; Harada, S.; Meier-Tackmann, D.; Ruofu, D.; Bienzle, V.; Kroger, A.; and Hussein, L. (1983). Population genetic studies on Aldehyde Dehydrogenase Isozyme deficiency and alcohol sensitivity. *Am. J. Hum. Genet.* 35:769–72.

Graves, R. M., and Magilavey, J. L. (1981). Increasing response rates to telephone survey: A door in the face or foot in the door? *Public Opinion Quarterly* 45:346–58.

Helzer, J. E. (1985). Cross-Cultural Applications of the DIS. DIS Newsletter. St. Louis, Mo.: Washington University School of Medicine, Department of Psychiatry. II-2:3–4.

Hsu, F. L. K. (1955). *Americans and Chinese.* London: Cressert Press.

Hwu, H. G.; Yeh, E. K.; Chang, L. Y.; Chen, C. C.; and Chen, T. Y. (1984). The Chinese Modification of NIMH Diagnostic Interview Schedule-Reliability study on assessment of psychiatric symptoms. *Psychol. Testing* 31:15–26.

Hwu, H. G.; Yeh, E. K.; and Chang, L. Y. (1986). Chinese Diagnostic Interview Schedule. I. Agreement with Physician's Diagnosis. *Acta Psychiatr Scand* 73:225–33.

Hwu, H. G.; Yeh, E. K.; Chen, C. T.; Chen, C. C.; and Chen, T. Y. (1983). An applicability of the Chinese Modification of Diagnostic Interview Schedule (DIS-CM). *Bulletin of Chinese Society of Neurology and Psychiatry* 9:30–38.

Lee, C. K. (1987). Alcoholism in Korea. Unpublished paper.

Lin, T. Y. (1953). A study of the incidence of mental disorders in Chinese and other cultures. *Psychiatry* 16:313–36.

Lin, T. Y., and Lin, D. T. C. (1982). Alcoholism among the Chinese: Further observations of a low risk population. *Cult. Med. Psychiatry* 6:109–116.

Mitchell, A. (1980). A comparison between a written and a Doorstep Approach in research interviewing. *Sociol. Rev.* 28:629–34.

Moser, C. A.; and Kalton, G. (1971). *Survey Methods in Social Investigation, second ed.* New York: Basic Books.

Omori, T.; Koyama, T.; Chen, C. C.; Yeh, E. K.; Reyes, B. V.; and Yamashita, I. (1986). The role of Aldehyde Dehydrogenase Isozyme variance in alcohol sensitivity, drinking habits formation and the development of alcoholism in Japan, Taiwan and the Philippines. *Prog. Neuropsychopharmacol. Biol. Psychiatry* 10:229–35.

Regier, D. A.; Meyers, M.; Kramer, M.; Robins, L. N.; Blazer, D. G.; Hough, R. L.; Eaton, W. W.; and Locke, B. Z. (1984). The NIMH Epidemiological Catchment Area Surveys. *Arch. Gen. Psychiatry* 41:934–41.

Rin, H., and Lin, T. Y. (1962). Mental illness among Formosan Aborigines as compared with the Chinese in Taiwan. *J. Ment. Science* 108:133–46.

Robins, L. N.; Helzer, J. E.; Croughan, J; and Ratcliff, K. S. (1981). National Institute of Mental Health Diagnostic Interview Schedule: Its history, characteristics and validity. *Arch. Gen. Psychiatry* 38:381–89.

Robins, L. N.; Helzer, J. E.; Ratcliff, K. S.; and Seyfried, W. (1982). Validity of the Diagnostic Interview Schedule, Version II: DSM-III Diagnosis. *Psychol. Med.* 12:855–70.

Robins, L. N.; Helzer, J. E.; Weissman, M. M.; Orvaschel, H.; Gruenberg, E.; Burke, J. D.; Weissman, M. M.; and Regier, D. A. (1984). Lifetime prevalence of specific psychiatric disorders in three sites. *Arch. Gen. Psychiatry* 41:949–58.

Singer, K. (1972). Drinking pattern and alcoholism in the Chinese. *Br. J Addict.* 67:3–14.

Singer, K. (1974). The choices of intoxicant among the Chinese. *Br. J. Psychiatry* 69:257–68.

Taipei City Psychiatric Center Annual Report 1970–1985.

Wang, R. P. (1968). A study of alcoholism in Chinatown. *Int. J. Soc. Psychiatry* 14:260–67.

Wolff, P. H. (1972). Ethnic difference in alcohol sensitivity. *Science* 175:449–50.

Wu, C. T., and Shen, W. W. (1985). An epidemiological note on Chinese alcoholism: Cases from Taiwan. Letter to Editor. *Alcohol & Alcoholism* 20: 81–82.

Taiwan Psychiatric Epidemiological Study Project. Department of Health, Executive Yuan, Republic of China. Yeh E. K., Principal Investigator, Hwu H. G., Collaborative Investigator, 1981–1986.

Yeh, E. K.; Yamamoto, J.; Wu E. C.; et al. (1980). Symptoms and Diagnosis in Taipei and Los Angeles. Paper presented at the Symposium on Transcultural Psychiatry. May, Manila: 2nd Pacific Congress of Psychiatry.

[14] Alcoholism in Korea

CHUNG KYOON LEE

The use of alcohol in Korea is as old as the country's long history. Alcoholic beverages have been used in traditional occasions and ritualistic activities such as birthdays, funerals, weddings, anniversaries of death, birthdays of ancients, promotions, and other landmarks and achievements. Alcohol is also considered a necessary means of promoting social communication.

Like other Eastern countries, Korea is a strongly male-oriented society. Men are encouraged to drink; women are not. The presence of a strong Confucian moral ethic discourages the exhibition of drunken behavior, but the Korean culture usually tolerates well and public attitudes are strikingly permissive. As a result, social regulations and constraints on drinking behavior are rather loose with a few exceptions, for example, driving a car while intoxicated.

A typical drinking situation is a private party or entertainment, usually held in a public restaurant, after one's daily work is over. There, not only alcoholic beverages but also a variety of foods are supplied. Rounds of drinks or "exchanging cups" are encouraged. The gathering may change locations for a second round of drinking, and this pattern of moving from place to place with heavy drinking at each spot often lasts until some of the members eventually become deeply intoxicated. Participants may insist that each other drink to their maximum ability. Any latecomer has to drink three full cups of alcohol in order to catch up, and is proud to be able to drink so much at once. Solitary drinking is very uncommon in the Korean culture, even in the case of heavy drinkers. Women drinkers are also notably rare. The beverage of choice varies with the region. In Korean rural areas, a kind of unrefined rice wine with low alcohol content, called "makkolli," is preferred; "so-ju," a distilled alcohol with 25 percent absolute alcohol, is more popular in the cities.

247

Recent reports (Cho et al., 1975; Kim & Lee, 1975) indicate that more than 70 percent of Korean adult males over 18 years of age drink at least occasionally and that half of them are "regular drinkers," that is drink at least weekly. Several epidemiological studies have examined the prevalence of alcoholism (Yoo, 1962; Kim, 1975; Woo, 1966). Rates vary depending on the definition used and a number of other factors. Rates for active, "hard-core" alcoholism range between 2.8 and 6.3 percent in most studies.

There are also no consistent data concerning per capita alcohol consumption, because unregistered alcohol is produced in many households in the rural areas, even though the law prohibits it. However, there has been a striking increase in the estimates of annual per capita alcohol consumption, from 0.7 liters of absolute alcohol in 1960 to 5.4 liters in 1981. There is also evidence that consumption of strong liquors or spirits together with beer is increasing substantially. Finally, surveys of hospital admission rates (Min, 1975; Park, 1985) show a gradual increment in the proportion of alcoholics as a percentage of all psychiatric inpatients over time, from 1.7 percent in 1960s to 6.4 percent in early 1980s.

Recently, coinciding with the great economic growth during the past few decades, mental health issues are getting increasing attention in Korea. Efforts are being made both at the political and academic level to obtain the necessary epidemiologic data and devising rational strategies regarding mental health problems. The survey to be presented here is one such effort, and has been undertaken because of the urgent need for estimating psychiatric morbidity, including alcohol-related disorders.

As the Dohrenwends (Dohrenwend & Dohrenwend, 1982) have pointed out, "second generation" epidemiological studies have many weaknesses in methodology and conceptual framework. Even when problems are recognized, it is often difficult to make corrections for them, making it difficult to estimate true prevalence of disorders. Because methods and diagnostic styles differ, it is also difficult to compare data across studies. In the hope of reducing such problems, the "third generation" studies—characterized by the use of standardized definitions, assessment tools, and advanced data processing—have emerged in the last decade.

During the past 5 years, stimulated by the establishment of the ECA project of the United States (Eaton et al., 1981; Eaton et al., 1984; Regier et al., 1984; Robins et al., 1984), a large scale epidemiological study patterned after the ECA has been carried out by a collaborative team of the Department of Psychiatry, Medical College of the Seoul National University. We have used a translated version of the DIS (Diagnostic Interview Schedule) (Robins et al., 1984; Robins et al., 1981), and have followed the same procedures of the ECA project, with the exception of the sampling technique. We believe this work makes it possible to obtain epidemiologic data relevant to our needs, as well as to compare the findings with other surveys done in similar fashion from around the world.

In this article, we present the prevalence of DIS/DSM-III ascertained alcoholism in Korea, its demographic correlates, and other pertinent findings together with an explanation of our sampling methodology. Cultural implications will also be discussed.

Methods

Selection of Designated Respondents

The Korean DIS study was designed to elicit rates of psychiatric morbidity in the total general population; therefore we needed a nationwide sample. To accomplish this, two component samples were selected. One representing the urban population was drawn from Seoul (the capital city of Korea), and the other from scattered rural locations over the entire country. A two stage cluster sampling method was used for each sample.

Using the 1980 census data as a guide to regional sociodemographic and cultural characteristics, we chose a group of large geographical administrative units as the primary (first-stage) sampling units (PSUs), using a probability proportionate to size (PPS) methodology.

The PSUs consisted of forty-seven Dongs in Seoul for the urban sample and twenty discrete Eubs or Myeons for the rural areas. (A "Dong" corresponds to a "subdistrict" or aggregation of "blocks" with a population grouping of 15,000 to 30,000, while "Eub" or "Myeon" corresponds to larger or smaller "town" or aggregation of "villages" with a population size of 10,000 to 50,000 respectively). Residents living in the outskirts of adjacent large cities were excluded in the rural sample. The readers should note that the population density of Korea is relatively high in both urban and rural regions. The population number of Seoul reaches to ten million currently.

Next, five smaller, secondary sampling units (SSUs) were drawn from each PSU by systematic random fashion. There were 235 SSUs in Seoul and 100 SSUs in rural areas. Each SSU was again a geographically determined administrative subunit called "Ban" in Seoul (twenty to thirty households) and "Ri" in rural areas (with thirty to fifty households). In terms of population size, the PSUs were 20 to 30 times larger than SSUs.

After screening out ineligible households, 2,645 households (1,645 in Seoul, 1,000 in rural areas) were selected randomly. There are some different points between our study and the U.S. (ECA) study in the methodology, most notably in the final selection of the designated respondents. As described elsewhere (Holzer et al., 1985), most ECA survey sites used the Kish selection method that randomized by age and sex within households, so that only one adult would be interviewed within each designated household. In our study, all family members living together for more than 3 months in a given household were regarded as designated respondents. In addition, we limited the respondent's age range from 18 to 65 years, unlike the ECA, which had no upper age limit.

Because average numbers of family members of one household were estimated at four or five in Korea, though the size of rural families was slightly larger than that of urban ones, and because approximately two-thirds of those in each household would be adults (Nat. Bur. Stat., 1985), approximately 6,200 respondents (4,000 in Seoul and 2,200 in rural areas) were expected to be identified for the field survey. Among them, 5,176 respondents (3,178 in Seoul and 1,998 in rural areas) completed the interview, giving completion rates of over 80 percent. We actually analyzed 5,100 data sheets (3,134 Seoul subjects and 1,966 rural ones) (Table 14–1).

Development of the DIS-IIIK (DIS-III Korean Version) (Lee et al., 1986)

In early 1982, adaptation of the DIS to the Korean culture was begun by a translation committee established in the Department of Neuropsychiatry at Seoul National University. It began its work after critical discussion about general applicability and acceptability of the DIS-III in the Korean culture. Staff psychiatrists participated in making initial translations of the instrument, based on the general guidelines proposed by Brislin (Brislin et al., 1973; Brislin, 1980). Several Korean Americans participated in this effort also. Back translation was carried out blindly by an independent, bilingual clinical psychologist who had studied in the United States. This was followed by expert review with item-by-item comparison and revision of the initial version. After pretesting with bilingual subjects and additional revision on preliminary field trial, the

Table 14–1 Completion Rates

	Korean Study		ECA Study		
	Seoul	Rural	New Haven	Baltimore	St. Louis
Died, language and other problem (%)	0.2	0.4	0.3	0.7	0.3
Refusal (%)	5.9	1.0	13.9	16.5	10.1
Never available (%)	5.4	7.0	1.1	0.7	2.2
Others (%)	8.5	2.3	9.1	4.2	7.9
No. of interviewed	3,178	1,998	3,058	3,481	3,004
Interview completion (%)	80.5	89.3	75.6	77.9	79.5
No. of analysis	3,134	1,966	3,058	3,481	3,004
Overall completion (%)	79.4	85.9	75.6	77.9	79.5

final draft of the Korean DIS version was prepared in early 1983. In general, the translation process of the DIS in Korea closely resembled that used for the Spanish DIS (Karno, 1983).

The validity of the Korean DIS was tested against clinicians with thirty-five psychiatric inpatients and thirty controls and resulted in moderate sensitivity (schizophrenia 0.69, overall affective disorders 0.78, anxiety disorders 0.80) and high specificity (schizophrenia 1.0, overall affective disorders 0.91, neurotic disorders 0.72). Test-retest reliability for twenty-one inpatients was measured by two trained interviewers. This resulted in nearly 90 percent agreement with kappa statistics that ranged from 0.36 to 1.0, with an average value of 0.70.

Field Survey

Seventy-eight lay interviewers were selected from volunteers from Seoul University. Over 60 percent were medical students. Training was similar to that of the ECA, with a full one-week course including homework, interview exercises, and several hours of practice sessions. During the actual field survey, each interviewer had unlimited access to his own supervisor or vice versa, and additional supervision was given at biweekly meetings. The survey was conducted from January to February 1984. It is worth noting that all interviewers assigned for the rural study stayed at their study areas throughout the survey period.

Items pertinent to psychosexual dysfunctions were omitted from the interview, since Korean mores would not permit discussing these items and asking them might have caused some undesirable effect to other interview items.

Older persons were oversampled, as in the case of several ECA sites, and we have weighted the data to correct for the oversample. However, in contrast to the ECA, a "one household, one respondent" method was not used in this study; weighting was done simply for age stratum, that is, to provide equal probability of respondent selection, regardless of age.

Demographic Composition of the Sample

Demographic profiles of the sample populations are shown in Table 14–2. In total there were 5,100 subjects (Seoul 3,134, rural 1,966). The Seoul sample is distributed more toward the younger aged groups and the rural sample toward the older groups. This reflects the age distribution of the country as a whole, according to the 1980 census data shown by comparison in Table 14–3. As noted earlier, those over 65 were excluded from our sample. For those included in the study, there are few differences in demographic profiles between sample and general population.

Table 14–2 Demographic Characteristics of Sample Population

Age	Seoul						Rural					
	Male		Female		Total		Male		Female		Total	
(yrs.)	N	(%)	N	(%)	N	(%)	N	(%)	N	(%)	N	(%)
18–24	299	(20.1)	339	(20.6)	638	(20.4)	146	(15.0)	114	(11.5)	260	(13.2)
25–34	412	(27.7)	504	(30.7)	916	(29.2)	179	(18.4)	206	(20.8)	385	(19.6)
35–44	385	(25.8)	403	(24.5)	788	(25.1)	199	(20.4)	222	(22.4)	421	(21.4)
45–54	264	(17.7)	263	(16.0)	527	(16.8)	257	(26.4)	274	(27.6)	531	(27.0)
55–65	130	(8.7)	135	(8.2)	265	(8.5)	193	(19.8)	176	(17.7)	369	(18.8)
Total	1,490	(100.0)	1,644	(100.0)	3,134	(100.0)	974	(100.0)	992	(100.0)	1,966	(100.0)

Table 14–3 Comparison of Sample with General Population

	Seoul		Rural	
	Sample	Census (1980)	Sample	Census (1980)
Size	3,134	5,119,647	1,966	8,401,261
Sex				
M	47.5%	49.2%	49.5%	50.6%
F	52.5%	50.9%	50.5%	49.4%
Age, yr.				
18–24	20.4%	29.1%	13.2%	24.2%
25–44	54.3%	51.8%	41.0%	42.8%
45–65	25.3%	19.1%	45.8%	33.0%

Lifetime Prevalence of Specific Psychiatric Disorders

The weighted lifetime prevalence of the specific psychiatric disorders we covered with the DIS are presented separately for the Seoul and rural samples in Table 14–4 (Lee et al., 1986). The diagnoses shown here are according to the DSM-III criteria and exclusion criteria were omitted so as to provide maximal comparability of our results with the ECA survey.

The lifetime prevalence of any DIS/DSM-III disorders (the proportion of respondents having at least one of those diagnoses listed in the table) was 39.8 percent in Seoul and 41 percent in rural areas. In both Seoul and the rural areas, the most common diagnoses were the substance use disorders. If tobacco dependence is excluded, total rates declined to 31.8 and 33 percent, respectively. In general, it is clear that there are remarkable similarities in the diagnostic rates across the two study samples (Seoul vs. rural) for most of the general and specific categories.

The two subcategories of alcoholism (abuse only and dependence) are additive, and thus it appears that about one adult out of every five was found to have alcohol abuse or dependence at some time in his or her life (Table 14–5). With respect to individual diagnostic categories of DSM-III alcoholism, the rates for alcohol abuse in Seoul were somewhat higher than those in rural areas, while rates for dependence were the opposite.

Demographic Correlates of Alcoholism

SEX.   As would be expected, the prevalence of alcoholism shows clear dominance for males, but the degree of dominance here is particularly striking, notably by 16–27 times that for females with no significant difference across the two sites, although rates of female alcoholics are a bit higher in Seoul areas (Table 14–6).

Table 14–4 Lifetime Prevalence Rate of DIS/DSM-III Disorders in Korea

	Seoul (%)		Rural (%)	
	(N = 3,134)		(N = 1,966)	
Any DIS disorder covered	39.81	(41.51)	41.05	(43.79)
Any DIS disorder except tobacco dependence	31.80	(33.22)	33.02	(35.09)
Any DIS disorder except substance use disorders	13.36	(13.40)	13.46	(14.24)
Substance use disorders	31.75	(32.83)	31.98	(34.49)
Alcohol abuse only	12.95	(13.59)	10.65	(10.63)
Alcohol dependence	8.76	(9.32)	11.74	(13.38)
Tobacco dependence	19.92	(20.80)	20.96	(22.74)
Drug abuse/dependence	0.88	(0.93)	0.49	(0.56)
Schizophrenic/Schizophreniform disorders	0.34	(0.35)	0.65	(0.56)
Schizophrenia	0.31	(0.32)	0.54	(0.46)
Schizophreniform disorder	0.03	(0.03)	0.11	(0.10)
Affective disorders	5.52	(5.49)	5.11	(5.39)
Manic episode	0.40	(0.35)	0.44	(0.36)
Major depression	3.31	(3.29)	3.47	(3.61)
Dysthymia	2.42	(2.48)	1.89	(2.09)
Anxiety disorders	9.19	(9.17)	9.85	(9.94)
Phobia(sum)	5.89	(5.87)	5.97	(6.31)
Agoraphobia	2.08	(2.17)	3.62	(3.71)
Social phobia	0.53	(0.51)	0.65	(0.56)
Simple phobia	5.35	(5.30)	4.67	(5.34)
Panic disorder	1.11	(1.21)	2.60	(2.90)
Agoraphobia with panic attack	0.65	(0.67)	1.27	(1.37)
Generalized anxiety disorder	3.56	(3.66)	2.89	(3.13)
Obsessive-compulsive	2.29	(2.23)	1.90	(1.88)
Somatoform disorder	0.03	(0.03)	0.18	(0.20)
Anorexia	0.03	(0.03)	0.00	(0.00)
Antisocial personality disorder	2.08	(2.07)	0.91	(0.76)
Gambling	1.02	(1.12)	0.98	(1.12)
Cognitive impairment mild	4.60	(5.42)	8.77	(10.58)
severe	0.16	(0.19)	1.85	(2.14)

( ): unweighted data.

AGE.   With regard to age specific estimates, lifetime alcoholism was generally found to be increasing with age in a linear fashion. However, the findings for total alcoholism in this regard are largely due to the prominence of alcohol dependence. In fact, rates for alcohol "abuse" in Seoul reach a plateau in the late 20s, while the highest prevalence of abuse in rural areas was noted in the 24–44-year-old group (Table 14–7).

EDUCATION.   A senior high school degree (10–12 years of education) appeared to be the most dominant educational status among male alcoholics, whereas a junior high school degree (7–9 years of education) was

Table 14–5 Lifetime Prevalence rate of DIS/DSM-III Alcohol Abuse/Dependence in Korea

	Seoul, % (N = 3,134)	Rural, % (N = 1,966)
Alcohol abuse only	12.95	10.65
Alcohol dependence	8.76	11.74
Alcohol abuse and dependence	7.87	10.76
Alcohol dependence only	0.89	0.98
Alcohol abuse/dependence (sum)	21.71	22.39

the most common among female ones. However, it may be that these findings do not reflect the true impact of education on alcoholism, but rather the educational patterns of the general population. In this sense, comparison of the relative frequency of educational level between alcoholics and general population is mandatory. By this approach, the results are further elaborated that college graduates are significantly more represented among male alcoholics ($p < .05$, chi-square test), while senior high school degrees are more represented among female ones.

OCCUPATION.   Roughly, alcoholism appeared to be prevalent among those engaged in skilled and semiskilled work (this may represent alcoholics in Seoul) as well as agricultural work (this may be due to alcoholics in rural areas). On the other hand, the "others" and "unemployed" groups also contributed major components to the group of alcoholics, items of which may denote those in parts with part-time workers and hard physical laborers or others with true alcoholic incompetents, although further validation is needed.

AGE OF ONSET.   The men were typically in their late 20s or early 30s when they manifested their first alcohol symptoms, whereas women did so in their mid- or late 30s (Table 14–8). Thus, women were invariably delayed in developing alcoholism compared to men, showing a consistent lag time of 6 years or more. This sex differential was consistent between Seoul and the rural areas. There was a general tendency for alcoholics in Seoul to develop symptoms at an earlier age than those in rural areas.

Table 14–6 Prevalence of Alcohol Abuse/Dependence by Sex

	Seoul, % Male / Female	Rural, % Male / Female
Alcohol abuse only	25.63/ 1.59	20.54/ 0.90
Alcohol dependence	17.23/ 1.04	22.39/ 0.67
Alcohol abuse/dependence	42.86/ 2.63	42.93/ 1.57

Table 14–7 Prevalence of Alcoholic Disorders by Age Group

	Yr., % 18–24	Yr., % 25–44	Yr., % 45–65
Alcohol abuse only			
Seoul	7.37	15.20	15.15
Rural	8.85	12.78	9.22
Alcohol dependence			
Seoul	5.96	8.45	13.89
Rural	5.00	10.30	18.56
Alcohol abuse/dependence			
Seoul	13.33	23.65	29.04
Rural	13.85	23.08	27.78

Severity of Alcoholism

The mean number of positive alcohol symptoms is shown in Table 14–9 and suggests that Korean alcoholics have, on an average, 4–6 positive lifetime DSM-III symptoms. In general, women appear to have slightly fewer symptoms than men, but the difference is not very great. Consistent with the findings shown in Table 14–5 of an excess of alcohol dependence in the rural areas, rural respondents are also shown here to have a slightly higher mean number of symptoms, and this is consistent for both men and women.

Symptom Frequencies

We can also examine the prevalence of specific symptoms of alcoholism with these data or the profile of symptom frequency. The DIS has seventeen symptom question items that ascertain the alcohol symptoms delin-

Table 14–8 Mean Age of Onset of First Alcohol Symptom

	Mean Age	Standard Deviation	Percentile 25%	Percentile 50%	Percentile 75%
Seoul					
All alcoholics (N = 574)	28	10	21	26	33
Male alcoholics (N = 538)	28	9	21	26	32
Female alcoholics (N = 36)	34	13	22	34	45
Missing age of onset N = 144					
Rural					
All alcoholics (N = 398)	30	9	24	30	37
Male alcoholics (N = 386)	30	9	24	30	36
Female alcoholics	38	11	26.5	37.5	47
Missing age of onset N = 74					

Table 14–9 *Mean Number of Positive Lifetime Alcohol Symptoms*

	Mean No. of Symptoms	Standard Deviation	Percentiles		
			25%	50%	75%
Seoul					
All alcoholics (*N* = 718)	5	3	3	5	7
Male alcoholics (*N* = 672)	5	3	3	5	7
Female alcoholics (*N* = 46)	4	3	2	4	6
Rural					
All alcoholics (*N* = 472)	6	3	3	5	8
Male alcoholics (*N* = 455)	6	3	4	6	8
Female alcoholics (*N* = 17)	4.5	3	3	3	5.5

eated in DSM-III. Table 14–10 shows the proportions of positive responses for the symptoms arranged by DSM-III group for nonalcoholics and those meeting criteria for alcohol abuse and dependence and separately for the Seoul and rural samples.

Even among those who were alcohol dependent, symptoms related to

Table 14–10 *Symptom Profile of Alcoholics in Korea*

Item No. of DIS		Nonalcoholics (%)		Abuse only (%)		Dependence (%)	
		Seoul / Rural		Seoul / Rural		Seoul / Rural	
(Pattern of pathological alcohol use)							
152	drank a fifth of alcohol in one day	8	/ 8	86	/ 91	92	/ 94
157	could not stop drinking	0.75	/ 0.93	27	/ 31	46	/ 53
158	tried to control drinking	1	/ 0.53	34	/ 25	45	/ 41
165 B	multiple day benders	0	/ 0.20	2	/ 7	12	/ 27
166	blackouts	0.29	/ 0.60	50	/ 48	58	/ 70
169	drank regardless of illness	0.21	/ 0.27	18	/ 18	39	/ 42
170	interfered with work	0	/ 0	0.47	/ 0.96	9	/ 20
(Impairment in social or occupational functioning)							
150	family objections	2	/ 0.93	80	/ 73	77	/ 78
156	warned of drinking problem	0.21	/ 0.13	31	/ 33	57	/ 61
160	job problem	0.41	/ 0.07	22	/ 29	39	/ 42
161	job loss	0	/ 0	0.23	/ 2	5	/ 3
162	driving problems	0.08	/ 0.07	3	/ 1	5	/ 3
163	arrested or held by police	0.25	/ 0.27	21	/ 8	28	/ 12
164	physical fights	1	/ 0.08	45	/ 36	53	/ 45
(Tolerance or withdrawal)							
153	excessive drinking (2 weeks)	0.04	/ 0.07	0	/ 0	72	/ 75
159	morning drinking	0.08	/ 0.27	0	/ 0	29	/ 43
167	had the shakes	0	/ 0	0	/ 0	30	/ 34

quantity of drinking were the most frequent. In fact, heavy daily drinking and drinking a fifth of alcohol in one day were the most frequent symptoms in every sample. Loss of job due to drinking was the least frequent symptom and "work interference" (being unable to do one's ordinary work well unless one had something to drink) was also very infrequent.

With respect to health consequences arising from drinking, about 20 percent of abusers and more than 40 percent of dependents experienced one or more medical complications, including liver problems, troubles with stomach or pancreas, peripheral neuropathy, or memory impairment (findings are not shown in the table). Furthermore, more than 30 percent of alcohol dependents had at least one episode of significant withdrawal symptoms such as "shakes," seizures and DTs. These findings suggest that in addition to the high prevalence rates, no small proportion of Korean alcoholics suffered from significant medical problems rather than simply troubles with social life. However, less than 10 percent of them had told a physician about the problems (item omitted from the table).

Relative Risk for Other Disorders

In order to learn about possible illness correlates with alcoholism, calculation of "relative risk (RR)" can provide useful information to us. To assess whether alcoholism is associated with other psychiatric disorders, and the extent of any association, we examined the relative risk ratio, that is, the prevalence of another disorder in alcoholics divided by its prevalence in nonalcoholics. The results are summarized in Table 14–11.

As has been found in studies done in other countries, diagnostic rates for antisocial personality disorder, mania, and drug use disorder are all well above 1.0 in both the Seoul and the rural samples. Major depression, obsessive-compulsive disorder, and schizophrenia are also above unity although not so high nor so consistently. The relative risk value for major depression is not as high as might have been expected from studies of clinical samples. On the other hand, the similarly high elevation in the case of obsessive-compulsive disorder was unexpected. Among those being virtually unaffected by the presence of alcoholism are dysthymia and cognitive impairment, and the anxiety laden disorders, panic disorder and phobia, are lower in alcoholics versus nonalcoholics (relative risk less than 1.0).

Discussion

Korea was divided into two parts—North and South—after the Second World War in 1945. The size of the Republic of Korea is 98,799 km.[2] and

Table 14–11 Prevalence of DIS/DSM-III Disorders Among Nonalcoholics and Alcoholics in Korea

DIS/DSM-III Diagnosis	Unweighted N's with Positive Diagnosis Seoul / Rural	Percent with Positive Diagnosis Among: Nonalcoholics Seoul / Rural	Alcoholics Seoul / Rural	Relative risk Seoul / Rural
Cognitive impairment	176 / 250	5.41% / 13.42%	6.38% / 10.57%	1.2 / 0.8
Mania	11 / 7	0.20 / 0.20	0.93 / 0.84	4.7 / 4.2
Depression	103 / 71	2.89 / 3.14	4.58 / 5.07	1.6 / 1.6
Dysthymic disorder	78 / 41	2.52 / 2.07	2.36 / 2.33	0.9 / 1.1
Any drug disorder	29 / 11	0.66 / 0.47	1.80 / 0.85	2.7 / 1.8
Schizophrenia	10 / 9	0.25 / 0.47	0.55 / 0.42	2.2 / 0.9
Schizophreniform disorder	1 / 2	0.04 / 0.07	0.00 / 0.21	— / 3
Phobic disorders	184 / 124	6.36 / 6.81	4.30 / 4.65	0.07 / 0.7
Somatization disorder	1 / 4	0.04 / 0.20	0.00 / 0.21	— / 1.1
Panic disorder	38 / 57	1.36 / 3.27	0.69 / 1.69	0.5 / 0.5
Antisocial personality	65 / 15	1.12 / 0.34	5.27 / 2.12	4.7 / 6.2
Anorexia	1 / 0	0.04 / 0.00	0.00 / 0.00	/ 0
Obsessive-compulsive disorder	70 / 37	1.98 / 1.74	3.05 / 2.33	1.5 / 1.3
Any above core diagnosis	523 / 447	16.30 / 23.43	17.75 / 20.30	1.1 / 0.9

Note: Data value is unweighted.

the population is about 40,000,000. The population density is 405 per km.², which makes it one of the most densely populated countries in the world.

Alcohol consumption of the Korean population has increased in parallel with the growth of industrialization and increased urbanization. Alcohol consumption per capita in 1960 was 0.7 liter of 100 percent alcohol (population over 15 was 1.2 liters) and 5.4 liters (population over 15 was 9.2 liters) in 1981. In 1960, the highest consumption country was the Soviet Union, which consumed 2.6 liters per capita. Furthermore, the quality of alcoholic beverages in Korea has also changed from low alcohol content to high content.

In the past 21 years, Korea has become one of the highest consumption countries in the world. This correlates very well with the high lifetime prevalence rate of alcohol abuse/dependence found using the DIS in Korea. Lifetime prevalence of alcohol abuse/dependence was 22 percent, making it the most prevalent psychiatric disorder of the ones we studied. Among the possible factors contributing to this high prevalence rate are the pattern of heavy consumption common among Korean men in social situations, the fact that alcohol is considered a food, evolution of the typical family model from extended to nuclear family, the rapid development of industrialization and modernization in Korea, the frequent opportunities to drink socially, social pressures toward competitive consumption at social drinking occasions, the inclusion of alcohol at most social events, and a generous attitude of the public toward open drunkenness.

Behavioral problems resulting from alcohol are well tolerated and accepted in Korean society and have been for a long time. There is a tendency to dismiss troubles or transgressions that have happened during a drunken state. The philosophy is that the problem was caused by alcohol, not by the individual, and alcohol is a "food." Furthermore, many Korean men think that ability to drink is a privilege and a source of pride.

Confucianism predominated over Korea for more than 5 centuries; therefore, like other Eastern countries, Korea is a strongly male oriented society. Women are not in a position to be resistant toward drinking by men, and they must obey and be submissive to men. Attitudes toward drinking by women are much less permissive, and this plus the expected submissiveness of women may help explain the large sex differences in the prevalence of alcoholism. Alcoholism was 16–27 times greater in men compared to women. This is quite a high sex differential compared to Western countries.

There were differences in the age of onset, too, with women having a later age of onset both in Seoul and in the rural areas. Men in their late 20s or early 30s were found to begin to manifest their alcohol symptoms, whereas women were delayed in developing alcoholism compared to men. Alcoholism was generally found to be increasing with age in a linear fashion, right up through the oldest age group. The rate of increase of alcohol abuse in Seoul appeared to reach a relative plateau in the late 20s, while in the rural sample this occurred in the 25–44-year-old group. But the lifetime prevalence of total alcoholism continued to increase with age in a linear fashion.

Alcoholism appeared to be prevalent among those engaged in skilled and semiskilled work in urban as well as in agricultural work in rural areas. The overall prevalence differed little between urban and rural areas. Abuse was more common in Seoul, but dependence was predominant in the rural sample and the sum was almost identical. There was a general tendency for alcoholics in the urban sample to show their symptoms at an earlier age than those in rural areas.

More than 30 percent of the alcohol dependents had at least one episode of withdrawal symptoms (e.g., shakes, seizures, or delirium tremens). This finding suggests that what we are dealing with is not a mild problem, since a high proportion have serious medical consequences as well as social and behavioral problems.

Lastly, the relationship between alcoholism and other psychiatric disorders is interesting because the relative risk figures are so low. Many of the relative risks are below or only slightly above 1. But even for those disorders that are known to be associated with alcoholism, the relative risk figures are not large. The relative risks for antisocial personality range from about 4 to 6, and those for drug abuse/dependence from about 2 to 3. Perhaps because it is so common and so well accepted, alcoholism does not seem to be strongly associated with other psychiatric disorders in Korea.

References

Brislin, R. W.; Lonner, W. J.; and Thorndike, R. M. (1973) *Cross-Cultural Research Methods.* New York: Wiley.

Brislin, R. W. (1980). Translation and content analysis of oral and written materials. In H. C. Triandis, and J. W. Berry (eds.), *Handbook of Cross-Cultural Psychology-Methodology,* vol. 2. Boston: Allyn & Bacon, pp. 389–444.

Cho, H. C.; Kim, J. W.; and Lee, S. H. (1975). Drinking patterns of Koreans. *J. Korean Neuropsychiat. Assn.* 14:1–14.

Cho, S. J., and Kim, J. S. (1983). A literature review study on mental disorders in Korea. *Korean Epid.* 5:118–139.

Choi, M. S. (1979). An epidemiological survey of major mental disorders in Korean rural areas. *J. Korean Neuropsychiat. Assn.* 18:15–21.

Chung, Y. G. (1977). An epidemiological survey of major mental disorders in the Yun Chun Area. *J. Korean Neuropsychiat. Assn.* 16:323–31.

Dohrenwend, D. P., and Dohrenwend, B. S. (1982). Perspectives on the past and future of psychiatric epidemiology (The 1981 Rema Lapouse Lecture). *Am. J. Public Health* 72:1271–79.

Eaton, W. W.; Regier, D. A.; Locke B. I.; and Taube, C. A. (1981). The Epidemiological Catchment Area Program of the National Institute of Mental Health. *Pub. Health Rep.* 96:319–25.

Eaton, W. W.; Holzer, C. E. III; Von Korff, M.; Anthony, J. C.; Helzer, J. E.; George, L.; Burnam, M. A.; Boyd, J. H.; Kessler, L. G.; and Locke, B. J. (1984). The design of the Epidemiological Catchment Area Surveys: The control and measurement of error. *Arch. Gen. Psychiatry* 41:942–48.

Hahn, S. U. (1965). Studies on the incidence of major mental disorders in a Korean rural area. *Med. Dig.* 4:2421–7.

Holzer, C. E. III; Spitznagel, E.; Jordan, K. B.; Timbers, D. M.; Kessler, L. G.; and Anthony, J. C. (1985). Sampling the household population. In W. W. Eaton and L. G. Kessler (eds.), *Epidemiologic Field Methods in Psychiatry: The NIMH Epidemiologic Catchment Area Program.* New York: Academic Press.

Hong, C. H. (1980). An epidemiological survey of major mental disorders in a Korean Rural Area, Keumku. *J. Korean Neuropsychiat. Assn.* 19:118–29.

Huh, C. H. (1965). The prevalence rate of major mental disorders in a Korean rural area. *Med. Dig.* 4:2428–37.

Joo, K.; Han, C. H.; Park, K. B.; Nam, K. H.; and Park, T. W. (1973). Studies on the prevalence of major psychoses in Korean rural area (Wu Chon Myun). *J. Korean Neuropsychiat. Assn.* 12:35–40.

Karno, M.; Burnam, M. A.; Escobar, J. I.; Hough, R. L.; and Eaton, W. W. (1983). Development of the Spanish-Language Version of the National Institute of Mental Health Diagnostic Interview Schedule. *Arch. Gen. Psychiatry* 40:1183–88.

Kim, C. K. (1961). Studies on the incidence of main psychoses in Korean farmers. *New Med. J.* (Korea) 4:1237–41.

Kim, G. S., and Rhi, B. Y. (1965). Studies on the incidence of major psychoses in Korean rural area (Ka Pa Do and Ma Ra Do), Collection of Scientific Papers in Commemoration of the Sixtieth Birthday on March 17, 1965, of Prof. C. W. Myung, vol. 2. Seoul: Seoul National University, pp. 68–78.

Kim, H., and Lee, S. I. (1983). An epidemiological survey of major mental disorders in a part of Korean urban communities. *J. Korean Neuropsychiat. Assn* 22:590–97.

Kim, J. H.; Kim, C. S.; Rhi, B. Y.; Lee S. B.; Kim, C. K.; Kim, H.; Lee, S. I.; and Nam, K. H. (1964). Studies of the incidence of main psychoses in Island Ul-Nung, Korea. *New Med. J.* (Korea) 7:65–75.

Kim, S. S., and Han, H. M. (1964). Studies of the incidence of main psychosis in the Korea rural area (Chin-Do). *J. Korean Neuropsychiat. Assn.* 3:378–84.

Kim, S. T. (1965). Studies on the incidence of major psychosis in a Korean rural area (Kue Jae Do), Collection of Scientific Papers in Commemoration of the Sixtieth Birthday on March 17, 1965 of Prof. C. W. Myung, vol. 2. Seoul: Seoul National University, pp. 114–27.

Kim, Y. S., and Lee, C. K. (1975). Drinking patterns of rural male residents in Korea. *J. Korean Neuropsychiat. Assn.* 14:376–88.

Kim, Y. S.; Kim, H. Y.; Lee, C.; Park, S. S.; Kim, H. W.; Kim J. K.; Choi, T. S.; Cho, D. Y.; Rhi, B. Y.; and Lee, C. K. (1975). An epidemiological survey of major mental disorders in Korean rural areas. *J. Korean Neuropsychiat. Assn.* 14:349–64.

Lee, C. G. (1965). Studies on the incidence of major psychoses in Korean rural area (Baik Hak Myun), Collection of Scientific Papers in Commemoration of the Sixtieth Birthday on March 17, 1965 of Prof. C. W. Myung, vol. 2. Seoul: Seoul National University, pp. 102–13.

Lee, C. K.; Kim, Y. S.; Han, J. H.; and Choi, J. O. (1986). The epidemiological study of mental disorders in Korea (VIII)—Development of DIS-III Korean Version. *Seoul J. Psychiatry* 11:235–96.

Lee, C. Y.; Kwack, Y. S.; Rhee, H.; Kim, Y. S.; Han, J. H.; Choi, C. W.; and Lee, H. Y. (1973). The epidemiological study of mental disorders in Korea (I)—Lifetime prevalence of urban and rural area. *Seoul J. Psychiatry* 1986 11:121–41.25. Zin, S. T. The study on the incidence of major mental disorders in an agricultural community in Korea. *J. Korean Neuropsychiat. Assn.* 12:25–34.

Lee, K. W. (1966). The survey on the incidence and actual status of the major mental disorders at a Korean rural area. *J. Modern Med.* 5:619–36.

Lee, S. K. (1974). Incidence of mental disorders in Korea. *J. Korean Med. Assn.* 17:164–70.

Lee, S. Y. (1975). Studies on the epidemiology of major psychoses. *J. Korean Neuropsychiat. Assn.* 14:189–97.

Lim, Y. J. (1982). A clinical study of admitted alcoholic mental disorders. *J. Korean Neuropsychiat. Assn.* 21:471–79.

Min, B. K.; Kim, C. N.; Lee, S. I.; Park, D. B.; Lee, C. W.; Kim, H. S.; Ahn, S. C.; Lee, K. H.; and Suk, J. H. (1975). A statistical survey on psychiatric inpatients. *J. Korean Neuropsychiat. Assn.* 14:171–83.

Nam, K. H. (1973). The Prevalence of mental disorders in a rural area, Korea. *Korean Pub. Health* 10:33–37.

National Bureau of Statistics (1985). Korea Statistical Yearbook 1985. Republic of Korea: Economic Planning Board.

Oh, S. W.; Park, C. Y.; Park, H. J.; Kim, C. S.; Lee, S. J.; and Lee, K. Y. (1973). A survey of the psychiatric in-patients at Busan University Hospital during past 10 years (Jan. 1962–Dec. 1971). *J. Korean Neuropsychiat. Assn.* 12:110–18.

Oh, Y. W., and Yoon, S. H. (1980). Alcoholic patients admitted to psychiatric department of General Hospital. *J. Korean Neuropsychiat. Assn.* 19:221–33.

Park, M. H. (1965). Studies on the incidence of major psychoses in Korean rural area (Mu An Myun), Collection of Scientific Papers in Commemoration of the Sixtieth Birthday on March 17, 1965 of Prof. C. W. Myung, vol. 2. Seoul: Seoul National University, pp. 54–67.

Park, M. H.; Lee, C. K.; Kim, Y. S.; and Chung, I. W. (1985). The epidemiological study of mental disorders in Korea. *Seoul J. Psychiatry,* Suppl 1985 10:28–29.3.

Regier, D. A.; Myers, J. K.; Kramer, M.; Robins, L. N.; Blazer. D. G.; Hough, R. L.; Eaton, W. W.; and Locke, B. Z. (1984). The NIMH Epidemiological Catchment Area Program: Historical context, major objectives and study population characteristics. *Arch. Gen. Psychiatry* 41:934–41.

Robins, L. N.; Helzer, J. E.; Croughan, J.; Williams, J. B. W.; and Spitzer, R. L. (1981). NIMH Diagnostic Interview Schedule: Version III (May 1981). Rockville, Md.: NIMH mimeo.

Robins, L. N.; Helzer, J. E.; Weissman, M.; Orvaschel, H.; Gruenberg, E.; Burke, J. D., Jr.; and Regier, D. A. (1984). Lifetime prevalence of specific psychiatric disorders in three sites. *Arch. Gen. Psychiatry* 41:949–58.

Robins, L. N.; Helzer, J. E.; Croughan, J.; and Ratcliff, K. (1984). National Institute of Mental Health Diagnostic Interview Schedule: Its history, characteristics and validity. *Arch. Gen. Psychiatry* 41:949–58.

Song, K. U., and Yoo, I. M. (1977). A study on the prevalence of major psychoses in Jindo Korea. *J. Korean Neuropsychiat. Assn.* 16:77–83.

Sung, K. D. (1965). Studies on the incidence of major psychoses in Korean rural area (Kang Nae Myun), Collection of Scientific Papers in Commemoration of the Sixtieth Birthday on March 17, 1965 of Prof. C. W. Myung, vol. 2. Seoul: Seoul National University, pp. 79–86.

Woo, J. I., and Cho, D. Y. (1966). The study on the prevalence of major mental disorders at a Korean rural area. *J. Modern Med.* 5:619–36.

Yeon, B. K.; Kim, Y. S.; Jung, K. I.; and Park, M. H. (1982). An epidemiological survey of major mental disorders in a Korean rural area. *Paing-Seong Eub Psych. Bulletin* 6:158–65.

Yoo, S. J. (1962). Mental Disorders in the Korean Rural Communities. *J. Korean Neuropsychiat. Assn.* 1:9–26

Yoo, S. J. (1962). Studies on the prevalence of mental disorders in two Korean rural communities. *J. Korean Neuropsychiat. Assn.* 1:113–22.

Zin, S. T. (1973). The study on the incidence of major mental disorders in an agricultural community in Korea. *J. Korean Neuropsychiat. Assn.* 12:25–34.

[15] Alcohol Use, Abuse, and Dependency in Shanghai

Chang-Hua Wang, William T. Liu,
Ming-Yuan Zhang, Elena S. H. Yu,
Zheng-Yi Xia, Marilyn Fernandez,
Ching-Tung Lung, Chang-Lin Xu,
and Guang-Ya Qu

The use of alcohol for social and ceremonial occasions was recorded in Chinese history as early as 1760 B.C. during the Yin Dynasty (Ci-Hai Encyclopedia, 1979:936). The cultural tradition of ancient China placed alcoholic beverages at the center of social occasions, which presumably was the origin of the adage: "Without wine, there is no *li* (or etiquette)." Thus, the use of alcoholic beverages has always been accompanied by the concept of propriety and the discharging of one's role obligations in social functions, rather than that of personal indulgence.

This study would not have been possible without the painstaking efforts of a team of dedicated interviewers in Shanghai whose assistance is gratefully acknowledged. Support for the research that led to this study was drawn from diverse sources: the Pacific/Asian American Mental Health Research Center under R01 MH 36408, the Faculty Research Grant of the University of Illinois at Chicago, and the support in kind of the Shanghai Psychiatric Hospital, as well as the Bureau of Public Health of the City of Shanghai. The study was conducted jointly by the Shanghai Psychiatric Hospital (SPH) under the direction of Chang-Hua Wang, M.D., and the Pacific/Asian American Mental Health Research Center (P/AAMHRC) under the leadership of William T. Liu, Ph.D. At the time the study began, Elena S. H. Yu was a U.S. Public Health Service's National Research Service Award (NRSA) Fellow at the Social Psychiatry Research Unit, Columbia University, as part of her career development grant from the National Institute of Mental Health. The following year, William T. Liu was a Mental Health Services Research Post-doctoral Trainee at Yale University, also under the support of NIMH. The authors are grateful to the aforementioned institutions, bureaus, and appropriate heads or representatives for their assistance in the study, direct or indirect. In addition, the authors are grateful to Philip Leaf, Ph.D., John Helzer, M.D., and Peggy Peterson, M. A., for their helpful comments and suggestions in an earlier draft of this paper.

Like any general statement, exceptions are recognized. Chinese literary writers are accorded creative works produced under the influence of alcohol. Huai Shu, a famous Chinese calligrapher, was known to write his "mad cursive" (or *Kuang-cao*) style as he drank. Li Bai (generally recognized as the God of poets in the Tang Dynasty), was known for his finest creations while under the influence of alcohol (*Li Bai dou jiu shi bai pian*), as was his contemporary, poet Du Fu. It is apparent from the biographies of these historical figures that drinking beyond moderation was sanctioned in traditional China under certain circumstances. Indeed, the violation of social norms on drinking by truly creative and talented individuals was a *social privilege*. The literati, being the most prestigious of the four social classes ("*Shi, Nong, Gong, Shang*" or "the Scholar, the Farmer, the Laborer, and the Merchant") that formed the traditional Chinese society, were accordingly granted that privilege. It was condoned and sustained by the belief that creative works were enhanced by the use of alcohol.

With the establishment of diplomatic relationships with the United States in 1979, and the subsequent liberalization of domestic economy in China, comes a more rapid accumulation of material wealth to individual households or families. A new "privileged" class has become visible in Socialist China—the *geti hu* or "individual household businessmen" whose singular income has far exceeded those of any other occupational categories since the Chinese revolution in 1949. With the emergence of a new privileged class in a mercantile economy has come an observable increase of alcohol use as a form of conspicuous consumption in China. Although the privileged still represent a very small percentage of the total population, their conspicuous consumptions has attracted attention. Psychiatric hospitals throughout the country have recently noted the increase of alcohol-related problems, confirming media warnings of excessive alcohol use, which started towards the end of the 1970s.

Alcohol Use and Abuse in Socialist China

Historically, little systematic research has been conducted on alcohol use, abuse, and dependency in China.[1] The few studies conducted on alcoholism in various parts of China after the Socialist Revolution have repeatedly shown low rates of alcohol use and abuse. Using community survey data reported in papers published between 1983 and 1986, by the Chinese and some unpublished data presented in conferences, Wang showed that in the provinces of Jilin, Shandong, Sichuan, Yunnan, Hubei, and in the City of Shanghai, the combined rates of alcohol abuse and "alcoholic psychosis" (called "psychosis due to alcoholic poisoning" in Chinese) have been reported to range from 0.04 percent to 3.5 percent of those surveyed (Wang, 1987). This is shown in Table 15–1.

In these separate studies in Jilin, Sichuan, Shandong, and Hubei, the criteria used for alcohol dependency and alcoholic psychosis were those published in 1985 in the *Chinese Psychiatric Epidemiological Survey Manual* (called *Jingshen Jibing Liuxingxue Diaocha Shouce* in Chinese). To qualify for alcohol dependency in these surveys, the subject must meet two criteria: (1) the presence of an uncontrollable craving for alcohol, that is, a desire to consume alcoholic beverages by any means and regardless of consequences; and (2) presence of withdrawal symptoms when deprived of alcohol, with or without alcoholic mental disturbances. Alcohol psychosis is diagnosed when: (1) there is a long history of alcohol intake; (2) withdrawal symptoms occur when alcohol intake is reduced or stopped; (3) the ICD-9 Criteria for an alcohol-related psychosis (291.0 to 291.9) are met;[2] and (4) there are no other psychiatric diagnoses.

Studies conducted in Yunnan Province, in Jilin Province, and the City of Shanghai were based on criteria specified on the Diagnostic Interview Schedule, Version III.[3] In the Hubei and Yunnan surveys, there was no distinction between alcohol dependency and alcoholic psychosis.[4]

Crude methodologies notwithstanding, survey after survey in China showed that alcohol use and abuse is almost exclusively a male phenomenon. There was no detailed breakdown in *rates* of alcoholism by

Table 15–1 Epidemiological Survey of Alcoholism in China

Characteristics	Jilin 1986	Shandong 1984	Sichuan 1985	Yunnan 1985	Hubei 1986	Yanbian 1986	Shanghai 1983
Diagnostic criteria	CPESM[a]	CPESM	CPESM	DIS	CPESM	DIS	DIS
Sample size							
Number of	500	29492	1000	N.A.	N.A.	N.A.	3000
households	3304	88822	3700	739	2571	1440	3098
Number of persons							
Positive cases of							
Alcohol dependence	13	32	14	26[b]	17[b]	44	14
in urban areas	—	6	N.A.	N.A.	N.A.	N.A.	N.A.
in rural areas	—	26	N.A.	N.A.	N.A.	N.A.	N.A.
Alcoholic psychosis	6	N.A.	N.A.	N.A.	N.A.	N.A.	N.A.
Percentages of persons							
w/alcohol dependence	0.393	0.036	0.378	3.518[b]	0.661[b]	3.056	0.452
in urban areas	0.323	0.030	N.A.	N.A.	N.A.	N.A.	N.A.
in rural areas	0.455	0.037	N.A.	N.A.	N.A.	N.A.	N.A.
Alcoholic psychosis	0.182	N.A.	N.A.	N.A.	N.A.	N.A.	N.A.

[a]The criteria for alcoholism was based on the CPESM—Chinese Psychiatric Epedimiological Survey Manual.

[a]The number represents the sum of cases of Alcohol Dependence and Alcoholic Psychosis.

Source: Wang (1987). Data have been compiled from unpublished papers (1986) prepared separately by Lu Qiu-Yun of Yunnan Province, Duan Cheng-Feng of Sicuan Province, Li Dong-Gen of Jilin Province, Ong Zheng Deng of Shangdong Province, and Wang Chang-Hua of Shanghai Psychiatric Hosptial.

occupation, even though counts of alcoholics by white- and blue-collar workers are available. The absence of population figures (which are needed as denominators for the calculation of rates) makes it difficult to interpret the number of reported cases, since these figures represent only the numerators. Similar difficulties were encountered with the data presented by income and marital status. Data obtained from drinkers suggest that, generally speaking, hard liquor (at least 50 percent proof) is the preferred drink among the abusers, with a "small" proportion drinking wine. But these estimates are woefully imprecise, and inadequate for cross-cultural comparisons of drinking problems. Thus far it appears that only the most severe cases of alcohol abuse and dependency have been recognized and counted in community surveys conducted in China. Clearly, more systematic studies should be conducted in the future.

In addition to the epidemiologic survey data, Wang juxtaposed pieces of information obtained from seventeen psychiatric hospitals in Shanghai, Ha'erbin and Changchun. From a combined total of 476 cases culled from these hospitals, he found a nearly sixfold increase in Shanghai between 1978 and 1985 in the percentage of alcoholic patients among all inpatients of mental hospitals; a nearly threefold increase in Ha'erbin between 1979 and 1985; and an almost fourfold increase in Changchun during a shorter time span, between 1981 and 1985. The data are shown in Table 15–2 (Wang, 1987). The predominance of males over females is readily observable from the date presented in Table 15–3.

The number of treated cases of alcohol abuse and dependence has increased dramatically compared to earlier reports of hospital cases between 1934 and 1937 at the Peking Union Medical College (Hsu, 1970). The number of cases reported in China is large compared to a comment attributed to Lin Tsung-Yi that "there had not been more than 10 cases of alcoholism in 17 years among the Chinese population in Taiwan"

Table 15–2 Number and Percentages of Alcoholic Patients in the Inpatient Department of Mental Hospitals: Selected Locations in China, 1978–1985

Year	1978	1979	1980	1981	1982	1983	1984	1985
Shanghai								
Number of cases	7	6	10	12	15	12	17	31
Percent alcoholic	0.19	0.16	0.29	0.36	0.47	0.40	0.59	1.10
Haerbin								
Number of cases	—	9	9	10	14	23	23	27
Percent alcoholic	—	0.58	0.51	0.59	0.83	1.30	1.26	1.58
Changchun								
Number of cases	—	—	—	1	0	1	6	13
Percent alcoholic	—	—	—	0.13	0	0.14	0.49	0.48

Source: Wang (1987). Data are compiled from unpublished papers (1986) prepared separately by Lu Qiu-Yun of Yunnan Province, Duan Cheng-Feng of Sicuan Province, Li Dong-Gen of Jilin Province, Ong Zheng Deng of Shandong Province, and Wang Chang-Hua of Shanghai Psychiatric Hospital.

Table 15–3 Sex and Age of Admission of Alcoholic Inpatients in China:
Selected Locations and Years

Location in China	Year	Number of Cases	Sex Male	Female	Age Minimum	Maximum
Jilin	1977	35	35	0	23	57
Haerbin	1979–1985	115	113	2	21	67
Beijing	1959–1979	35	33	2	25	73
Yanbian, Jilin[a]	1960	80	80	—	—	—
Shanghai	1958–1981	83	80	3	21	72
Changchun, Jilin	1981–1985	60	57	3	16	72
Shengli	1974–1985	6	6	0	—	—
Qingdao	1984–1986	18	18	0	—	—
Liao-Ning	Latest	26	25	1	27	72
Shan-Xi	1966	3	3	0	30	47
Heilongjiang	1966	1	1	0	—	54
Zhejiang	1962–1982	14	14	0	30	61

[a]Large number of Korean minorities reside in this part of China.

Source: Wang (1987). Data are compiled from unpublished papers (1986) prepared separately by Lu Qiu-Yun of Yunnan Province, Duan Cheng-Feng of Sicuan Province, Li Dong-Gen of Jilin Province, Ong Zheng Deng of Shandong Province, and Wang Chang-Hua of Shanghai Psychiatric Hospital.

(Chafetz, 1964). Obviously, times have changed, and there are clear differences in drinking disorders by geographic area. What was it about the changes in time that result in differential rates of alcoholism?[5] What is it about the different places in China that result in differential rates of alcohol use, abuse, and alcoholism? These are important questions to pursue in future epidemiologic studies.

Limitations of Existing Data

Chinese statistics on drinking are imprecise for a number of reasons: First, there is lack of standardized measures for frequency and quantity, as well as lack of criteria as to what constitutes problem drinking. Second, lack of sophistication in epidemiologic concepts has often resulted in population-based rates of alcohol use, abuse, and alcoholism not being reported. Third, there are considerable cultural variations in the norms of alcohol use and abuse across the broad expanse of China. Despite these differences, however, the Chinese share a common belief that drinking is a part of good food, and that alcoholic beverages should be consumed slowly to enhance the "pleasure of drinking" (*fong-qu*). They are best enjoyed when taken in moderation. The combined principles of moderation and proper occasions for drinking generally has served as the basis for separating alcohol use and alcohol abuse in China, as in other societies. However, the lack of precise statistics on alcohol use, abuse, and alcoholism comparable to those that have been collected routinely in the United States and other countries, have rendered it almost impossible to make cross-cultural comparisons.

The absence of precise statistics was addressed when, in 1983, the Shanghai Psychiatric Hospital, in collaboration with the Pacific/Asian American Mental Health Research Center at the University of Illinois, adopted standardized procedures and criteria by using the DIS-III as the principal instrument in their psychiatric epidemiologic survey in Shanghai.

The Shanghai Diagnostic Interviews

Translation of the DIS into Chinese was undertaken by a binational research team from Shanghai Psychiatric Hospital and the Pacific/Asian American Mental Health Research Center at the University of Illinois at Chicago. The reader is referred to a separate paper for a detailed description of the process (Yu et al., 1987).

The Research Site

Interviews were conducted in 1983 among 3,108 persons selected from Xuhui District, one of the ten administrative districts in Shanghai, with a total population in the 1982 Census of more than half a million. Historically a market port, sections of Xuhui became a part of the French and the English concessions during the first half of the century. Today, it is the site of several famous educational and research institutions in Shanghai, such as the Jiaotong University, College of (Traditional) Chinese Medicine, the Shanghai First Medical College (considered one of the finest in the nation), the Shanghai Psychiatric Hospital (the leading psychiatric hospital in Shanghai), the Shanghai Institute of Mental Health (one of only two WHO Collaborating Centers in China for Research and Training in Mental Health at that time), and research institutes of the Academia Sinica.

The Shanghai Psychiatric Hospital—which serves the entire metropolis of Shanghai—and the Shanghai Institute of Mental Health jointly housed the project, and are both located there. Thus, because of the unprecedented nature of the DIS study, the choice of Xuhui as the DIS research site was made to maximize community cooperation and reduce the cost of conducting the survey by minimizing travel time for interviewers.

Sampling Procedures

Each district in the City of Shanghai consists of about ten *jiedao's* or Street Committees. Two sample *jiedao's* were chosen with a total population in 1982 of 138,179 persons. Within each *jiedao* a random cluster sampling procedure was used to select households. Lists of computer-generated random numbers, stratified by household size, were used to select one eligible person per household for interview. Eligibility criterion consists of all persons between the ages of 18 and 64 years, inclusive. The sample proportion of households corresponded closely to the household distribution found in the two *jiedao*'s. A total of 3,350 households was identified for interview.

Use of Household Registry Records

Permission was obtained from the Bureau of Public Security to copy the household information, which included age and sex of all members in that household. The list, stratified by household size, provided the basis of pre-identifying the sample persons for the study through a process of random selection.

Details about the complex processes of training more than 50 interviewers recruited from the staff of the Shanghai Psychiatric Hospital, its affiliative-network hospitals and clinics in Metropolitan Shanghai, and the field work procedures are described in a separate report (Liu et al., 1984).

The Response Rate

The DIS Survey, being the first nongovernmental sociomedical collaboration in a large-scale community study between a major research hospital in China and individual researchers from the United States, required extreme caution in many respects. Our concern over a possibly high noncompletion rate proved unfounded because, as it turned out, some 92.8 percent of the pre-identified sample persons were successfully interviewed. The reasons for not interviewing 252 of the sample households were:

Failure to meet the age-eligibility criterion 137

"Empty" household register(i.e, unoccupied household address)......... 46

Household was moved but register not yet updated.................... 17

The eligible person was outside of Shanghai 13

Person never home when the interviewer came....................... 12

Psychotic, severe mental disturbance or retardation 10

Hepatitis, still contagious 9

Explicitly refused to be interviewed................................. 8

From the above data, it appears that the Shanghai Household Registration System has been diligently maintained. Only 1.4 percent of 3,350 sampled households were deliberately "empty" registers (called "*kong-gua hu-kou*"), i.e., no one actually lived at the stated address. This is because some people who have moved out of Shanghai are unwilling to cancel their household registration records—the basis for the *per-capita* rationing of *liang-piao* (i.e., "grain stamps" to buy rice, flour, or noodles) and cotton materials in China. An additional 0.5 percent of the sample households had moved out of Shanghai but the official registration of their departure was delayed. Insofar as the interviewers could determine, these are true delays and not disguised empty registers.

Since it was not possible to know beforehand which households have a person between the ages of 18 and 64, inclusive, we have a total of 137 households that failed to meet the age-eligibility criterion after the clusters of households were drawn. These 137 households cannot form a part of the denominator used to calculate the response rate. Even if we consider the twelve sample persons who were not home whenever the interviewer arrived as having "passively" refused to be interviewed, the noncooperation rate totals only 0.6 percent—an impressively low figure compared to the experience of survey researchers in the United States and elsewhere.

The Sample

The sample reported in this paper consists of 3,098 persons, with males representing 46.7 percent of the total and the median age was 36 years. About 15 percent were between 18–24 years of age, 30 percent between 25–34 years, and 23 percent between 35–44 years, with a total of 32 percent between 45–64 years (see Table 15–4).

The combined percentage of illiterates and those with less than 4 years of primary school education is large—about 1 in 4 of the entire sample, chiefly clustered around the older age group. Those who had completed junior high school education accounted for about one third of the sample. Some 37 percent had either a senior high school or technical vocational education. Only a little over 12 percent of the sample had college-level or higher education.

Income variations were relatively small at the time of interview, which was to be expected of that historical period when the salaries of most individuals were determined by the State rather than by market conditions.

Using the procedure for determining occupational prestige reported by Hollingshead and Redlich (1958), exactly one-third of the sample can be classified as falling in the upper one-third, some 40 percent in the middle third, and 27 percent in the bottom third. This distribution would be expected of Xuhui because of the preponderance of professional and technical personnel living in the area. Just about one-quarter of the sample were never married, exactly 70 percent were married, and 4 percent were either widowed, separated, or divorced. The percentage of respondents who had been married more than once was quite small.

Table 15–4 Demographic Characteristics of the Xuhui Sample

	Frequency	Percent
Sex		
Male	1,446	46.70
Female	1,652	53.30
Total	3,098	100.00
Age		
18–24	456	14.70
25–34	937	30.20
35–44	708	22.90
45–54	593	19.10
55–65	404	13.10
Total	3,098	100.00
Sex by Age		
Male		
18–24	212	14.66
25–44	761	52.63
45–65	473	32.71
Female		
18–24	244	14.77
25–44	884	53.51
45–65	524	31.72
Education		
Illiterate/Primary	598	19.32
Junior High	976	31.52
Senior High	700	22.61
Technical	447	14.44
College + Grad School	375	12.22
Income		
0–50 Yuan	865	28.60
51 Yuan or more	2,160	71.40
Total	3,025	100.00
Occupational status prestige		
score in		
Upper $^1/_3$	1,006	33.0
Middle $^1/_3$	1,218	40.0
Lower $^1/_3$	822	27.0
Occupation		
Farming, labor, and other	1,483	48.4
Clerks, sales, and service	556	18.2
Professional, technical, and		
managerial	1,022	33.4
Total	3,061	100.0
Marital status		
Never married	802	25.9
Currently married (including		
cohabitation)	2,165	70.0

(*continued*)

Table 15-4 (Continued)

	Frequency	Percent
Widowed, separated, and divorced	128	4.1
Total	3,095	100.0
Number of marriages		
0	802	25.9
1	2,219	71.8
2+	71	2.3

Lifetime Prevalence of Mental Disorders

Table 15-5 presents the lifetime prevalence of mental disorders (using the DIS/DSM-III Criteria) in the total sample of 3,098 persons.[6] The data indicate that the specific rates of mental disorders are low, compared to those reported in the United States. However, as in the United States, the frequency for phobic disorders ranks first among the disorders covered in the Chinese DIS interviews, followed by alcohol abuse/dependence, and dysthymia. Major depression and schizophrenia occurred in equal frequency and appear to be uncommon in the Xuhui sample. Only 2.13 percent of the sample had at least one diagnosis (excluding alcohol abuse or dependence).

Because of the small number of alcohol abuse and/or dependence cases, efforts to determine the extent to which these diseases may serve as a risk factor for other types of mental disorders resulted in null findings. We report below our findings on drinking status and frequency of drinking.

Table 15-5 Lifetime Prevalence of Specific Disorders in the Total Sample: Xuhui, Shanghai[a]

	Frequency	(%)
Mania	—	—
Depression	6	0.19
Dysthymia	9	0.29
Schizophrenia	6	0.19
Schizophreniform	1	0.03
Phobia	46	1.48
Somatization	1	0.03
Panic	2	0.06
Obsessive-compulsive	2	0.06
Alcohol abuse/dependence	14	0.45
Any Core Diagnosis[b] except alcohol	66	2.13

[a]The prevalence rates are based on the total sample ($N = 3,098$).

[b]Any core diagnosis refers to any of the above nine diagnoses.

Drinking Patterns

The DIS alcohol section only assesses alcohol abuse, dependence, and patterns of problem drinking. There was concern that these problems may be relatively rare in China as the literature had suggested. At the recommendation of the Institutional Review Board, a question was added in the Shanghai DIS Study to determine just what percentage of the population drinks and how often the responders drink.[7] Table 15–6 shows that the majority of the Chinese (77 percent of 3,098 respondents) are nondrinkers. Among those who drink, most (88.5 percent of 699 persons) are "sometimes" or "occasional" drinkers, rather than "frequent" drinkers. When cross-tabulations were made between frequency of drinking and the lifetime prevalence of specific disorders, few variations were found in the number of cases with specific mental disorders.

Table 15–6 also shows a lack of overlap between alcohol abuse and dependence cases with lifetime prevalence cases of other specific mental disorders. The lack of overlap is, as mentioned earlier, most likely a result of the extremely small number of prevalence cases of mental disorders found in the study, and the paucity of drinkers in the sample. As a group, drinkers (which include the occasional, sometimes, and often drinkers) compared with nondrinkers do show some risks for specific mental disorders, particularly panic disorders (risk ratio = 3.5).

Symptoms of Alcoholism

Tables 15–7a, b, and c examine the symptom-specific prevalences. Of 3,098 respondents in Xuhui, only 52 persons (or 1.7 percent) reported ever drinking daily for a month or more (Table 15–7a). Among the latter, some 38 percent reported daily or weekly heavy drinking, and 29 percent admitted to drinking as much as a fifth of liquor in one day or

Table 15–6 Lifetime Prevalence of Specific Disorders Among Alcoholics: Xuhui, Shanghai

	Alcohol Dependence/ Abuse (N = 14) Prevalence	Drinkers: Occasional, Sometimes, Often (N = 699) Prevalence	Drinkers: Occasional, Sometimes (N = 619) Prevalence	Drinkers: Often (N = 80) Prevalence
Mania	—	—	—	—
Depression	—	0.14 (1)[a]	0.16 (1)	—
Dysthymia	—	0.29 (2)	0.32 (2)	—
Schizophrenia	—	0.14 (1)	0.16 (1)	—
Schizophreniform	—	—	—	—
Phobia	—	0.86 (6)	0.97 (6)	—
Somatization	—	0.14 (1)	0.16 (1)	—
Panic	—	0.14 (1)	0.16 (1)	—
Obsessive-compulsive	—	—	—	—
Any core diagnosis except alcohol	—	1.57 (11)	1.78 (11)	—

[a]Number in parentheses are frequencies.

Table 15–7a Individual Symptom Frequencies For Those Ever Drunk Daily for a Month or More: Xuhui, Shanghai[a]

Dis Item Number	Symptom	Proportion of Those Drinking Daily for a Month or More Who Endorsed This Item		
		%	Freq.	N
150	Family objected to respondent's drinking	11.54	6	52
151	Respondent thought himself an excessive drinker	23.81	5	21
152	Fifth of liquor in one day, 4 bottles of beer	28.85	15	52
153	Daily or weekly heavy drinking	38.46	20	52
155	Told physician about drinking problem	15.38	8	52
156	Friends or professionals said drinking too much	15.38	8	52
157	Wanted to stop drinking but couldn't	7.69	4	52
158	Efforts to control drinking	3.85	2	52
159	Morning drinking	0.00	0	52
160	Job troubles due to drinking	3.85	2	52
161	Lost job	0.00	0	52
162	Trouble driving	0.00	0	52
163	Arrested while drinking	0.00	0	52
164	Physical fights while drinking	0.00	0	52
165	Two or binges	0.00	0	50
166	Blackouts while drinking	4.00	2	50
167	Any withdrawal symptom	0.00	0	50
168	Any medical complication	6.00	3	50
169	Continued to drink with serious illness	8.00	4	50
170	Couldn't do ordinary work without drinking	6.00	3	50

[a]Please see footnote 7 in the text.

four bottles of beer. Some 24 percent of those who drank daily thought of themselves as being an excessive drinker. In 15 percent of the cases, the respondent had told a physician about his drinking problem, and in yet another 15 percent of the cases, the respondent had received warnings from friends and professionals about his drinking problems. In 12 percent of the cases, the respondent's family objected to his drinking.

Of those who had ever drunk daily for a month or more, 38 persons are without alcohol disorders (Table 15–7b). About 16 percent of these 38 persons drank heavily on a daily or weekly basis. In 11 percent of the cases, the respondent drank as much as a fifth of liquor in one day or 4 bottles of beer. In 16 percent of the cases, the respondent had told a physician about his drinking problem.

Among those who had ever drunk daily for a month or more and developed alcohol disorders, all drank heavily on a daily or weekly basis. In two-thirds of these cases, families objected to the respondent's drinking. As well, a similar percentage of friends or professionals thought the respondent was drinking too much. Spearman correlation of symptom rankings between those with alcohol disorders (Table 7c) and those without alcohol disorders equals 0.49, which is statistically significant at the .05 level.

Table 15–7b Individual Symptom Frequencies Among Ever Daily Drinkers Without Alcohol Disorders: Xuhui, Shanghai[a]

| DIS Item Number | Symptom | Proportion of Those Without Alcohol Disorders Who Endorsed This Item | | |
		%	Freq.	N
150	Family objected to respondent's drinking	0.0	0	38
151	Respondent thought himself an excessive drinker	0.0	0	7
152	Fifth of liquor in one day, 4 bottles of beer	10.53	4	38
153	Daily or weekly heavy drinking	15.79	6	38
155	Told physician about drinking problem	15.79	6	38
156	Friends or professionals said drinking too much	5.26	2	38
157	Wanted to stop drinking but couldn't	0.0	0	38
158	Efforts to control drinking	0.0	0	38
159	Morning drinking	0.0	0	38
160	Job troubles due to drinking	0.0	0	38
161	Lost job	0.0	0	38
162	Trouble driving	0.0	0	38
163	Arrested while drinking	0.0	0	38
164	Physical fights while drinking	0.0	0	38
165	Two or binges	0.0	0	38
166	Blackouts while drinking	0.0	0	38
167	Any withdrawal symptom	0.0	0	38
168	Any medical complication	0.0	0	38
169	Continued to drink with serious illness	0.0	0	38
170	Couldn't do ordinary work without drinking	0.0	0	38

[a]This refers to respondents who reported having drunk daily for a month or more in their lifetime.

Lifetime Rates of Various Drinking Categories

Among those who had ever drunk daily for a month or more, only one was a total abstainer at the time of the interview (Table 15–8). Forty percent are classified as nonheavy/nonproblem (social) drinkers, nearly 20 percent (19.23) are problem drinkers even though they are not alcoholic—that is, they have had at least one alcohol-related problem in their lives, even though they have not had enough to qualify for a DSM-III diagnosis of alcoholism. The latter group may be mostly sporadic drinkers, or they may have been (recent) drinkers who have not yet developed symptoms. Another 12 percent are classified as heavy/nonproblem drinkers—that is, they have had a period when they regularly consumed seven or more drinks at least one evening a week but have never had any social, legal, or medical problems related to alcohol and no withdrawal symptoms. Helzer et al. (1986) suggest that "it would appear that most of those who consume that much alcohol are destined to have at least some problems from it." Some 27 percent of the cases fit the category of "Dependence with or without abuse" and not one case of alcohol abuse only was found in the Xuhui sample, even though it is considered the less severe form of the alcohol disorders.

Table 15–7c Individual Symptom Frequencies Among Ever Daily Drinkers With Alcohol Disorders: Xuhui, Shanghai[a]

DIS Item Number	Symptom	Proportion of Those with Alcohol Disorders Who Endorsed This Item		
		%	Freq.	N
150	Family objected to respondent's drinking	66.67	6	9
151	Respondent thought himself an excessive drinker	55.56	5	9
152	Fifth of liquor in one day, 4 bottles of beer	66.67	6	9
153	Daily or weekly heavy drinking	100.00	9	9
155	Told physician about drinking problem	22.22	2	9
156	Friends or professionals said drinking too much	66.67	6	9
157	Wanted to stop drinking but couldn't	44.44	4	9
158	Efforts to control drinking	22.22	2	9
159	Morning drinking	0.0	0	9
160	Job troubles due to drinking	22.22	2	9
161	Lost job	0.0	0	9
162	Trouble driving	0.0	0	9
163	Arrested while drinking	0.0	0	9
164	Physical fights while drinking	0.0	0	9
165	Two or binges	0.0	0	7
166	Blackouts while drinking	28.57	2	7
167	Any withdrawal symptom	0.0	0	7
168	Any medical complication	42.86	3	7
169	Continued to drink with serious illness	57.14	4	7
170	Couldn't do ordinary work without drinking	42.86	3	7

Spearman Correlation of Symptom Rankings Between Those
With and Without Alcohol Disorders ($N = 20$) $r = 0.492; p = 0.0275$

[a]This refers to respondents who reported having drunk daily for a month or more their lifetime.

The Course of Alcoholism

Table 15–9 examines the course of alcoholism. Out of 43 persons for whom data on intoxication are available, 56 percent (or 24 persons) reported having ever been intoxicated. The mean age of first intoxication for men is 26.26 years. Alcoholics, on average, experienced their first intoxication at a much younger age (23.71 years) compared with nonalcoholics (28.38 years). In both cases, these ages are much higher in China than those reported by Helzer et al. based on data from the ECA studies conducted in the United States.

The age of onset of alcoholism is also somewhat delayed in China (33.5 years) as compared with findings obtained from the United States. The course of illness, however, appears to be of similar duration in China as in the United States in that 8.83 years elapsed in the Shanghai study between the time of first intoxication to first alcohol symptom, compared to about 8 years in the United States. The mean number of lifetime symptoms is just over 5 in China, as in the United States.

We found only one case of "alcoholic in remission," that is, absence of

Table 15–8 Lifetime Rates of Various Drinking Categories Among Ever Daily Drinkers for a Month or More: Xuhui, Shanghai

Lifetime Drinking Category[a]	%	Freq.	N	Mean Ages
Nonheavy/nonproblem (social) drinkers	42.31	22	52	51.64
Heavy/nonproblem drinkers	11.54	6	52	49.17
Problem drinkers (not alcoholic)	19.23	10	52	52.30
Alcohol abuse only	0.00	0	52	—
Dependence with or without abuse	26.92	14	52	50.71
Total	100.00	52		51.23
6-Month Prevalence of Alcoholism (abuse and/or dependence combined)	11.36	5	44	—

(Mean Age of the entire sample is 38.13 years)

[a]One case of total abstention at the time of interview was found among the respondents who admitted having ever drunk daily for a month or more in their lifetime. That person's age was 38 years. The respondent is counted in the nonheavy/nonproblem (social) drinkers category.

Table 15–9 Onset, Severity, and Course of Alcoholism in Xuhui, Shanghai

	Men	Total
Mean Age First Intoxicated (If Ever)		
Total sample	26.26 (23)[a]	26.21 (24)
Alcoholics only[b]	23.71 (7)	23.88 (8)
Nonalcoholics[c]	28.38 (13)	28.38 (13)
Mean value among alcoholics		
Age of onset of alcoholism	33.50 (6)	33.50 (6)[d]
Number of years from first intoxication to first alcohol symptom	8.83 (6)[e]	8.83 (6)
Mean number of lifetime symptoms	5.25 (8)	4.89 (9)
Mean values among alcoholics in remission[f]		
Age last symptom	47.00 (1)	47.00 (1)
Duration of alcoholism in years	2.00 (1)	2.00 (1)
Mean number of lifetime symptoms	4.00 (1)	4.00 (1)
Mean number of lifetime alcohol symptoms for duration of alcoholism 0–10 years	4.00 (1)	4.00 (1)
Mean values among alcoholics not in remission		
Mean number of lifetime symptoms	6.40 (5)	6.40 (5)
Mean number of lifetime symptoms 0–10 years	5.33 (3)	5.33 (3)
Mean number of lifetime symptoms 11+	8.00 (2)	8.00 (2)
	(%)	Freq.
Ever Intoxicated	55.8	24
Never Intoxicated	44.2	19
Total number of persons with data	100.0	43

[a]Numbers in parentheses are frequencies. Data for women not presented because there was only one case.

[b]There was one male alcoholic with missing data on age.

[c]Some persons who fall in this category have missing data on age of first intoxication.

[d]Three persons had missing data.

[e]Two persons had missing data.

[f]Remitted Alcoholic = No alcohol symptoms for at least one year prior to interview.

alcoholic symptoms for at least 1 year prior to the interview. For this one person, the age of the occurrence of last symptom was in the late 40s, a pattern rather consistent with a delayed ónset in China as compared to the United States. The occurrence of the first and last symptoms is only 2 years. The average number of lifetime symptoms for this one case of alcoholic in remission compared with those not in remission differed somewhat in that the symptom count is higher among the latter than the former group. In the case of alcoholics not in remission, the symptom count increases with duration of illness.

Risk Factors and Correlates of Alcoholism

Data on risk factors for alcohol disorders (abuse and/or dependence) in Shanghai are presented in Table 15–10. First, gender differences in alcohol abuse/dependence are rather striking. Drinking disorders are associated with being male rather than female. Additional data collected separately from the same sample show that while only 7.45 percent of Xuhui women (18–64 years old) drink, some 40 percent of the men in that same age group are drinkers, either occasionally, sometimes, or often (table not presented due to space limitations). Drinking is a predominantly male practice. Second, the percentage who drink (26%) is highest for the oldest age group in the study, those 45–64 years of age. The two younger age groups (18–24 and 25–44 years) appear to have similarly low percentages of drinkers (21%). On the whole, the data suggest the possibility that drinking behavior may not have been part of the early adulthood socialization of Xuhui citizens. This conjecture makes sense in the context of the spartan life that characterized China from 1949 when the People's Republic was established, to 1979 when contact with the West was finally permitted as a result of the "normalization" of the U.S.–China relationship. Those 45–64 years old in 1983 were 11–30 years old in 1949. For the next younger age group (25–44 years), the oldest member would have been only 10 years old when the People's Republic of China was established. As these age cohorts of Chi-

Table 15–10 Lifetime Prevalence of Alcoholism by Sex and Age: Xuhui, Shanghai (N = 52)[a]

Age Group	Men (%)	Women (%)	Total (%)
18–24	— (0/0)	— (0/0)	— (0/0)
25–44	42.86 (3/7)[b]	0.00 (0/2)	33.33 (3/9)
45–65	23.81 (10/42)	100.00 (1/1)(1)	25.58 (11/43)
Total	26.53 (13/49)	33.33 (1/3)	26.92 (14/52)

[a]Data available only on fifty-two persons who reported having ever drunk daily for a month or more. See footnote 7 in the text for clarification.

[b]Numbers in parentheses are the numerators and denominators used in the calculation of rates.

nese entered early and young adulthood, they would have experienced the austere life required of a country that has had to heal from the wounds of 8 years of Sino-Japanese War (1937–1945) and 3 years of Civil Wars (1946–1949), followed by periods of poverty and tremendous food shortage such that few families or individuals could afford the luxury of drinking alcoholic beverages on a regular basis. In epidemiologic parlance, exposure to the agent (i.e., alcoholic beverages) may have been unusually minimal, or may have occurred much later in life for most Chinese under 64 years of age in 1983, and certainly for those in the 25–44-year age group, because of peculiar sociohistorical contexts.

Note, however, that when lifetime prevalence of alcoholic disorders by sex and age are calculated using the method suggested by Helzer et al. (Table 15–10), the prevalence rate for the males in the oldest age group (23.81 percent) is lower than that for the 25–44-year age group (42.86 percent). Notwithstanding the small number of cases in Xuhui who reported ever drinking daily for a month or more, this drop in lifetime prevalence with age is similar to that reported by Helzer et al. in the United States. It occurs even though there are more drinkers in the oldest age group of the Shanghai sample (26 percent among the 45–64-year age group, compared with 21 percent for 25–44-year age group). Problems of recall during the interview and/or higher chances of early deaths among the alcoholics are likely reasons for the observed pattern.

The argument of an age-cohort effect in alcoholism remains to be tested and, we suspect, will possibly be found in future studies in China because of the rapid changes the country is experiencing. Such changes have made it possible for more people to find work even though their wages may be low. They have also resulted in the greater availability of alcoholic beverages for domestic consumption. The result is that more and more people can afford to purchase alcoholic drinks now than in the past. For those in the 44–65-year age group, the economic employability of their grown children has resulted in their having a little more cash than in the past to spend on things for sheer pleasure. Alcoholic drinks are a privilege to be enjoyed by the older folks. For those in the 25–44-year age group, the new economy has created a sense of optimism and expansiveness such that going out drinking with friends for fun is no longer "decadent." But the older group may be much more able to control their drinking to a moderate level, compared to the younger ones. The net effect of these forces may result in more instances of problem drinking, and higher lifetime prevalences of alcoholism for the 25–44-year age group (compared with those in the 45–64-year age group) that were beginning to emerge in the 1980s, despite their presumably low and later exposure to alcoholic beverages.

Table 15–11 shows that more than half of all daily drinkers in Xuhui are heavy drinkers (58.82 percent). Close to half (46.67 percent) of all

Table 15–11 Risk Factors and Correlates for Heavy Drinking and Alcoholism: Xuhui, Shanghai

	Proportion of All Daily Drinkers Who Are Heavy Drinkers		Proportion of Heavy Drinkers Who Are Alcoholic	
	Percent	(Cases)	Percent	(Cases)
Total sample	58.82	(30/51)[a]	46.67	(14/30)
Risk factor or correlate				
Number of marriages				
0	100.00	(2/2)	50.00	(1/2)
1	59.09	(26/44)	46.15	(12/26)
2+	40.00	(2/5)	50.00	(1/2)
Years of education				
Illiterate/primary	63.33	(19/30)	36.84	(7/19)
Junior high	60.00	(6/10)	50.00	(3/6)
Senior high	100.00	(4/4)	75.00	(3/4)
Technical/vocational	33.33	(1/3)	100.00	(1/1)
College/graduate school	—		—	
Occupational status				
Upper ⅓	38.46	(5/13)	60.00	(3/5)
Middle ⅓	53.85	(7/13)	71.43	(5/7)
Lower ⅓	72.00	(18/25)	33.33	(6/18)
Residence at time of interview[b]	N.A.		N.A.	
Childhood conduct group positive[c]	N.A.		N.A.	
Intoxicated before age 15				
No	56.10	(23/41)	52.17	(12/23)
Yes	100.00	(1/1)	100.00	(1/1)

[a]One person in the denominator has missing data on heavy drinking.

[b]The study was conducted entirely in the urban area.

[c]This section of the DIS was not included in the Shanghai DIS study because it required extensive modifications and testing of the individual items to ensure that they are culturally appropriate.

heavy drinkers are alcoholic. Examination of the risk factors or correlates of drinking indicate that the number of marriages is not associated with heavy drinking or with alcoholism among those who drink heavily. This is because the social conditions in China are different than in the United States. Divorce is less prevalent and more difficult to obtain in China than in the United States. Likewise, multiple marriages are rare. Second, age of first intoxication and the course of illness occurs about a decade later than in the United States, with the result that the occurrence of the first symptoms in China is likely to emerge in the context of (the first and only) marriage for most people. As the young delay marriage longer, more frequent and heavy drinkers may be found among the never-married group in the future. The data in Table 15–11 suggest the possibility of such a trend.

Education shows an intriguing pattern in that close to two-thirds of drinkers with primary education or less, as well as drinkers with only junior high school education, are heavy drinkers. Only one person with a vocational or technical school education was classified as a heavy drinker. All of the drinkers who have a senior high school education are heavy drinkers, suggesting that in China, higher education is associated with heavy drinking. Likewise, among the heavy drinkers, having a higher education seems to be associated with being an alcoholic. Seventy-five percent of the heavy drinkers with senior high school education are alcoholic, while only 37 percent of the heavy drinkers with primary education or less are alcoholic. Caution is warranted in the interpretation of the data because the number of cases is too small. It may be important in future studies to examine the concept of power and social privilege in alcohol use and abuse across cultures. It would seem that, in China, the highly educated, the businessmen, and the old have the opportunities to drink regularly as a form of social privilege. Among these drinkers, we hypothesize that the psychological need for power and the growing acceptance of alcohol as a coping mechanism for life stress may explain why some develop drinking problems while others do not.

Inconsistent results are obtained when one examines occupational status. There seems to be an inverse association between heavy drinking and lower occupational prestige. Some 72 percent of all drinkers in the lower-third of occupational status are heavy drinkers compared to only 38 percent in the upper-third category, whereas, among the heavy drinkers, a higher occupational prestige is associated with becoming an alcoholic. Data on age of intoxication provides strong evidence of a much later age of intoxication for the Chinese sample compared with the U.S. data.

Questions on residence at the time of interview were not asked in the Shanghai Study because the sample is a uniformly urban one. Information on childhood conduct disorders are not available because that section of the DIS required major modifications before it could be used in China and was not included in the study.

Discussion

The Shanghai data present a composite picture of drinking habits among the Chinese that is distinctly different from those of Americans. First, a large majority of Chinese do not drink at all. But when they do, we hypothesize that the change from nondrinking to drinking status may be associated with the concept of power and social privilege, in the sense that it is men and not women who drink heavily and, among heavy drinkers, those whose education was low or whose occupations are more prestigious appear to have higher chances of becoming an alcoholic. The classic examples of several literary figures in China have been mentioned. The DIS data collected in Xuhui suggests to us a possible avenue for future research into the relationship between drinking behavior in China and the concept of social power and social privilege. In ancient China, being a literary figure was accorded the highest social status. In socialist China undergoing modernization in the 1980s, being a *geti hu* or an individual household businessman has become socially desirable and for which conspicuous consumption is necessary in order to demonstrate one's newly acquired economic power and social entitlements. In both instances across different time spans, a greater incidence of public intoxication has been observed to be associated with these socially prestigious occupations. That drinking frequency was low in the past is credible in light of the near absence of conspicuous consumption in a population struggling to move beyond sheer subsistence level. As the individual possesses more cash to spend beyond the basic necessities of life, avenues for pleasure-seeking will be pursued by those who desire to assert their newly gained social status. The principle of moderation embedded in the Confucian concept of "the way of the mean" and the notion that drinking is a social privilege may have served to keep problem drinking in relatively low frequencies in China, although that will change. Clearly, what is needed in future studies is further validation of our observations and conjectures.

Second, there has been a tendency for past researchers to consider all Chinese as alike and to ignore the possibility of geographic variations in drinking behavior among the different Chinese populations. The recent review of data in Wang's unpublished paper suggests the need to conduct surveys in different parts of China in order to understand better the regional differences in drinking status and alcoholism. The reported rates that Wang found in his review of data for internal use only are certainly much higher than those we obtained in the first DIS survey in Shanghai. The educational and occupational mix of the Xuhui population needs to be carefully considered before one draws any firm conclusions about drinking behaviors in China. This is especially important in light of the interesting relationships we uncovered between education and occupation with heavy drinking as compared with alcoholism. Xuhui, after all, is not Shanghai; it is certainly not China.

Third, there may have been cultural variations in the public sensitivity as to what is reportable alcoholic symptoms. Thus, persons who drink heavily on weekends or at regular intervals spaced further apart because of financial constraints may possibly have reported themselves and be viewed by others as mild drinkers if not nondrinkers. This may account for the public as well as professional (mis)perceptions among Chinese psychiatrists themselves that problem drinking is rare in Chinese populations. The changes that were made in the DIS questions as they were used in Shanghai resulted in the absence of information on episodic problem drinkers and mild cases of alcohol abuse or dependency.

Fourth, drinking behaviors are socialized at later ages in Shanghai than in the United States. This delay of as much as 10 years has beneficial consequences in that it shifts the age of first intoxication upwards from early teens to mid-20s, the onset of alcoholism to the 30s, and the mean age of alcoholics in remission to the 40s. Differences in the availability of treatment opportunities in Shanghai may be associated with the different levels of public sensitivity to problem drinkers.

Fifth, it is remarkable that the average number of symptoms reported by alcoholics and the course of illness in China, are almost identical to the U.S. patterns, thereby suggesting a possible course of illness that is, perhaps, more biophysiologically than socially determined. Alternatively, the similarity in the course of illness may be an artifact of the methodology used in extracting information on psychiatric disorders. It behooves future researchers to examine this issue further.

Notes

1. Alcohol research based on data collected among the ethnic Chinese is available, and generally falls into two categories: (1) studies concerned with reactions to alcohol, and (2) studies focusing on ethnic patterns of alcohol consumption and abuse. The physiological studies have been greatly influenced by the work of Wolff, who reported in 1972 that 83 percent of the Asian subjects in his study showed a marked flushing response that was observed in fewer than two percent of the Caucasian subjects (Wolff, 1972). Since then, evidence to support Wolff's earlier findings continue to accumulate (Ewing et al., 1974; Stamatoyannopoulous et al., 1975; Reed et al., 1976; Hanna, 1978; Seto et al., 1978). Studies focusing on ethnic patterns of alcohol consumption and abuse, which include samples of the Chinese population rather than anecdotal observations, have reported inconsistent findings.

2. These are: delirium tremens (291.0); Korsakov's psychosis, alcoholic (291.1); other alcoholic dementia (291.2); other alcoholic hallucinosis (291.3); pathological drunkenness (291.4); alcoholic jealousy (291.5); other (291.8); unspecified (291.9).

3. In addition, the Yunnan Interview Schedule also contained the Self-Administered Alcoholism Screening Test (SAAST) as screening instrument.

4. The data collected in the border town of Jilin Province where large numbers of Korean minority populations reside cannot always be compared with those obtained elsewhere in China because of cultural and genetic differences between these two groups. Reported studies of alcoholics among Korean minorities in China found that they consume alcohol frequently and in large quantities, as well as at an earlier age.

5. One thing is quite clear: the emergence of frequent drinking and the risk of alcoholic disorders are more likely in societies that have moved beyond the level of sheer subsistence. China in the 1930s was characterized by massive poverty. Conspicuous consumptions occurred only in an extremely small segment of the total population.

6. Ten of the 3,108 persons interviewed suffered from mental illness or mental retardation so severe that they could not be interviewed directly. Although a proxy interview was conducted with the respondent's caretaker in the same household, the latter's lack of precise information about the specificity of some symptoms, the age of onset for reported clusters of symptoms, and the course of illness made it impossible to subject their interview

protocols to the same computer algorithms which were used in generating diagnostic information from the remaining 3,098 completed interviews.

7. The inclusion of this question represents a compromise solution between two groups of decision makers: the Institutional Review Board that supervised the survey, which wanted to shorten different sections of the DIS instrument (such as the somatization, depression, phobia, schizophrenia, and other questions) for fear of negative consequences from respondents as yet unaccustomed to this type of structured interview; and the researchers who wanted to keep all the DIS questions identical to those used in the ECA survey in the United States in order to facilitate cross-cultural comparisons. Since knowledge of the magnitude of alcohol problems in several populations abroad was to come only after the results of the ECA studies in the United States was published, and existing reports within China conveyed the picture of extremely low prevalence of alcohol problems at the time the study was about to begin, it was thought that the alcohol section would be a "safe" place to demonstrate the researchers' willingness to heed advice while the rest of the DIS questions used in Shanghai remained unaltered. Thus, a decision was made to introduce a skip question to the DIS-Alcohol section, which translates into English as follows: "Do you drink?" Respondents who indicated that they do drink—even if only a little or only rarely—were then asked (N=699 persons because two other persons had missing data on this first question) a second question: "Have you ever drunk daily for a month or more?" those who reported in the negative (N=644 because two more persons had missing data) were not asked the DIS alcohol questions. The decision to use the latter question as a criterion for asking the DIS alcohol questions was made after consulting the criteria for alcohol abuse and/or dependence described in the DSM-III published by the American Psychiatric Association. The data in this paper are thus based on a total of only fifty-two persons (one other person eligible for the question had missing data) who admitted that they drink and had ever drunk daily for a month or more. Moreover, it was thought that DIS Q.154 is impolite to ask if the respondent already answered "no" to DIS Q.153. Q.154 was therefore eliminated. Page restriction in printing the instrument led to the dislocation of the question order for DIS Q.151, which ended up following Q.153 instead of preceding it as it is in the English version. This change in question order led to fewer respondents for Q.151 than for Q.152 or Q.153. The objective of keeping the DIS interviews within reasonable limits was made at a great cost—the loss of valuable information about a social behavior that appears to be a growing problem in certain parts of China.

References

Anonymous (1979). *Ci-Hai Encyclopedia*. Shanghai: Shanghai Ci-Dong Publishing Co.

Chafetz, Morris E. (1964). Consumption of alcohol in the Far and Middle East. *N. Eng J. Med.* 271,6:297–301.

Duan, Cheng-Feng (1986). An epidemiologic survey of alcohol dependency in Chong-Qing (in Chinese). Unpublished paper read at the Conference on Alcohol Dependency and Related Problems held in Beijing in October 1986.

Ewing et al. (1974). Alcohol sensitivity and ethnic background. *Am. J. Psychiatry* 131, 2 (February): 206–210.

Hanna, Joel M. (1978). Metabolism responses of Chinese, Japanese and Europeans to Alcohol. *Alcoholism: Clinical and Experimental Research*, 2, 1 (January):89–92.

Helzer et al. (1986). Alcoholism—North America and Asia: Comparison of population surveys with the DIS. First draft.

Hollingshead, A. B. and Redlich, F. C. (1958). *Social Class and Mental Illness*, a Community Study. New York: Wiley.

Hsu, Francis L. K. (1970). *Chinese and Americans*. New York: The Natural History Press.

Li, Dong-Gen (1986). Use of the DIS and the diagnostic criteria in diagnosing alcohol dependency. Unpublished paper read at the Conference on Alcohol Dependency and Related Problems held in Beijing in October 1986.

Liu, William T., et al. (1984). The 1983 Shanghai Psychiatric Epidemiologic Survey: Research objectives, procedures, and field operations. Working Paper No. 103b of the Shanghai Project. Chicago: P/AAMHRC.

Lu, Qiu-Yun (1986). Report of a sample survey of alcohol-dependency and related problems in Yunnan's Simao and Xishuangbanna areas (in Chinese). Unpublished paper read at the Conference on Alcohol Dependency and Related Problems held in Beijing in October 1986.

Ong, Zheng-Deng (1986). Report of an epidemiologic study of alcohol and drug abuse in Shandong (in Chinese). Unpublished paper read at the Conference on Alcohol Dependency and Related Problems held in Beijing in October 1986.

Reed, T. Edward, et al. (1976). Alcohol and acetaldehyde metabolism in Caucasians, Chinese and Amerinds. *CMA Journal* 6 (November 6):851–55.

Seto, A., et al. (1978). Biochemical correlates of ethanol-induced flushing in Orientals." *Journal Stud. Alcohol* 39:1–11.

Stamatoyannopoulous, G.; Chen, Shi-Han; and Fukui, Miyoshi (1975). Liver alcohol dehydrogenase in Japanese: High population frequency of atypical form and its possible role in alcohol sensitivity. *Am. J. Hum. Genet.* 27:789–96.

Wang, Chang-Hua (1987). Alcohol dependency and alcohol abuse in parts of China (in Chinese). Unpublished. Copies available on request.

Wolff, P. H. (1972) Ethnic differences in alcohol sensitivity. *Science* 175:449–50.

Yu, Elena; Ming-Yuan Zhang; Zheng-Yi Xia; and William T. Liu (1987). Translation of instruments: Procedures, issues, and dilemmas. In William T. Liu (ed.), *The Pacific/Asian American Mental Health Research Center. A Decade Review of Mental Health Research, training, and Services. A Report to the National Institute of Mental Health.* Chicago: P/AAMHRC, pp. 75–86.

[V] Conclusions

[16] Comparative Analysis of Alcoholism in Ten Cultural Regions

JOHN E. HELZER AND GLORISA J. CANINO

The Cross-Cultural Appropriateness of DSM-III

The advantages for cross-national comparisons of having the same set of diagnostic criteria and the same interview structure are obvious and have been highlighted by the preceeding chapters. It is a premise of this book that the DSM-III criteria are appropriate to the multiple cultural contexts in which we have applied them. In order to draw conclusions from the intercultural similarities and differences these chapters identify, we need assurance that the interview and diagnostic methods used here are appropriate to the task.

Perhaps the best evidence that the DSM-III, and by extension the DIS, are appropriate is that the investigators involved in these studies have chosen to apply them. This series of studies did not begin as a coordinated effort. No doubt the size and visibility of the ECA survey, and the advance it represented for psychiatric epidemiology, generated much of the concurrent interest in replicating that effort elsewhere. The fact that the DIS interview can be administered by nonclinicians and the consequent economy was no doubt an attraction also. But it hardly seems likely that such large epidemiologic investigations would have been undertaken if the DSM-III criteria on which the DIS is based had been considered inappropriate to the culture in which it was to be applied. Since the DSM-III illness definitions are relatively specific, use of this taxonomy connotes more than simple acceptance of its diagnostic labels and general illness concepts, as might be the case with a less specific taxonomy such as DSM-II or the ICD-9.

There is also previous evidence of the cross-national acceptability and utility of DSM-III. Spitzer et al. (1983) reported commentary and

289

some data on DSM-III usage from investigators and clinicians in eighteen countries in a volume published 3 years after DSM-III. Contributors' comments at that point, though mostly of a general nature, were largely favorable. Especially interesting was a survey of more than fifty senior psychiatrists throughout the People's Republic of China. Even at that early date, most of these Chinese psychiatrists had studied DSM-III, were favorably disposed toward it, and had applied it in clinical and research work. All of the respondents felt it had already had a marked influence on psychiatric diagnosis in China (Kuo-Tai and Shan-Ming, 1983).

In 1985, Mezzich et al. reported the results of a survey sponsored by the World Psychiatric Association of 175 "expert diagnosticians" in fifty-two countries spanning all continents. Nearly as many of the respondents used DSM-III as used ICD-9, and 46 percent rated DSM-III high on "usefulness," whereas only 29 percent so rated the ICD-9. This preference was found in every region of the world except Africa, and even there only 14 percent rated DSM-III as of low usefulness, compared to 27 percent for the ICD-9.

The above studies imply that the DSM-III illness definitions are utilitarian in many cultures. However, some of the above positive responses may be based not so much on the particular illness definitions per se, but the fact that the definitions provided are highly specified rather than descriptive as most previous taxonomies have been. In an effort to test definitional appropriateness, we conducted a cross-national survey of clinicians and investigators in the countries represented in this volume and others. A questionnaire was devised that included questions about ownership or access to DSM-III, the contexts in which it might be used, and the appropriateness and preferability of the major Axis I illness definitions.

We mailed the questionnaire to psychiatric colleagues in twenty-seven countries. As in the previous international surveys on DSM-III, the sampling design was one of convenience. We sent five copies to each correspondent and asked him to distribute them to practitioners known to be acquainted with DSM-III. A self-addressed envelope was attached to each questionnaire so the completed form could be returned directly to us, although the original recipients were invited to copy and distribute more forms if they wished. So far as we could tell, only our colleague in Taiwan did so. He was especially generous, and we received fifty-two returns for the five that we sent him. We received no response from colleagues in Lebanon, East Germany, and Colombia and do not know whether these requests were ever received. Setting aside the three countries from which we had no response and counting the generous response from Taiwan separately, we received eighty-eight questionnaires from the twenty-three remaining countries (a response rate of 77%). Including the Taiwan data, the tables and figures described below are based on 140 responses from twenty-four countries. (The Taiwan data were analyzed separately, but since rates differed little from overall rates, they were merged.)

This survey confirmed previous impressions of the international popularity of DSM-III, since 93 percent of the respondents owned their own copy of the manual. Although most clinicians were required to use ICD to code their clinical diagnoses, the DSM-III was preferred either as the exclusive nomenclature, or in concert with other diagnostic systems (Table 16–1).

We next asked the respondents to give their preferred diagnostic system for three contexts: clinical work, teaching, and research (Figure 16–1). Thirty-seven percent indicated an exclusive preference for the DSM-III definitions for clinical work, and an additional 60 percent preferred the DSM for some disorders, leaving only 3 percent who preferred some other system for all diagnoses. Exclusive preference for DSM-III rises to 56 percent for teaching and to 69 percent for research work. Exclusive preference for some other taxonomy is 5 percent or less in all three types of usage. Eighty-two percent of the respondents said they "often" refer to the DSM-III definitions.

Perceived Appropriateness of DSM-III Illness Definitions

The possible survey responses regarding the appropriateness of specific DSM-III definitions included two indicating the definition is appropriate in the respondent's cultural context, and two indicating questionable or outright inappropriateness (Figure 16–2). It is clear that most respondents considered the DSM-III definitions to be appropriate in their

Table 16–1 Ownership and Use of DSM-III(R) Cross-Nationally[a]

Question	Positive (%)
Do you own a copy of DSM-III?	93
Do you have access to a copy?	100
Are you required to code diagnoses using a particular nomenclature?	84
Which one?	
ICD	68
DSM-III	32
Other	0
Which is your preferred nomenclature?	
ICD	18
DSM-III	50
Mixture of DSM-III and others	32

[a]N = 140 responses from 24 countries.

Of those required to use ICD exclusively, 65% said they preferred DSM-III for their own clinical work.

Source: Reprinted from Helzer et al., 1989.

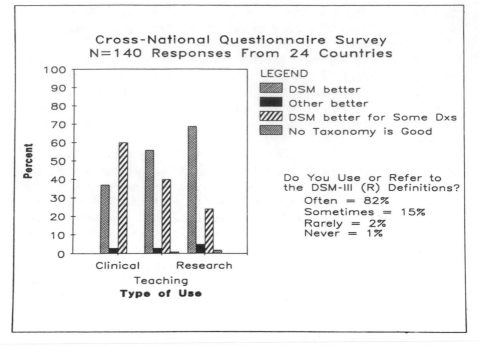

Figure 16–1 Comparison of DSM-III-R and Other Taxonomies for Clinical Work, Teaching, and Research. Cross-national Questionnaire Survey. *N* = 140 responses from 24 countries.

country, whether or not they personally preferred a different definition. The sum of these two "appropriate" categories is 90 percent or above for a majority of the diagnoses and 80 percent or higher for all of them. The "clearly inappropriate" category was less than 1 percent for eight diagnoses, and less than 5 percent for all. The four with the lowest appropriateness ratings were alcohol, drugs, antisocial personality, and somatization disorders. For the first three, socially disapproved behaviors play a major role in diagnosis, and it is not surprising that social disapproval varies by culture. The fourth diagnosis, somatization disorder, was found inappropriate primarily in Germany, Sweden, and Puerto Rico. It was found acceptable in Asia and other Latin American countries.

It should be emphasized that this survey did not consist of a random sample of respondents, and the participants may have been more enthusiastic about DSM-III than other clinicians. However, the main point of this opinion survey was to ascertain whether practicing clinicians interested in diagnostic issues felt that the DSM-III definitions were appropriate in their various countries. On this score the results were overwhelmingly positive and highly consistent from country to country. This plus the other evidence cited above of the popularity of DSM-III would

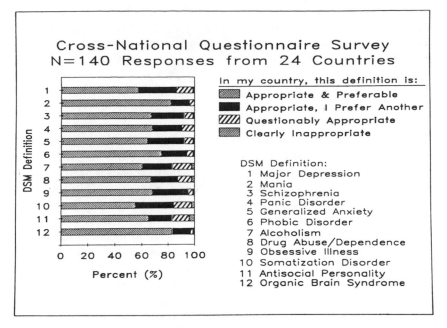

Figure 16–2 Appropriateness of DSM-III-R Diagnostic Definitions. Cross-national Questionnaire Survey. *N* = 140 responses from 24 countries.

seem to leave little doubt that these definitions are utilitarian in a wide range of cultures.

Comparison of Results Across Ten Regions

In this comparative summary of the findings, we will focus mainly on the ten regions in which studies were based on general population samples, but draw comparisons with findings in American Indians (Chapter 8) and the French/North American comparison study (Chapter 11) where appropriate.

Prevalence Findings

The lifetime prevalence rates of alcohol abuse and/or dependence varied considerably among sites represented here. The highest lifetime prevalence rates were found in U.S. native Mexican Americans at 23 percent (Chapter 9), and in the Korean survey, where the total sample rate was about 22 percent (Chapter 14). There is about a fiftyfold difference in lifetime prevalence between these two samples and Shanghai, where the lowest lifetime prevalence of .45 percent was found (Chapter

15). Shanghai was a clear outlier, and if we exclude it, the prevalence range is not as dramatic, but still considerable at over fourfold. The remaining rates clustered around the high teens: Christchurch (Chapter 12)—18.9 percent and Edmonton (Chapter 7)—18.0 percent; Rates in the mid-teens were the ECA (Chapter 6)—13.7 percent; U.S. immigrant Mexican Americans (Chapter 9)–13 percent; Munich (Chapter 10)—12.6 percent; and Puerto Rico (Chapter 9)—12.6 percent; and the three Taiwan sites (Chapter 13) ranged from 5 to about 9 percent.

Since the demographic structure of the populations studied here may differ and since rates of alcoholism vary by sex and age, differences in prevalence between sites could be due to differences in demographic composition. To correct for this possibility, elsewhere (Helzer et al., 1990) we age-standardized by sex to the St. Louis ECA sample the prevalence rates of four of the regions (Edmonton, Puerto Rico, Taiwan, and Korea) reported in this book. The age and sex standardization produced little change in prevalence rates across sites, suggesting that the intersite differences reported were not due to demographic differences in the samples. Since this standardization effort included sites with one of the highest (Korea) and one of the lowest (Taiwan) prevalence rates, it is likely that results would be similar if the standardization were to be repeated with all of the regions reported here.

Some of the high prevalence rates reported here strain credibility, especially rates by sex. Lifetime prevalence among Korean men, for example, is over 42 percent. Even the U.S. rate for men of 24 percent (Helzer et al., 1991) is still dramatic. Is it plausible that one in four U.S. males is alcoholic? It is important to clarify what these rates represent. First, it is important to recognize that the rates reported at all of the sites are lifetime prevalence, so that anyone who ever accrued the requisite number of symptoms would be included regardless of how long ago symptoms might have occurred. For example, the 6-month prevalence rate for alcoholism in Edmonton (Chapter 7) is 5.4 percent, while lifetime prevalence is 18 percent. Second, the DSM-III criteria have a relatively low threshold for alcoholism: a minimum of two alcohol problems for abuse or only one problem, with evidence of tolerance or withdrawal, for dependence. DSM-III also requires no temporal overlap of symptoms. Thus, a single occurrence of one symptom followed by a single occurrence of a second symptom, even years later, could be sufficient for a diagnosis.

Although as Wang et al. (Chapter 15) point out, there has been little systematic research on alcohol use in China; previous reports suggest very low rates of drinking and alcohol-related problems in China, Taiwan, and Hong Kong. Low rates for the former two are certainly borne out here, and a DIS-based survey in Hong Kong confirms a similarly low rate there (Chen et al., 1986). The low rates compared to Western cultures have been attributed to the Confucian moral ethic, which discourages the exhibition of drunken behavior; the fact that alcohol is seen as appropriate for meals and ceremonial occasions, rather than for personal indulgence; and to biological reasons (the flushing phenomenon).

Since these factors are presumably all present in both Taiwan and China, the considerable difference in prevalence rates is of interest. Wang et al. mentions that there have actually been three DIS-based population surveys in China since 1983; the other two resulted in life-time prevalence estimates of 3 and 3.5 percent, figures that are more similar to but still lower than the 5 to 9 percent rates reported in the three Taiwan surveys reported here in Chapter 13. Wang et al. (chapter 15) speculate that relative cultural isolation and the subsistence economic level of much of the population may have kept rates of alcohol use low. There is an interesting consistency between Mexican American immigrants (Chapter 9) and the Shanghai sample (Chapter 15) in that more highly educated heavy drinkers have higher rates of alcoholism than heavy drinkers with low education. Since they also probably have more disposable income, it is tempting to conclude that income may be an important factor in groups close to the subsistence level. However, the numbers are very small and any conclusions must be tentative.

The authors from Taiwan (Chapter 13) and China (Chapter 15) express concern about increasing rates of alcohol consumption and increasing hospitalization rates for alcohol related problems. Both feel this may be related to increasing exposure to Western culture and improved economic conditions. It is interesting to note the increase in alcohol use and problems in the growing Chinese business class, and the parallels Wang et al. draw between this and the privileged literary class in previous centuries. It would be even more interesting to know the relationship of this to flushing. It may be that social acceptance and perhaps demand characteristics of privilege overcome any deterrent value of flushing.

Flushing is known to occur widely in Koreans also, but among the men, at least, it seems to have little impact on alcohol consumption. Park et al. (1984) reported that an alcohol-related flush does occur in Koreans, but that it tends to be a slower onset, less noxious phenomenon as compared to flushing in Taiwanese. This could render flushing ineffective as a deterrent to drinking in Korea.

There is also a much more tolerant attitude toward drinking among men in Korea (Chapter 14). In fact, heavy consumption is encouraged, even demanded, in certain social contexts. As Lee describes, drinking with coworkers at the end of the work day is a common practice, and this frequently evolves to consumption contests lasting until some of the contestants have to be carried home. On the other hand, the culture is less tolerant of solitary drinking. Alcohol is a potentially addicting substance and heavy drinking that is socially condoned carries the risk of progressing to the point that the individual is no longer able to remain within social boundaries. As Skog (1985) has suggested, this social permissiveness toward excessive drinking may explain the high prevalence of alcoholism in the culture. However, the fact that the prevalence of dependence in Korean men is lower than abuse, suggests that social sanctions (especially against solitary drinking) continue to exercise a role even where alcohol consumption is high.

Despite the fact that alcoholism rates were low in China and Taiwan, in both sites it was more prevalent than most of the other psychiatric disorders that were ascertained, that is, its prevalence compared to other disorders was similar to the other sites. This finding is inconsistent with the "substitution hypothesis" of corresponding higher prevalence in some other disorder(s). The substitution hypothesis suggests an underlying consistency in some populational diathesis toward mental illness. There is also little evidence elsewhere to support this concept.

The similar relative prevalence ranking of alcoholism that we have found here extends to other disorders as well. We have reported a mean rank order correlation for lifetime prevalence of psychiatric disorders across eleven cultural regions of .82, and only a slightly lower mean correlation between Asian centers and the ECA in the U.S. of .73 (Helzer & Canino, 1989). This might suggest that Taiwan and China are more psychiatrically healthy, with lower rates of all the psychiatric disorders we asked about. Another possibility, however, is a response effect. These Asian countries may be less psychologically minded or less willing to endorse psychiatric symptomatology to an anonymous interviewer. At least one of the participants in the Shanghai study (Chapter 15) feels the latter is the case (W. T. Liu, personal communication). However, alcoholism is among the most reliable diagnoses, and while there may be a negative response bias in both Taiwan and Shanghai, prevalence differences between the two countries are still striking.

It has long been held that modernization and industrialization also have an impact on alcohol consumption and alcoholism (Chafetz, 1962). It is interesting to note that technological progress has been particularly strong in both South Korea and Taiwan in recent years, and that growth in manufacturing in these two countries has been faster than in the United States (Abelson, 1987). Decades ago Bales (1946) proposed that a combination of sociocultural stress, such as might occur with technological modernization, and cultural attitudes toward drinking could account for cross-national differences in drinking. Such a mechanism could be relevant to the patterns seen here of increases over past drinking levels in both Taiwan and Korea, but a much greater prevalence rate in the latter country. There is also much evidence of sociocultural stress in Edmonton (Chapter 7), the Western site with the highest levels of alcohol dependence among both men and women. Edmonton has the second highest per capita income in Canada, but is a petroleum-based, boom/bust economy. It has the highest female participation in the labor force, but high rates of unemployment, divorce, single parent families, and suicide compared to the rest of Canada.

The Course and Symptomatic Expression of Alcoholism

Despite the dramatic difference in prevalence rates across the studies reported here, there was considerable similarity in the symptoms and course of alcoholism. For most of the sites, the mean age of onset of first symptom was in the early to mid-20s. There is a somewhat later mean onset in four of the sites, Puerto Rico (Chapter 9), Korea (Chapter 14), Shanghai (Chapter 15), and Munich (Chapter 10). The later onset of alcohol symptoms in Shanghai and Korea may be related to the fact that drinking behaviors are socialized at a later age in these countries. In Puerto Rico, there is a great tolerance of the society for intoxication and alcoholic behavior; it may be that symptomatic behavior is not endorsed until it is more severely expressed. In Munich, the later onset may be also related to the greater tolerance of the society for alcohol-related behavior. In any event, even in these countries, the mean age of onset only rises to the late 20s to early 30s. The age of onset is quite consistent in countries where alcoholism was rare compared to where it was common.

The mean number of positive alcohol symptoms among alcoholics ranged from four to six, and like age of onset showed no consistent difference in sites with low prevalence compared to those with high prevalence. For example, the mean number of symptoms among alcoholics in Shanghai (Chapter 15) was four, but it was only 4.3 in Christchurch (Chapter 12), where the prevalence rate of alcoholism was much higher. The only site showing variance from this narrow range is Munich where the mean number of symptoms ranged from about eight in those with alcohol dependence to an even higher 10.5 in those with abuse. However, as the authors point out, many of the original DIS symptom questions for the alcohol section were modified quite considerably. Therefore it is difficult to compare the symptom results in Munich with the other surveys.

The duration of alcoholism among those in remission for a year or more was based on the mean number of years from the first to the most recent symptom. Among the sites reporting this figure, it ranged from 8 to 10 years. This figure is lower in Shanghai, but is based on only one remitted alcoholic! Duration is somewhat lower in the Munich sample also, but again is based on small numbers. Duration tends to be higher for men than women in all sites where this distinction is reported.

The pattern of symptoms is also similar across sites. Heavy daily drinking and drinking a fifth of alcohol in one day were among the four most frequent symptoms in every site. Among those who are alcohol dependent, quantity symptoms are invariably the most frequent. Health consequences due to drinking are infrequent in most Western regions except Munich, but more common in Taiwan, where the proportion of alcoholics reporting damage to health ranks relatively high. In Munich, 75 percent of alcoholics scored positive on this item, well above other sites. Wittchen and Bronisch suggest two possible explanations for this. First, the method of ascertainment of this item by the Munich study was different. In this site, health consequences were not assessed by self reports but by checking health insurance records and clinic data. This could account for the higher rates of health consequences if alcoholics tend to underestimate their alcohol-related physical problems in comparison to actual physical examinations. Second, this was the third wave of a longitudinal study, and the average age of the Munich sample was greater. Therefore the overall risk of physical illness was higher.

Job troubles due to drinking were among the least frequently endorsed symptoms in most sites. An exception to this was again Munich, where job troubles and job loss were much more frequently endorsed. Wittchen and Bronisch attribute this to particular societal influences, like the beer festival, which may promote absenteeism from jobs.

In order to empirically assess the degree to which alcoholic symptoms varied across sites, we rank ordered symptoms according to frequency of occurrence in alcoholics at each site and then did rank order correlations between sites (Table 16–2). Despite the obvious differences in cultural context between the regions described, the expression of alcoholism in terms of relative frequency of alcohol symptoms among alcoholics is similar between sites. Unfortunately the Munich site could not be included, since many of the symptoms ascertained at the other sites were not included in the Munich survey.

Generally correlations are higher between sites within the same region of the world. Correlations between various cultural groups in North America are nearly all .80 or better and many exceed .90. Similarly, correlations between the various Asian sites are nearly all above .80, and while those between the three sites in Taiwan (Chapter 13) are higher than those between Taiwan and Korea (Chapter 14), the latter correlations don't fall by very much. The exception to this finding are the correlations between Shanghai (Chapter 15) and the other Asian sites, which however are still fairly substantial at the .60 to .70 range. New Zealand is geographically distant from the West, but Christchurch (Chapter 12) is a highly Westernized city and the pattern of symptom correlations looks very similar to that seen for the North American sites.

What perhaps is even more remarkable, however, is the similarity of symptom frequency rankings across highly diverse cultural regions. For example, except for Shanghai, the correlations between Puerto Rico and the Asian sites are all above .70 and most approach .80. Even the Shanghai correlation is substantial at .61. Correlations between the ECA data in the United States (Chapter 6) and the sites in Korea and Taiwan are all

Table 16–2 DIS Symptoms of Alcohol Abuse and/or Dependence Across Thirteen Sites (Spearman Rank Order Correlations)

	Site 1	Site 2	Site 3	Site 4	Site 5	Site 6	Site 7	Site 8	Site 9	Site 10	Site 11	Site 12	Site 13
United States (Site 1)	1.0	.84	.89	.96	.85	.95	.38[a]	.96	.63	.59	.73	.54	.63
Puerto Rico (Site 2)		1.0	.80	.85	.69	.86	.61	.82	.73	.79	.84	.78	.77
Mex American Immigrants (Site 3)			1.0	.94	.83	.86	.36[a]	.88	.57[a]	.55[a]	.77	.59	.69
Native Mexican Americans (Site 4)				1.0	.87	.91	.38[a]	.92	.66	.61	.79	.62	.73
American Indians (Site 5)					1.0	.80	.16[a]	.86	.56[a]	.48[a]	.70	.50[a]	.59
Christchurch (Site 6)						1.0	.33[a]	.96	.64	.59	.70	.56	.59
Shanghai (Site 7)							1.0	.29[a]	.58	.70	.65	.74	.69
Edmonton (Site 8)								1.0	.58[a]	.54[a]	.70	.49[a]	.56
Seoul (Site 9)									1.0	.94	.82	.83	.79
Rural Korea (Site 10)										1.0	.85	.85	.80
Taipei City (Site 11)											1.0	.92	.95
Taiwan Townships (Site 12)												1.0	.96
Taiwan Villages (Site 13)													1.0

[a]Denotes those correlations that are not significant at the .01 level or better.

above .54 and most are in the .6 to .7 range. The correlation between Puerto Rico and Taipei City is higher than that between Seoul and Taipei City. Except for Shanghai, virtually all of these correlations are statistically significant and most at the .01 level or better. As noted, the Shanghai data are difficult to interpret because of the small number of alcoholics, but even here the similarities in symptom ranking with other Asian sites are quite high, with the correlations ranging from .58 to .74, all but one being above .65, and all being significant at the .01 level or better.

Thus, in terms of the symptoms specified in the DSM-III definition of alcohol abuse and dependence, there is great similarity in the relative frequency of symptoms between alcoholics in such diverse cultural regions as Canada, Puerto Rico, Korea, and Taiwan. This finding suggests two things. First, it tends to validate the appropriateness of the types of symptoms used in the DSM-III definition as being cross-culturally appropriate. Not only do the specified symptoms occur in alcoholics in various parts of the world, but they occur in frequency patterns that are highly similar. Second, it suggests that alcoholism is a disorder with considerable consistency, whether it occurs in the highly industrialized major cities of the United States and Canada or the agrarian economies of rural Korea and rural Taiwan. Despite major differences in the prevalence of alcoholism and in the relative frequency of abuse versus dependence, the symptomatic picture among those who pass the minimum threshold of alcohol involvement is highly similar.

Risk Factors and Correlates of Alcoholism

SEX: Not only is there similarity in the symptomatic expression of alcoholism between different cultural regions, but the risk factors and correlates also follow a similar pattern. Sex is a major risk factor for alcoholism in every culture; rates for alcohol abuse and/or dependence in men are substantially above those for women in all ten cultural regions. Second, rates for men are strikingly high, up to nearly one-third of the male population in Edmonton and over 40 percent in Korea.

In all the cultures studied, excessive drinking and alcoholism were predominantly male activities, but the male/female ratio for alcoholism varies considerably across cultures. It is particularly high in the Asian and Hispanic cultures (where alcoholism is considerably more common in men) compared to Western and Anglo Saxon cultures. In the five U.S. communities (Chapter 6), Munich, Edmonton, Christchurch, and among the American Indians (Chapter 8), alcoholism is from 4 to 6 times greater in men than in women. In Seoul, Puerto Rico and among the U.S. Mexican American immigrants, alcoholism is between 12 to 25 times greater in men. Possible explanations for this include differential

genetic risk, lower tolerance for alcohol among women, and gre[
social stigma attached to their drinking. The fact that this ratio is abo[
in Mexican Americans native to the United States, and about 25 in
Mexican American immigrants to the United States (Chapter 9) suggests
an important societal effect.

In Figure 16–3 we have disaggregated sex as a risk factor for heavy
drinking and for alcoholism among heavy drinkers in order to explore
possible reasons for these sex differences in a different way. This information is not available for the French sample and was not provided for
the three Asian countries, presumably because heavy drinking in women
was so rare that the results were not considered meaningful. For example, in Shanghai there were only three women who reported drinking
consistently, and only one of these met criteria for alcoholism. Therefore
the results for rates by sex are not useful.

The seven groups for which we have usable, relevant data on heavy
drinking and alcoholism are presented in Figure 16–3. There is considerable variation in the male/female ratio for heavy drinking, ranging
from a low of 1.7 among American Indians to 6.3 in Puerto Rico. This
range of sex ratios would be even greater if the Asian data were included. The ratio is greatest in Puerto Rico where excessive drinking by
women is strongly disapproved. Once the exposure variable is equalized
by considering only those who drink heavily, alcoholism rates by sex are
more similar and more cross-culturally consistent, as evidenced by the

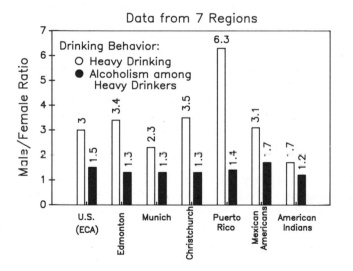

Figure 16–3 Sex Ratios for Heavy Drinkers and Alcoholism Among Heavy
Drinkers. Data from 7 regions.

lower and more constant sex ratios. The sex ratio in Puerto Rico, for example, is in the same range as other sites. We interpret this set of findings to mean that cross-cultural differences in social disapproval of drinking by women has a major impact on alcoholism rates. Once the social stigma regarding heavy drinking has been overcome, alcoholism rates are higher and more similar cross-culturally. However, even among heavy drinkers the sex ratio for alcoholism in all cultures is still greater than 1. This would suggest that biological or social factors continue to have some impact even among those women who drink heavily, and that the impact is consistent across cultures with quite different attitudes toward drinking by females.

AGE: The lifetime prevalence of alcoholism by age show interesting differences between regions. In the United States, Christchurch, Taipei, Edmonton, Shanghai, and among American Indians and Mexican Americans, the lifetime prevalence of alcoholism is higher in the younger cohorts and decreases after age 45. In contrast, in Puerto Rico, Seoul, rural Korea, and Munich, the lifetime prevalence increases with age. Population data in these latter sites were only collected up through the age of 64, but the fall in lifetime prevalence does not appear in the 45–65-year-old cohort as it does in the other sites.

Lifetime prevalence is cumulative over the entire age of risk, and since some risk of alcoholism continues into old age, the fall in lifetime prevalence with age seen in most of the sites seems counterintuitive, prevalence by age group should continue to rise. There are several possible explanations for the fall in prevalence with age.

One logical explanation is that this is the result of a differentially high mortality rate among older alcoholics. Since severe alcoholism leads to early death, this is likely to be part of the explanation. But, there is evidence from the present comparison that differential mortality is not the entire explanation. As we have seen, alcohol-related health problems are more common among alcoholics in Taipei relative to the other sites, but the proportional fall in prevalence in older ages is about the same in Taipei compared to Edmonton and actually lower than in the United States.

Diminished recall of early drinking problems by older respondents or decreased willingness to admit such difficulty could also explain the lower lifetime prevalence in older respondents. However, if this is the reason, it is difficult to explain why it occurs at some sites and not others. Admission of alcohol problems would seem to be just as sensitive an issue in Puerto Rico as in the United States, for example, perhaps more so. Similar findings regarding the lifetime prevalence of major depression by age are reported by Klerman and Weissman (1989) for seven different regions, including Seoul, Puerto Rico, United States, Edmonton, and

Mexican Americans. The replications of findings for another psychiatric disorder in some of the same regions and the inconsistencies among sites makes it unlikely that differential failure of older persons to report drinking problems is the sole explanation of the lower lifetime prevalence.

Another possible contributing factor to this pattern is a cohort effect, that is, that alcoholism is becoming more prevalent in younger age groups than it was among their elders. This seems likely to be an operative factor and one that most of the authors have identified as occurring in their own countries. This interpretation is consistent with the rising per capita consumption of alcohol that has been observed in many countries and that began in the United States in the 1950s. It is understandable how a liberalization of attitudes toward alcohol consumption would differentially affect the young. The drinking habits of young persons are not yet established, and the attitudes of the society are likely to have a profound influence on the evolution of personal habits.

How then might we explain the lack of a cohort effect in some sites such as Munich and Korea? One possible explanation is a more long-standing liberal attitude toward drinking such that older members of the society have also been exposed to heavy drinking from an early age and thus have higher cumulative rates of alcoholism.

Another explanation is offered by Wang et al. for Shanghai (Chapter 15). They suggest that the lack of disposable income has been a deterrent to drinking and has helped to keep the prevalence of alcoholism low among the young. However, older people are beginning to enjoy a bit of disposable income now that the Chinese economy is improving. This enables them to buy alcohol, whereas before drinking was out of their income range. The extent to which such an economic factor might apply to more affluent cultures is unclear.

OTHER PSYCHIATRIC DISORDERS: The DIS interview ascertains diagnostic information on the major Axis I DSM-III diagnoses, and several of the chapters in this volume offer an opportunity to examine the prevalence of other psychiatric disorders. Prevalence information for other illnesses is available for five of the participating centers: the ECA (Chapter 6), Edmonton (Chapter 7), Puerto Rico and Mexican Americans in the United States (Chapter 9), Christchurch, New Zealand (Chapter 12), and Shanghai (Chapter 15). In addition, Munich (Chapter 10) and Korea (Chapter 14) data sets provide separate prevalence rate data for those with and without alcoholism.

Major depression is a diagnosis of general interest. The lifetime prevalence rate in the ECA sample as reported here is 6.4 percent. The rate is somewhat higher in the Edmonton sample (8.6%) and lower in Puerto Rico (4.6%). Depression is higher in the Christchurch sample at 12.5

percent. The rate is so exceedingly low in the Shanghai sample (.19%) that it again raises the question whether an anonymous personal interview method is appropriate in mainland China.

Surprisingly, the lifetime rate of major depression is lower in Mexican American immigrants to the United States (3.1%) than in Mexican American natives (6.5%) (Chapter 9). However, this preponderance in native Mexican Americans is seen with nearly every other diagnosis as well, except cognitive impairment, which is over three times higher in Mexican American immigrants. This latter is not surprising given the likely educational bias of the Mini-mental Status examination and the probable educational disadvantage of immigrants.

At all the sites for which we have diagnostic specific prevalence data, alcoholism is the most frequent or nearly the most frequent diagnosis. Even in Shanghai where the absolute rate is very low, alcoholism is second in prevalence only to phobic disorder. At each of the sites, alcoholism and phobic disorders have a high prevalence, the affective, anxiety, and antisocial personality disorders are intermediate, and schizophrenia, mania, somatization, and anorexia all have quite low prevalences. As noted above, a previous analysis (Helzer & Canino, 1989) has shown a substantial correlation in the ranking of disorders by prevalence across various cultures. Disorders that are prevalent in one culture tend to be similarly prevalent in the others.

Another question of interest regarding diagnosis is the relationship between alcoholism and other psychiatric disorders. Most of the chapters in this book provide information on the risk ratios for other diagnoses among alcoholics. The risk ratio is a measure of the likelihood that other diagnoses will be seen at a higher rate among alcoholics compared to nonalcoholics. This is a measure of association without implying any causal direction. A risk ratio greater than one indicates that a particular disorder was more prevalent among alcoholics than among nonalcoholics.

Depression is well known to be associated with alcoholism among patients in treatment settings. In examining the findings from the various sites reported here, major depression has a relative risk that is typically around 2—depression is about twice as likely to be diagnosed in alcoholics as in nonalcoholics. Dysthymic disorder shows a relative risk that is near or greater than unity in most of the samples but not strikingly high for any of them. Thus the relative risks for affective illnesses in alcoholism are generally elevated, but not dramatically so.

The modest relative risk for depressive illness among alcoholics is consistent with recent work suggesting that depression and alcoholism are independent disorders (Shuckit, 1986). Depressive disorder does not appear to be strongly associated with alcoholism in any of the sites studied here. The impression, based on persons coming to treatment, that alcoholism and depression are more consistently associated may be a result of the fact that while most alcoholics don't seek medical treatment, those that do so are more likely to also be having trouble with depression, the latter being a motivator to seek help.

The diagnoses that show the highest risk ratios (are most strongly associated with a diagnosis of alcoholism) are drug abuse and dependence and antisocial personality disorder. Many of the sites also show a strong association between alcoholism and mania. The latter diagnosis is rare, but the elevated risk ratio is reasonably consistent across the various sites. There is also some correlation between the relative risk rates for antisocial personality disorder and the population prevalence rate of alcoholism—in those cultures where alcoholism is prevalent, such as Korea, alcoholism is five to six times more common among those with antisocial personality disorder. Where the rate of alcoholism is low, such as in Metropolitan Taipei, alcoholism is 240 times more common in those with antisocial personality disorder. This does not imply that antisocial personality is common in Taipei; in fact, the lifetime population prevalence is quite low at under 0.1 percent (Helzer et al., 1990). But what antisocial personality disorder does exist is strongly associated with alcoholism. In a previous analysis (Helzer et al. 1990), we found that the likelihood of an association between alcoholism and the occurrence of any of the other psychiatric disorders ascertained in the DIS tended to be higher if the population prevalence of alcoholism was rare compared to countries where alcoholism was more common. This suggests that where social sanctions against alcoholism are strong, the occurrence of other diagnoses plays a greater role in the development of alcoholism.

Concluding Remarks

We feel the present volume is an important step in the direction of greater consistency and interpretability of cross-national psychiatric data, but only a step. For one thing, the DIS is an interview that was developed in one culture and adapted to others. This is not necessarily inappropriate and in fact may be a practical necessity (Sen and Mari, 1986). However, a more recent effort, the Composite International Diagnostic Interview (CIDI), which is in part sparked by the DIS and its widespread international use, has had cross-national input from its earliest developmental stages.

Another issue in the present volume is the coordination of data analyses. As we noted, this was largely done by each of the sites replicating on their own data a set of analyses originally conducted on the U.S. (ECA) data set. This has several drawbacks, perhaps the most serious of which is the relative lack of opportunity for a broad group of scientists to have ongoing input into the analyses. Some input was possible through joint discussions prior to embarking on the analyses, but the result would have been much richer if a broad spectrum of investigators could have had access to a cross-national data bank.

A further advantage of a data bank is that exact replications of data analyses are difficult to achieve. Minor differences in analysis due to the inability of any single investigator to control all aspects of the analysis lead to differences in results that are methodological rather than substantive. Furthermore, the replication difficulty is compounded as the sophistication of the analyses increases, that is, multivariate analyses, path analytic approaches, and so on. A single data bank that is available to multiple contributors is a much more powerful data tool. Recently we have been working to develop such a resource and have created a multinational bank consisting of the five ECA study sites (Chapter 6) and the three Taiwan sites (Chapter 13) and have begun to use it for cross-national comparisons (Compton et al., 1991). Cross-national efforts that are designed from the outset with the idea of a data bank in mind would greatly reduce the problems inherent in merging intersite data.

Another limitation of the present effort is the relative lack of systematic information about social variables that may be relevant to the development and/or maintenance of alcoholism. All of the sites collected information regarding social variables, but this was not done in a uniform way across sites, since there is relatively little in the way of social variables in the DIS other than those used for diagnosis. Because of the lack of uniformity, it is difficult to incorporate data on social variables into cross-site analyses.

Finally, the chapters in this book are based on prevalence, not incidence data. The latter is preferable for epidemiologic investigation, since prevalence is a function of both the occurrence of illness and its duration as expressed in the formula: Prevalence = Incidence × Duration. Thus correlates of illness identified in a prevalence study may relate to the duration of illness and not necessarily to the onset or etiology of the illness per se. Since the primary goal of epidemiologic research is to discover clues to etiology through examining correlates of illness, clues based on prevalence data may not be relevant to this primary goal. The study and quantification of incidence in psychiatric disorder is still in its infancy, and progress in this still needs to be made before we would be in a position to examine incidence of illness cross-nationally.

These caveats aside, it is gratifying to see how influential the ECA survey has been in sparking widespread international interest in large-scale diagnostic specific epidemiologic surveys. This holds promise for the development of greater cross-cultural consistency in the approach to psychiatric diagnosis generally as well as for cross-national psychiatric epidemiology. It is clear that this is beginning to occur. For example, the International Classification of Disease in its newest iteration (ICD-10) will include highly specific, "operational" illness definitions as in DSM-III and DSM-III-R. Furthermore, the newest iteration of the DSM system, DSM-IV, is developing collaterally with ICD-10 and there is an attempt between the groups constructing these two sets of criteria to keep the definitions as consistent as possible.

Furthermore, as the diagnostic definitions are developed, there is a simultaneous effort to develop a highly structured diagnostic interview, the Composite International Diagnostic Interview (CIDI) mentioned earlier. This interview is patterned after the Diagnostic Interview Schedule (DIS) used in the series of studies reported here. This codevelopment of criteria and interviews strengthens both, since proposed criteria are constantly being tested against the practical reality of having to phrase symptom questions in a way that respondents can understand them. Invariably it is found that while certain criteria seem conceptually sound in the abstract, conceptual vagueness becomes apparent when authors deal with the issue of asking the questions necessary to ascertain the occurrence of a specific event or symptom (Robins, 1989).

These developments are very hopeful for cross-natonal psychiatric research and for psychiatric nosology in general. Without a common nomenclature, science lacks a foundation, a language for communication (Kendell, 1975). Only in the last decade or so has the field of psychiatry begun to universally accept this proposition. The attitude toward classification that was most prevalent in the United States in the 1950s and 1960s and in much of the rest of the world was that psychiatric states were unique from one individual to the next, influenced by the particular personality and the experiences of that individual. Thus, while illness might be ranked on some severity continuum, categorical classification was inappropriate. Another predominant idea was that psychiatric states were culturally indigenous, and that the mores, beliefs, and characteristics of each culture determined the development and expression of illness in ways that were unique from other cultures. Thus, while it might be possible to define a set of disorders for one culture, any attempt to develop a universal set of definitions would be misguided.

The publication of a set of specific criteria for sixteen psychiatric disorders by a group of investigators in St. Louis, the so-called "Feighner" criteria (Feighner et al., 1972), found rapid acceptance, and indeed this became the most cited article in the psychiatric literature for many years. The almost immediate and worldwide acceptance of DSM-III after its publication in 1980 demonstrated that a consistent nomenclature was an idea whose time had come, not only in the United States, where DSM-III was developed, but in other parts of the world as well. This sequence of developments challenged both the above propositions about categorical diagnoses and their universality. In only a few years the field of psychiatry has moved from widespread scepticism of the appropriateness of carefully defined illness states to almost universal acceptance. The evidence from previous studies we've reviewed here and the findings from the various sties participating in this project give further evidence of the appropriateness of a universal taxonomy, not only for alcoholism but for the other major psychiatric disorders as well. International participation in the development of the DSM-IV, the ICD-10, and the CIDI will greatly enhance progress toward a universal diagnostic language for the science of psychiatry.

References

Abelson, P. H. (1987). United States trade. *Science* 235–829.

Bales, R. F. (1946). Cultural differences in rates of alcoholism. *A. J. Stud. Alcohol.* 6:480–99.

Chafetz, M. E., and Demone, H. W. (1962). *Alcoholism and Society.* New York: Oxford University Press.

Chen, C. N.; Wong, J.; Lee, N.; and Lai, P. (1986). An On-Going Study of Alcoholism in Hong Kong. Paper presented at Symposium 109 on Alcoholism with the DIS: America, Europe, and Asia. Washington, D.C.: 139 Annual Meeting of the American Psychiatric Association.

Compton, W. M.; Helzer, J. E.; Hwu, H-G.; Yeh, E-K.; Spitznagel, E. L.; McEvoy, L.; and Tipp, J. E. (1991). New Methods in Cross-Cultural Psychiatry: Psychiatric Illness in Taiwan and the United States. *Am. J. Psychiatry* 148, 12 (December): 1697–1704.

Feighner, J. P.; Robins, E.; Guze, S. B.; Woodruff, R. A.; Winokur, G.; and Munoz, R. (1972). Diagnostic Criteria for Use in Psychiatric Research. *Arch. Gen. Psychiat.* 26:57–63.

Helzer, J. E., Burnam, A., and McEvoy, L. T. (1991). Alcohol abuse and dependence. In L. N. Robins and D. A. Regier (eds.), *Psychiatric Disorders in America.* New York: Free Press.

Helzer, J. E., and Canino, G. J. (1989). The implications of cross-national research for diagnostic validity. In L. N. Robins and J. E. Barrett (eds.), *The Validity of Psychiatric Diagnosis.* New York: Raven Press.

Helzer, J. E.; Canino, G. J.; Yeh, E. K.; Bland, R. C.; Lee, C. K.; Hwu, H. G.; and Newman, S. (1990). Alcoholism-North American and Asia. *Arch. Gen. Psychiatry* 47: 313–19.

Kendell, R. E. (1975). *The Role of Diagnosis in Psychiatry.* Oxford, London, Edinburgh, Melbourne: Blackwell Scientific Publications.

Klerman, G. L., and Weissman, M. M. (1989). Increasing rates of depression. *J. Am. Med. Assoc.* 261:2229–35.

Kuo-Tai, T., and Shan-Ming, Y. (1983). The impact of DSM-III on Chinese psychiatry. In R. L. Spitzer, J. B. W. Williams, and S. E. Skodol (eds.), *International Perspectives on DSM-III.* Washington, D.C.: American Psychiatric Press.

Mezzich, J. E.; Fabrega, H.; Mezzich, A. C.; and Coffman, G. A. (1985). International experience with DSM-III. *J. Nerv Ment Dis.* 173:738–41.

Park, J. Y.; Huang, Y-H.; Nagoshi, C. T.; Yuen, S.; Johnson, R. C.; Ching, C. A.; and Bowman, K. S. (1984). The flushing response to alcohol use among Koreans and Taiwanese. *J. Stud. Alcohol.* 45:481–85.

Robins, L. N. (1989). Diagnostic grammar and assessment: Translating criteria into questions. In L. N. Robins and J. E. Barrett (eds.), *The validity of Psychiatric Diagnosis.* New York: Raven Press, Ltd, pp. 263–78.

Schuckit, M. A. (1986). Genetic and clinical implications of alcoholism and affective disorder. *Am. J. Psychiatry* 143:140–47.

Sen, B., and Mari, J. D. J. (1986). Psychiatric research instruments in the transcultural setting: Experiences in India and Brazil, *Soc. Sci. Med.* 23:277–81.

Skog, O-J. (1985). The collectivity of drinking cultures: A theory of the distribution of alcohol consumption. *Br. J. Addict.* 80:83–99.

Spitzer, R. L.; Williams, J. B. W.; and Skodol, A. E. (eds.) (1983). *International Perspectives on DSM-III.* Washington, D.C.: American Psychiatric Press.

Appendix 1

Alcohol Section of the Diagnostic Interview
Schedule (DIS-III)

```
                    CODE
  1 = no          4 = med. exp.
  2 = below crit.  5 = yes
  3 = drugs or alc.
```

149. Now I am going to ask you some questions about using alcohol. **How** old were you the **first** time you ever drank enough to get drunk? (NEVER = 00; BABY, INFANT = 02)

    ENTER AGE: ☐☐ ⓪ ① ② ③ ④ ⑤ ⑥ ⑦ ⑧ ⑨
                    ⓪ ① ② ③ ④ ⑤ ⑥ ⑦ ⑧ ⑨   11/

    ┌───┐
    │ **INTERVIEWER:** IF 15 OR OLDER, SKIP TO Q. 150 │
    │ IF LESS THAN 15, ASK B.   │
    │ IF "DK," ASK A.   │
    └───┘

    A. Do you think it was before or after you were 15?

       Before 15 (RECORD 01 ABOVE & ASK B)
       15 or older (RECORD 95 ABOVE & SKIP TO Q. 150)
       Still DK   (RECORD 98 ABOVE & SKIP TO Q. 150)   13/

    B. Did you get drunk more than once before you were 15?

       No ....①
       Yes ....⑤   14/

150. Has your family ever **objected** because you were drinking too much?

    No ....①
    Yes, but volunteers they object to
      moderate drinking by **anyone** ....②
    Yes ─────────────────────────────→ ⑤ *   15/

    ┌───┐
    │ IF R **VOLUNTEERS** HE HAS **NEVER** HAD A DRINK, SKIP TO Q. 172 │
    └───┘

151. Did you ever think that you were an **excessive** drinker?

    No ....①
    Yes ─────────────────────────────→ ⑤ *   16/

152. Have you ever drunk as much as a fifth of liquor in one day, that would be about 20 drinks, or 3 bottles of wine or as much as 3 six-packs of beer in one day? IF VOLUNTEERS ONLY ONCE: CODE 2.

    No .... ①
    Only once .... ②
    Yes .... ⑤   17/

309

153. Has there ever been a period of two weeks when every day you were drinking 7 or more beers, 7 or more drinks or 7 or more glasses of wine?

No ....(SKIP TO Q. 154)............. ①
Yes ....(ASK A) .... ⑤   18/

A. How long has it been since you drank that much or do you still?

CODE MOST RECENT TIME POSSIBLE

Still or within last 2 weeks ....(SKIP TO Q. 155) ...... ①
Within last month ....(SKIP TO Q. 154A)..... ②
Within last 6 months ....(SKIP TO Q. 154A)..... ③
Within last year ....(SKIP TO Q. 154A)..... ④
More than 1 year ago ....(SKIP TO Q. 154A)..... ⑤   19/

154. Has there ever been a couple of months or more when at least one evening a week, you drank 7 drinks, or 7 bottles of beer or 7 glasses of wine?

No ......(SKIP TO Q. 155) ....①
Yes ....(ASK A) ....⑤   20/

A. How long has it been since you drank 7 or more drinks at least once a week, or do you still?

CODE MOST RECENT TIME POSSIBLE

Still or within last 2 weeks ....①
Within last month ....②
Within last 6 months ....③
Within last year ....④
More than 1 year ago ....(ASK B)....⑤   21/

B. **IF MORE THAN 1 YEAR AGO:** How old were you then?

ENTER AGE: ⬚⬚   ⓪ ① ② ③ ④ ⑤ ⑥ ⑦ ⑧ ⑨
⓪ ① ② ③ ④ ⑤ ⑥ ⑦ ⑧ ⑨
22/

155. Have you ever told a doctor about a problem you had with drinking?

No ....①
Yes ....⑤   24/

156. Have friends, your doctor, your clergyman, or any other **professional** ever said you were **drinking too much** for your own good?

No, or only to lose weight ....①
Yes ——————————————→ ⑤ *   25/

157. Have you ever wanted to stop drinking but couldn't?

No ....①
Yes ——————————————→ ⑤ *   26/

158. Some people promise themselves not to drink before 5 o'clock or never to drink alone, in order to **control** their drinking. Have you ever done anything like that?

No ....①
Yes ——————————————→ ⑤*   27/

159. Did you ever need a drink just after you had gotten up (that is, before breakfast)?

No ....①
Yes ——————————————→ ⑤ *   28/

160. Have you ever had job (or school) **troubles** because of drinking—like missing too much work or drinking on the job (or at school)?

No .... ①
Yes ——————————————→ ⑤ *   29/

161. Did you ever lose a job (or get kicked out of school) on account of drinking?

No .... ①
Yes ⎯⎯⎯⎯⎯⎯⎯⎯⎯⎯⎯⎯⎯⎯⎯▶⑤ *   30/

162. Have you ever gotten into **trouble driving** because of drinking—like having an accident or being arrested for drunk driving?

No .... ①
Yes ⎯⎯⎯⎯⎯⎯⎯⎯⎯⎯⎯⎯⎯⎯⎯▶⑤ *   31/

163. Have you ever been **arrested** or held at the police station because of drinking or for disturbing the peace while drinking?

No .... ①
Yes ⎯⎯⎯⎯⎯⎯⎯⎯⎯⎯⎯⎯⎯⎯⎯▶⑤ *   32/

164. Have you ever gotten into physical **fights** while drinking?

No .... ①
Yes ⎯⎯⎯⎯⎯⎯⎯⎯⎯⎯⎯⎯⎯⎯⎯▶⑤ *   33/

```
┌──────────────────────────────────────────────────────────────┐
│ INTERVIEWER: HAVE ANY 5*'s BEEN CODED IN Qs. 150-164?        │
│   [Y]        NO .............(SKIP TO Q. 172) ........ ①      │
│              YES ............. (ANSWER A).......... ③         │
│   A. HAS ONLY ONE 5* BEEN CODED?                             │
│  [Y₁]        ONLY ONE 5* .........(ANSWER B)............ ①    │
│              MORE THAN ONE 5* ...(GO TO Q. 165)........ ⑤     │
│                                                              │
│   B. HAVE EITHER Q. 153 OR 154 BEEN CODED "5"?              │
│              NO ............(SKIP TO Q. 172)......... ①       │
│  [Y₂]        YES ........... (GO TO Q. 165) ........ ⑤        │
└──────────────────────────────────────────────────────────────┘
```

165. Have you ever gone on binges or benders, where you kept drinking for a couple of days or more without sobering up?

No ....(SKIP TO Q. 166)................ ①
Yes ...(ASK A AND B)................. ⑤   37/

A. Did you neglect some of your usual responsibilities then?

No ....①
Yes ⎯⎯⎯⎯⎯⎯⎯⎯⎯⎯⎯⎯⎯⎯⎯▶⑤*   38/

B. How many times have you gone on benders that lasted at least a couple of days?

BENDERS: ☐ ☐ ⓪ ① ② ③ ④ ⑤ ⑥ ⑦ ⑧ ⑨
             ⓪ ① ② ③ ④ ⑤ ⑥ ⑦ ⑧ ⓪   39/

```
┌──────────────────────────────────────────────────────────────┐
│ INTERVIEWER:  IF R SAYS 96 OR MORE, CODE 96 AND GO TO Q. 166.│
│               IF R SAYS "DK": ASK C                          │
└──────────────────────────────────────────────────────────────┘
```

C. Was it just once or more often than that?

Just once ....(RECORD 01 ABOVE)
More than once ..(RECORD 95 ABOVE)
Still DK ....(RECORD 98 ABOVE)   41/

166. Have you ever had **blackouts** while drinking, that is, where you drank enough so that you couldn't remember the next day what you had said or done?

No ....①
Yes ⎯⎯⎯⎯⎯⎯⎯⎯⎯⎯⎯⎯⎯⎯⎯▶⑤*   42/

167. Have you ever had **"the shakes"** after stopping or cutting down on drinking (for example, your hands shake so that your coffee cup rattles in the saucer or you have trouble lighting a cigarette)?

No ....(ASK A)....................①

Yes _____(GO TO Q. 168)_____⑤*   43/

A. Have you ever had **fits or seizures** after stopping or cutting down on drinking?

No .... (ASK B) .... ①

Yes _____(GO TO Q. 168)_____⑤*   44/

B. Have you ever had the **DT's** (hallucinations and fever) when you quit drinking?

No .... (ASK C) .... ①

Yes _____(GO TO Q. 168)_____⑤*   45/

C. Have you ever **seen or heard things** that weren't really there after cutting down on drinking?

No .... ①

Yes _____⑤*   46/

168. There are several health problems that can result from long stretches of pretty heavy drinking. Did drinking ever cause you to have:

A. liver disease or yellow jaundice?

No ....(ASK B)....................① 47/

Yes _____(GO TO Q. 169)_____⑤*

B. vomiting blood or other stomach troubles?

No ....(ASK C)....................① 48/

Yes _____(GO TO Q. 169)_____⑤*

C. trouble with tingling or numbness in your feet?

No ....(ASK D)....................① 49/

Yes _____(GO TO Q. 169)_____⑤*

D. memory trouble when you **haven't** been drinking (**not** blackouts)?

No ....(ASK E)....................① 50/

Yes _____(GO TO Q. 169)_____⑤*

E. inflamation of your pancreas or pancreatitis?

No .... ① 51/

Yes _____⑤*

169. Have you ever continued to drink when you knew you had a serious physical illness that might be made worse by drinking?

No ....①   52/

Yes ....⑤

170. Has there ever been a period in your life when you could not do your ordinary daily work well unless you had had something to drink?

No ....①   53/

Yes ....⑤

171. I'm going to mention some things you told me about drinking. I'll be asking how old you were the first time any one of these things happened. You mentioned (LIST ALL CODED 5* ITEMS IN Qs. 150-168). What's the **earliest** age **any** of these things happened?

ENTER AGE: ⬚⬚   ⓪ ① ② ③ ④ ⑤ ⑥ ⑦ ⑧ ⑨   54/
            ⓪ ① ② ③ ④ ⑤ ⑥ ⑦ ⑧ ⑨

A. When was the last time any of these (STARRED) things happened?

CODE MOST RECENT TIME POSSIBLE	Within last 2 weeks ....① 56/ Within last month ....② Within last six months ....③ Within last year ....④ Within 3 years ....⑤ More than 3 years ago ....(ASK B)....⑥

B. **IF MORE THAN 3 YEARS AGO:** How old were you the last time?

ENTER AGE: ⬚⬚   ⓪ ① ② ③ ④ ⑤ ⑥ ⑦ ⑧ ⑨   57/
            ⓪ ① ② ③ ④ ⑤ ⑥ ⑦ ⑧ ⑨

Appendix 2

Computer Scoring for Alcohol Section of DIS-III

DSMIII DIAGNOSTIC PROGRAMS FOR THE NIMH DIAGNOSTIC
INTERVIEW SCHEDULE VERSION III

****

DSMIII ALCOHOL ABUSE AND DEPENDENCE—DSMALC

THE FOLLOWING VARIABLES ARE CONSTRUCTED TO MAKE THE
DIAGNOSIS AND PROVIDE OTHER INFORMATION:

DSMALCA THE DSMIII A CRITERIA FOR ALCOHOL ABUSE: PATTERN
OF PATHOLOGICAL USE. MISSING IS DRINKING NON-
BEVERAGE ALCOHOL.

DSMALCB THE DSMIII B CRITERIA FOR ALCOHOL ABUSE:
IMPAIRMENT IN SOCIAL OR OCCUPATIONAL
FUNCTIONING.

DSMALCD THE DSMIII B CRITERIA FOR ALCOHOL DEPENDENCE:
TOLERANCE OR WITHDRAWAL.

DSMALC THE DSMIII DIAGNOSIS OF ALCOHOL ABUSE AND
ALCOHOL DEPENDENCE:
 FOR ALCOHOL DEPENDENCE, DSMALCD MUST BE
POSITIVE ALONG WITH DSMALCA OR DSMALCB. FOR
ALCOHOL ABUSE, DSMALCB AND DSMALCA ARE BOTH
POSITIVE.
 A CODE OF 2 INDICATES ABUSE WITHOUT
DEPENDENCE. A CODE OF 3 INDICATES DEPENDENCE
WITHOUT ABUSE. A CODE OF 4 INDICATES ABUSE AND
DEPENDENCE ARE BOTH PRESENT.

FSTDMALP THE AGE FIRST ALCOHOL PROBLEM IF EVER MET
CRITERIA FOR THE DSMIII DIAGNOSIS OF ALCOHOL
ABUSE (DSMALC=2 OR 4).

FSTDMALD THE AGE FIRST ALCOHOL PROBLEM IF EVER MET

314

CRITERIA FOR DSMIII DIAGNOSIS OF ALCOHOL
DEPENDENCE (DSMALC=3 OR 4).

FSTDMALC   THE AGE FIRST ALCOHOL PROBLEM IF EVER MET
            CRITERIA FOR THE DSMIII DIAGNOSIS OF ALCOHOL
            ABUSE OR DEPENDENCE (DSMALC=2-4).

LSTDMALP   THE AGE LAST ALCOHOL PROBLEM IF EVER MET
            CRITERIA FOR THE DSMIII DIAGNOSIS OF ALCOHOL
            ABUSE (SEE NOTE) (DSMALC=2 OR 4).

LSTDMALD   THE LAST AGE ALCOHOL PROBLEM IF EVER MET
            CRITERIA FOR DSMIII DIAGNOSIS OF ALCOHOL
            DEPENDENCE (SEE NOTE) (DSMALC=3 OR 4).

LSTDMALC   THE AGE LAST ALCOHOL PROBLEM IF EVER MET
            CRITERIA FOR THE DSMIII DIAGNOSIS OF ALCOHOL
            ABUSE OR DEPENDENCE (SEE NOTE) (DSMALC=2-4).

            AT THE END OF ALL THE FSTDMAL_ AND LSTDMAL_
            CONSTRUCTIONS, YOU WILL NOTE THAT A '.' IS
            CONVERTED TO 99. THIS IS NECESSITATED BY AN
            ERROR IN THE INTERVIEW. CODE 5'S IN Q.152 AND
            Q.153 SHOULD HAVE BEEN STARRED (*) LIKE Q.156-
            168, SO THAT THEY WOULD HAVE BEEN INCLUDED IN
            COUNTING 5'S IN INTERVIEWER BOXES Y AND Y1.
            BECAUSE OF THIS ERROR, IT IS POSSIBLE FOR SOMEONE
            MEETING DIAGNOSTIC CRITERIA, NOT TO BE ASKED
            AGES OF ONSET AND TERMINATION.

DSMALCSX   THE TOTAL NUMBER OF SYMPTOMS OF ALCOHOL ABUSE
            OR DEPENDENCE. THIS IS NOT USED FOR DIAGNOSIS
            BUT CONTRIBUTES TO A TOTAL SYMPTOM COUNT WHEN
            ADDED TO SIMILAR COUNTS FOR OTHER DIAGNOSES.

NOTE: IF THE MOST RECENT EPISODE OF THIS DIAGNOSIS ENDED
MORE THAN 1 YEAR AGO AND THE RESPONDENT IS AGED 91-96, AGE
IS CODED 90. IF THE MOST RECENT SYMPTOM OF THIS DIAGNOSIS
WAS WITHIN THE LAST THREE YEARS THE DATE OF LAST SYMPTOM IS
CODED AS FOLLOWS:

            91—LAST SYMPTOM WITHIN LAST TWO WEEKS
            92—LAST SYMPTOM TWO WEEKS TO ONE MONTH AGO
            93—LAST SYMPTOM ONE MONTH TO SIX MONTHS AGO
            94—LAST SYMPTOM SIX MONTHS TO ONE YEAR AGO
            95—LAST SYMPTOM WITHIN LAST THREE YEARS

****

DSMALCA=0;
IF DIS157 EQ 5 OR DIS158 EQ 5 OR DIS152 EQ 5 OR DIS166 EQ 5

```
      OR (DIS165B GE 2 AND DIS165B LE 96) OR DIS169 EQ 5 OR DIS170
      EQ 5 THEN DSMALCA=1;

DSMALCB=0;
IF  DIS150 EQ 5 OR DIS156 EQ 5 OR DIS160 EQ 5 OR DIS161 EQ 5
    OR DIS162 EQ 5 OR DIS163 EQ 5 OR DIS164 EQ 5 THEN
    DSMALC3=1;

DSMALCD=0;
IF  DIS153 EQ 5 OR DIS159 EQ 5 OR DIS167 EQ 5 THEN DSMALCD=1;

DSMALC=1;
IF  DSMALCB EQ 1 AND DSMALCA EQ 1 THEN DSMALC=2;
IF  DSMALC=1 AND DSMALCD=1 AND (DSMALCA=1 OR DSMALCB=1)
    THEN DSMALC=3;
IF  DSMALC=2 AND DSMALCD=1 THEN
    DSMALC=4;

FSTDMALP=DIS171;
IF  DSMALC=1 OR DSMALC=3 THEN FSTDMALP=00;
IF  FSTDMALP=. THEN FSTDMALP=99;

FSTDMALD=DIS171;
IF  DSMALC=1 OR DSMALC=2 THEN FSTDMALD=00;
IF  FSTDMALD=. THEN FSTDMALD=99;

FSTDMALC=DIS171;
IF  DSMALC=1 THEN FSTDMALC=00;
IF  FSTDMALC=. THEN FSTDMALC=99;

LSTDMALP=DIS171B;
IF  LSTDMALP GE 91 AND LSTDMALP LE 96 THEN LSTDMALP=90;
IF  DIS171A GE 1 AND DIS171A LT 6 THEN LSTDMALP=DIS171A+90;
IF  DSMALC=1 OR DSMALC=3 THEN LSTDMALP=00;
IF  LSTDMALP=. THEN LSTDMALP=99;

LSTDMALD=DIS171B;
IF  LSTDMALD GE 91 AND LSTDMALD LE 96 THEN LSTDMALD=90;
IF  DIS171A GE 1 AND DIS171A LT 6 THEN LSTDMALD=DIS171A+90;
IF  DSMALC=1 OR DSMALC=2 THEN LSTDMALD=00;
IF  LSTDMALD=. THEN LSTDMALD=99;

LSTDMALC=DIS171B;
IF  LSTDMALC GE 91 AND LSTDMALC LE 96 THEN LSTDMALC=90;
IF  DIS171A GE 1 AND DIS171A LT 6 THEN LSTDMALC=DIS171A+90;
IF  DSMALC=1 THEN LSTDMALC=00;
IF  LSTDMALC=. THEN LSTDMALC=99;

DSMALCSX=0;
IF  DIS152 EQ 5 THEN DSMALCSX+1;
IF  DIS157 EQ 5 THEN DSMALCSX+1;
IF  DIS166 EQ 5 THEN DSMALCSX+1;
IF  DIS158 EQ 5 THEN DSMALCSX+1;
```

```
IF   DIS165B GE 2 AND DIS165b LE 96 THEN DISMALCSX+1;
IF   DIS150 EQ 5 THEN DSMALCSX+1;
IF   DIS156 EQ 5 THEN DSMALCSX+1;
IF   DIS159 EQ 5 THEN DSMALCSX+1;
IF   DIS160 EQ 5 THEN DSMALCSX+1;
IF   DIS161 EQ 5 THEN DSMALCSX+1;
IF   DIS162 EQ 5 THEN DSMALCSX+1;
IF   DIS163 EQ 5 THEN DSMALCSX+1;
IF   DIS164 EQ 5 THEN DSMALCSX+1;
IF   DIS153 EQ 5 THEN DSMALCSX+1;
IF   DIS167 EQ 5 THEN DSMALCSX+1;
IF   DIS169 EQ 5 THEN DSMALCSX+1;
IF   DIS170 EQ 5 THEN DSMALCSX+1;
```

Appendix 3

U.S. Apparent Consumption of the Drinking-Age Population in Gallons per Year, 1850–1983

Year	Beer Volume	Beer Ethanol	Wine Volume	Wine Ethanol	Spirits Volume	Spirits Ethanol	All Beverages Ethanol
1850	2.70	0.14	0.46	0.03	4.17	1.88	2.05
1860	5.39	.27	.57	.10	4.79	2.16	2.53
1870	8.73	.44	.53	.10	3.40	1.53	2.07
1871–80	11.26	.56	.77	.14	2.27	1.02	1.72
1881–90	17.94	.90	.76	.14	2.12	.95	1.99
1891–95	23.42	1.17	.60	.11	2.12	.95	2.23
1896–1900	23.72	1.19	.55	.10	1.72	.77	2.04
1901–05	26.20	1.31	.71	.13	2.11	.95	2.39
1906–10	29.27	1.47	.92	.17	2.14	.96	2.60
1911–15	29.53	1.48	.79	.14	2.09	.94	2.56
1916–19	21.63	1.08	.69	.12	1.68	.76	1.96
(*Prohibition*)							
1934	13.58	.61	.36	.07	.64	.29	.97
1935	15.13	.68	.50	.09	.96	.43	1.20
1936	17.53	.79	.64	.12	1.20	.59	1.50
1937	18.21	.82	.71	.13	1.43	.64	1.59
1938	16.58	.75	.70	.13	1.32	.59	1.47
1939	16.77	.75	.79	.14	1.38	.62	1.51
1940	16.29	.73	.94	.16	1.43	.67	1.56
1941	17.97	.81	1.02	.18	1.58	.71	1.70
1942	20.00	.90	1.11	.22	1.89	.85	1.97
1943	22.26	1.00	.94	.17	1.46	.66	1.83
1944	25.22	1.13	1.03	.18	1.00	.76	2.07
1945	25.97	1.17	1.13	.20	1.95	.88	2.25
1946	23.75	1.07	1.34	.24	2.20	.99	2.30
1947	24.56	1.11	.90	.16	1.69	.76	2.03
1948	23.77	1.07	1.11	.20	1.56	.70	1.97
1949	23.48	1.06	1.21	.22	1.55	.70	1.98
1950	23.21	1.04	1.27	.23	1.72	.77	2.04
1951	22.92	1.03	1.13	.20	1.73	.78	2.01
1952	23.20	1.04	1.22	.21	1.63	.73	1.98
1953	23.04	1.04	1.19	.20	1.70	.77	2.01
1954	22.41	1.01	1.21	.21	1.66	.74	1.96
1955	22.39	1.01	1.25	.22	1.71	.77	2.00

(continued)

318

Appendix 3: (Continued)

Year	Beer Volume	Beer Ethanol	Wine Volume	Wine Ethanol	Spirits Volume	Spirits Ethanol	All Beverages Ethanol
1956	22.18	1.00	1.27	.22	1.31	.81	2.03
1957	21.44	.97	1.26	.22	1.77	.80	1.99
1958	21.35	.96	1.27	.22	1.77	.80	1.98
1959	22.15	1.00	1.28	.22	1.86	.84	2.06
1960	21.95	.99	1.32	.22	1.90	.86	2.07
1961	21.47	.97	1.36	.23	1.91	.86	2.06
1962	21.98	.99	1.32	.22	1.99	.90	2.11
1963	22.51	1.01	1.37	.23	2.02	.91	2.15
1964	23.08	1.04	1.41	.24	2.01	.95	2.23
1965	23.07	1.04	1.42	.24	2.21	.99	2.27
1966	23.52	1.06	1.40	.24	2.26	1.02	2.32
1967	23.81	1.07	1.46	.25	2.34	1.05	2.37
1968	24.33	1.09	1.51	.26	2.44	1.10	2.45
1969	24.90	1.12	1.62	.26	2.51	1.13	2.51
1970	25.23	1.14	1.71	.27	2.48	1.11	2.52
1971	25.63	1.15	1.93	.31	2.50	1.12	2.59
1972	25.91	1.17	2.10	.30	2.52	1.09	2.56
1973	26.77	1.20	2.13	.31	2.57	1.10	2.62
1974	27.75	1.25	2.13	.31	2.59	1.11	2.67
1975	28.09	1.26	2.22	.32	2.58	1.11	2.70
1976	28.14	1.27	2.23	.32	2.56	1.10	2.69
1977	28.72	1.29	2.28	.29	2.57	1.06	2.65
1978	29.44	1.32	2.40	.31	2.61	1.07	2.71
1979	30.39	1.37	2.48	.32	2.58	1.06	2.75
1980	30.59	1.38	2.63	.34	2.53	1.04	2.76
1981	30.91	1.39	2.72	.35	2.49	1.02	2.76
1982	30.77	1.38	2.76	.36	2.39	.98	2.72
1983	30.47	1.37	2.80	.36	2.33	.96	2.69
1984[a]	29.99	1.35	2.88	.37	2.28	.94	2.65
1985	29.56	1.33	2.98	.38	2.20	.90	2.62
1986	29.78	1.34	3.03	.39	2.04	.85	2.58
1987	29.78	1.34	2.95	.38	2.01	.83	2.54
1988	29.56	1.33	2.79	.36	1.92	.80	2.49

Source: Data updated from Horton M. Hyman, Marilyn A. Zimmerman, Carol Gurioli, and Alice Helrich, Drinkers, Drinking and Alcohol—Related Mortality and Hospitalizations: A Statistical Compendium [1980 Edition]

U.S. Alcohol Epidemiologic Data Reference Manual, Vol. 1., Sept., 1985, DBE, NIAAA, PHS, HHS

[a] Volume statistics for 1984–1988 computed from Table 1 in Surveillance Reports #2, 7, 10, 13 & 16 from NIAAA, Division of Biometry and Epidemiology and Alcohol Epidemiologic Data System.

Appendix 4

Compilation of Surveys Assessing Drinking Patterns, 1971–1985[a]

Drinking category	1971	1972	1973	1973	1974	1975	1976	1979	1983	1988[b]
ALL										
Abstainer	36	36	34	37	36	36	33	33	39	43
Lighter	34	32	29	30	28	31	38	34	30	30
Moderate	20	23	23	21	28	21	19	24	21	19
Heavier	10	10	14	11	11	12	10	9	10	8
MALES										
Abstainer	30	28	25	26	24	27	26	25	28	32
Lighter	29	29	24	29	24	27	33	29	28	30
Moderate	26	28	29	26	34	26	24	31	28	25
Heavier	15	15	22	19	18	20	18	14	16	13
FEMALES										
Abstainer	42	44	42	47	42	45	39	40	50	53
Lighter	40	34	35	32	32	35	44	38	30	30
Moderate	13	18	17	17	21	15	15	18	15	14
Heavier	5	4	6	4	5	4	3	4	4	3

Sources: 1971–1979 surveys: Clark and Midanik (1982), p. 9.
   1983: Malin et al. (1986), p. 49.
[a] By percent in each category.
[b] Unpublished data, Alcohol Epidemiologic Data System, NIAAA, 1991.

Index